Sourcebook of Adult Assessment Strategies

APPLIED CLINICAL PSYCHOLOGY

Series Editors:
Alan S. Bellack
Medical College of Pennsylvania at EPPI, Philadelphia, Pennsylvania
Michel Hersen
Nova Southeastern University, Fort Lauderdale, Florida

Current volumes in this Series

BEHAVIOR ANALYSIS AND TREATMENT
Edited by Ron Van Houten and Saul Axelrod

A BEHAVIOR ANALYTIC VIEW OF CHILD DEVELOPMENT
Henry D. Schlinger, Jr.

CASEBOOK OF THE BRIEF PSYCHOTHERAPIES
Edited by Richard A. Wells and Vincent J. Giannetti

CLINICAL PSYCHOLOGY SINCE 1917
Science, Practice, and Organization
Donald K. Routh

ETHNIC VALIDITY, ECOLOGY, AND PSYCHOTHERAPY
A Psychosocial Competence Model
Forrest B. Tyler, Deborah Ridley Brome, and Janice E. Williams

FUNDAMENTALS OF BEHAVIOR ANALYTIC RESEARCH
Alan Poling, Laura L. Methot, and Mark G. LeSage

GUIDEBOOK FOR CLINICAL PSYCHOLOGY INTERNS
Edited by Gary K. Zammit and James W. Hull

PERSPECTIVES AND PROMISES OF CLINICAL PSYCHOLOGY
Edited by Anke Ehlers, Wolfgang Fiegenbaum, Irmela Florin, and
Jürgen Margraf

SEXUAL BEHAVIOR
Problems and Management
Nathaniel McConaghy

SOURCEBOOK OF ADULT ASSESSMENT STRATEGIES
Nicola S. Schutte and John M. Malouff

THERAPEUTIC CHANGE
An Object Relations Perspective
Sidney J. Blatt and Richard Q. Ford

A Continuation Order Plan is available for this series. A continuation order will bring delivery of each new volume immediately upon publication. Volumes are billed only upon actual shipment. For further information please contact the publisher.

Sourcebook of Adult Assessment Strategies

NICOLA S. SCHUTTE and
JOHN M. MALOUFF
Nova Southeastern University
Fort Lauderdale, Florida

Plenum Press • New York and London

Library of Congress Cataloging-in-Publication Data

Schutte, Nicola S.
    Sourcebook of adult assessment strategies / Nicola S. Schutte and
John M. Malouff.
        p.   cm. -- (Applied clinical psychology)
    Includes bibliographical references and index.
    ISBN 0-306-45029-1
    1. Psychiatric rating scales.   I. Malouff, John M. II. Title.
III. Series.
    [DNLM: 1. Mental Disorders--diagnosis. 2. Psychiatric Status
Rating Scales.   WM 141 S396s 1995]
RC473.P78S38 1995
616.89'075--dc20
DNLM/DLC   95-9524
for Library of Congress   CIP

ISBN 0-306-45029-1

© 1995 Plenum Press, New York
A Division of Plenum Publishing Corporation
233 Spring Street, New York, N. Y. 10013

10 9 8 7 6 5 4 3 2 1

Printed in the United States of America

Foreword

Assessment is a topic that is central to psychology. In the case of clinical psychology, assessment of individual functioning is of keen interest to individuals involved in clinical practice as well as research. Understanding the multiple domains of functioning, evaluating characteristics of individuals in relation to others (normative assessment) as well as in relation to themselves (ipsative assessment), and charting progress or change over time all require well-developed assessment tools and methods. In light of the importance of the topic, books, journals, and monographs continue to emerge in large numbers to present, address, and evaluate diverse measures. Keeping informed about measures, identifying the measures in use, and obtaining the necessary information for their interpretation make the task of Sisyphus look like a vacation. In this book, the editors provide information that eases the task remarkably.

The overriding goal of this book is to provide concise, useful, and essential information about measures of adult functioning. To that end, this is a sourcebook, a format that is particularly noteworthy. The measures are presented and organized according to diagnostic categories, as derived from the *Diagnostic and Statistical Manual of Mental Disorders* (DSM-IV). The categories are broad (e.g., substance-related disorders, anxiety disorders, mood disorders, schizophrenia and related disorders) in recognition that those who develop measures and those who use them in clinical research or practice usually do not have narrowly defined diagnostic entities in mind. Also, the categories include more general domains of adult functioning (e.g., relationship problems, impulse control, global functioning) and selected characteristics (e.g., to measure irrational beliefs, reasons for living, pleasant events) that are likely to be of interest in clinical work. Within a domain, multiple measures are presented.

The editors have provided us with a very special resource by the format in which the measures are presented and reviewed. First and foremost, the individual measures are reproduced. Along with each measure, critical information is provided related to different types of reliability and validity, samples to whom the measure has been applied, cutoff scores and their meaning, the use and availability of different versions of the scale, including translations. Selected references provide support for various psychometric properties; further readings direct the reader to other resources related to individual measures as well as assessment practices and standards in general.

The book is designed to be of practical use. That criterion alone could foster presentation of as many measures as possible, with little attention to how they are used and whether there are any supporting data in behalf of their reliability and validity. To the editors' credit, they describe each instrument and present the reader with basic material to permit critical evaluation. In addition, the reader is cautioned in general about reliance on any single measure and to seek additional resources to facilitate test evaluation.

The book redresses many of the issues that occur in research and practice in relation to obtaining and using measures including, but extending well beyond, practical issues. Certainly the practical issues are important. For example, it is very difficult to obtain many measures that are of interest and even to identify the source from which they may be obtained. Encyclopedic measurement manuals and handbooks are available in principle but accessible to few in practice. Second, evaluation of individual measures is not an easy task. We know through our training how to evaluate measures and the importance of various criteria. Yet, spending the time to procure this information, which is spread over time and scores of publication outlets, is a mini-career. Third, and perhaps more weighty, is that there are many versions of a given measure. In the evolution of a measure, standardized or not, a mutation emerges as an investigator or practitioner shortens the form, deletes a few items that are not pertinent, or rewords the instructions in light of special characteristics of the sample or clients. This version of the measure then circulates from colleague to colleague, faculty to student, and so on. Eventually, separate species of the scale have emerged and further evolve. The original standardization and normative data and subsequent evaluations of various forms of validity and reliability may be cited as the bases of the evolved scale, but the connections become more strained as the departure increases. Even our most commonly used measures in clinical work, or perhaps especially these measures, show this type of evolution. Witness, as one example, the Hamilton Rating Scale for Depression which might be viewed more as a family of measures than as a single scale (see Grundy et al., 1994). The advantage of this sourcebook is in providing a common resource for original versions of the scales or the most commonly used versions, as well as making explicit information about other versions that are available. A common resource for the scales is invaluable.

Overall, the editors are to be commended for providing a sourcebook of assessments for adult functioning. The domains and measures included will be of widespread interest. By addressing researchers and practitioners and by focusing on assessment of domains of clinical relevance, the book contributes enormously to uniting clinical research and practice. Apart from research and clinical work, the book can play a pivotal role in graduate training in psychology and mental health professions more generally where integration of systematic assessment in practice is encouraged.

ALAN E. KAZDIN
Yale University
New Haven, Connecticut

REFERENCE

Grundy, C. T., Lunnen, K. M., Lambert, M. J., Aston, J. E., & Tovey, D. R. (1994). The Hamilton Rating Scale for Depression: One scale or many. *Clinical Psychology: Science and Practice, 1,* 197–205.

Preface

Practitioners, researchers, and instructors who seek scales measuring a certain aspect of psychopathology often are frustrated. Even though many excellent scales measuring mental disorders exist, it is sometimes difficult or impossible to find the actual scale, instructions for its use, or a current review of the psychometric properties of the scale. *Sourcebook of Adult Assessment Strategies* responds to a need in the mental health field for this information.

ORGANIZATION OF THE BOOK

The presentation of scales in the book corresponds to the order of related diagnostic categories in *Diagnostic and Statistical Manual of Mental Disorders*, Fourth Edition (DSM-IV) (American Psychiatric Association, 1994). Information about each scale is broken into the following sections: purpose and development, administration and scoring, sample and cutoff scores, reliability, validity, and the actual scale items. Information in each of these sections is designed to allow practitioners and researchers to judge whether the particular scale meets their needs.

The section on purpose and development gives information about the realm of use of the scale and the procedures used to develop the scale. Some of the scales may be of help in making a diagnosis. Others are intended to give information about the exact symptomology, the antecedents, or the consequences of a disorder. This section also provides information about subscales, other versions of the measure, and translations of the scale into other languages.

The administration and scoring section gives step-by-step directions on how to administer and score the scale. Sample scores give a standard of comparison, allowing clinicians and researchers to judge whether the scores they obtain are relatively high or low. Whenever cutoff scores were available, we present these and give the diagnostic accuracy of the cutoff scores. The next chapter contains suggestions about how to evaluate cutoff and sample scores. Because weighing the reliability and validity information about a scale is crucial in the decision of whether to use a scale, we discuss these issues at length in the next chapter. The actual scale items and scale instructions are generally presented in their original format. For a few scales, we made and noted minor changes in format. Changes in societal conditions have dated some items pertaining to gender roles in a few of the scales; we did not modify these items, but scale users may wish to do so.

SCALE SELECTION

We searched the relevant literature and reviewed many hundreds of scales assessing various disorders and characteristics related to disorders. On the basis of this review we selected those scales that had good psychometric properties and covered the range of DSM-IV adult mental disorders. We excluded some excellent scales because they are exceptionally lengthy, require extensive training for their use, are beyond the scope of this book, or are quite similar to scales that have more extensive psychometric data. Finally, we were unable to obtain permission to include some popular scales (usually ones that are sold commercially), but in each case we found psychometrically sound alternatives to include.

Because the book contains actual scale items, we obtained permission from the copyright holders to present this material in its original form. If the scale items and instructions for use were published in a journal article or book, we obtained permission from the publisher holding the copyright. If only the psychometric properties of a scale were described in the published literature, we obtained permission from the developer of the scale and asked for a copy of it. If the actual scale was published but a copyright notice named an author as having rights to the scale, we obtained permission from that author.

OTHER SOURCES OF INFORMATION FOR READERS

We refer readers who wish to find information about mental health scales not included in this volume to the following useful review books:

Mental Measurements Yearbooks (e.g., Kramer & Conoley, 1992), *Dictionary of Behavioral Assessment Techniques* (Hersen & Bellack, 1988), *Measuring Human Problems* (Peck & Shapiro, 1990), *The Instruments of Psychiatric Research* (Thompson, 1989), and *Measuring Mental Illness: Psychomeiric Assessment for Clinicians* (Wetzler, 1989). These books do not give actual scales or instructions for their use; however, the *Mental Measurements Yearbooks* give the addresses of the companies that sell the scales reviewed and the *Dictionary of Behavioral Assessment* gives detailed information on where to find the noncommercial scales reviewed. The following sources provide reviews and actual scales from other fields: *Measures of Personality and Social Psychological Attitudes* (Robinson, Shaver, & Wrightsman, 1991) and *Handbook of Marketing Scales* (Bearden, Netemeyer, & Mobley, 1993).

ACKNOWLEDGMENTS

Many dedicated researchers and clinicians created the scales reviewed and presented in this book and many others carried out further reliability and validity studies. We are very pleased to be able to present their work. As well as giving us permission to use their scales, a number of researchers also provided us with further references or as yet unpublished information.

Dr. Michel Hersen, Dr. Alan Bellack, and Mr. Eliot Werner gave us expert guidance. Dr. Lilith Schutte provided helpful editing advice. Ms. Joan Edelman gave valuable assistance in processing the actual scales. Many thanks to them all.

REFERENCES

American Psychiatric Association (1994). *Diagnostic and statistical manual of mental disorders* (4th ed.). Washington, DC: Author.

Bearden, W. O., Netemeyer, R. G., & Mobley, M. F. (1993). *Handbook of marketing scales.* Newbury Park, CA: Sage.

Hersen, M., & Bellack, A. S. (Eds.). (1988). *Dictionary of behavioral assessment techniques.* New York: Pergamon.

Kramer, J., & Conoley, J. C. (Eds.). (1992). *The eleventh mental measurements yearbook.* Lincoln, NE: University of Nebraska Press.

Peck, D. F., & Shapiro, C. M. (Eds.). (1990). *Measuring human problems.* New York: John Wiley.

Robinson, J. P., Shaver, P. R., & Wrightsman, L. S. (Eds.). (1991). *Measures of personality and social psychological attitudes.* New York: Academic Press.

Thompson, C. (Ed.). (1989). *The instruments of psychiatric research.* New York: John Wiley.

Wetzler, S. (Ed.). (1989). *Measuring mental illness: Psychometric assessment for clinicians.* New York: American Psychiatric Press.

Contents

CHAPTER 1

The Psychometric Properties and Clinical Use of Scales

The appropriate clinical or research use of the measures in this book requires a certain amount of psychometric knowledge. For instance, in order to interpret research findings relating to a measure, readers need to understand the usual ways of testing reliability and validity, as well as how to use sample or cutoff scores. The appropriate clinical use of the measures also requires knowledge about clinical assessment strategies in general and ethical standards. In this chapter we provide this basic information for scale users and provide references for more detailed information.

RELIABILITY

Reliability is the ability of a scale to consistently measure a construct. Each scale review in this book includes data on one or more of three types of reliability.

Internal Consistency. The first type involves the internal consistency (homogeneity) of the scale. The usual statistic reported is Cronbach's alpha, which is based on the intercorrelations of the items and represents an estimate of the correlation of the scale with an imagined parallel form. The Kudor–Richardson 20 formula sometimes used for dichotomous items is merely a variant of alpha. Sometimes researchers calculate a split-half correlation (e.g., total of odd-numbered items with the total of the even-numbered items) and use the Spearman–Brown formula to estimate the correlation of the whole scale with an imagined parallel form (Cohen, Montague, Nathanson, & Swerdlik, 1988). Occasionally, researchers report only correlations between items and total scores. If these are fairly uniformly high (say, .50 and above), one can roughly estimate that the items are fairly consistent with each other.

Test–Retest. For this method researchers administer the scale to the same individuals once and then again sometime in the next few days or weeks. The correlation between scores provides an estimate of how consistently the scale measures a construct over time. As the period of time becomes longer, say a few months, the term "test–retest stability" becomes more appropriate because now the correlation may reflect as much about changes in the characteristics measured as it does about the ability of the scale to measure it.

Interrater. For scales that involve clinical judgment the burden lies with the scale developer to show that clinicians will assign similar scores to the same person. A typical study of this sort involves one clinician interviewing a client and both that clinician and another observer rating the client on scale items, with neither rater aware of the other's ratings. The Pearson's correlation, kappa, or intraclass correlation of the clinician ratings of a group of clients provides an estimate of how consistent raters are in using the scale. See Cicchetti (1994) for differences among these statistics.

Reliability in General. For clinician rating scales, all three types of reliability have value. For self-report measures, only internal consistency and test–retest reliability make sense.

Because reliability coefficients for published scales are virtually always high enough to be statistically significant, researchers often do not use space to report a level of significance. We concur in this approach.

All else being equal, it makes sense for clinicians to use scales with high reliability, but for some disorders there are no methods of assessment available with very high reliability. Hence, scale users often wonder what minimal level of reliability is needed to justify use of a scale. No one can provide a simple answer to that because different uses may require different levels. For many uses of scales, Nunnally (1978) and Kline (1993) recommend a minimal internal consistency or test–retest reliability of .70. For clinical uses, we believe that this standard can suffice as long as no important decisions are based solely on the scores of a single measure. For kappa and the intraclass correlation coefficient, both of which can be used for evaluating interexaminer agreement, Cicchetti (1994) suggested a minimal level of .40.

Clinicians concerned about errors in measurement may want to calculate confidence intervals for scores. See Nunnally (1978) for the details of how to do this.

VALIDITY

Validity involves the issue of whether a scale measures what it is intended to measure. Researchers have presented many types of data to support or disconfirm the validity of psychological measures. We will describe the logic of the most common types of validity in the order we will present them in each review. In the actual reviews we will not characterize each type of validity findings as "construct," "concurrent," and so on because we believe that these jargon terms serve more to confuse (or at least distract) scale users than to aid them.

Convergent Validity. A significant correlation between a new scale and a previously validated scale for measuring the same or a related construct provides evidence of validity. For instance, developers of new depression measures generally test them against the Hamilton Depression Rating Scale, which is sometimes called the gold standard of depression assessment. Valid measures of a characteristic should also produce scores that correlate with measures of related characteristics. For instance, measures of dementia ought to correlate with intelligence test scores, with signs of brain disease at autopsy, and with other indicators of mental decay.

Discriminant Validity. Measures should not correlate highly with supposedly unrelated variables. For instance, a measure of psychosis should not correlate highly with social desirability responding or anxiety.

Distinct-groups Validity. Scales that validly measure a construct should produce higher scores in some groups of persons than in others. For instance, as a group, clients entering an alcohol treatment program should have higher scores on a measure of alcoholism than patients of similar age and gender who are beginning treatment for depression or psychosis.

Sensitivity to Treatment. A valid measure of a disorder will show a decrease after appropriate, generally successful treatment. For instance, a measure of mania should show a group decrease after first-time lithium treatment begins with manics.

Predictive Validity. A valid measure of a disorder should predict future behavior or results. For instance, a measure of Alzheimer's disease should predict future worsening of cognitive abilities.

Validity in General. The more types of validity evidence a scale has, the safer it is to conclude that it measures a specific construct. Hence, all else being equal, it is best to use scales with the most evidence of validity. For some scale uses, however, one specific type of validity may be especially important. For instance, in choosing a scale for treatment research, evidence of sensitivity to treatment may be paramount. For diagnostic purposes, ability to discriminate between specific groups may be more important. At a minimum though, it makes sense for researchers and clinicians to require that a scale have at least some replicated evidence of validity.

CUTOFF AND SAMPLE SCORES

This book provides cutoff scores and score distributions for individuals without a diagnosis and clinical groups. Clinicians and researchers often want this information when deciding whether individuals might have a disorder, might benefit from treatment, or require further evaluation. However, caution is appropriate in using cutoff scores and sample means because the information may be inappropriate for a person who differs in an important way from the individuals in the research sample. For instances, errors may occur if a poorly educated individual is compared to samples of college students, if a medical patient in one culture is compared to medical patients in another, or if an older person is compared to a sample of young people. Likewise, optimum cutoff scores sometimes change radically from one group (e.g., medical patients) to another (e.g., college students).

Although some commercially sold measures, such as intelligence tests, have nationally representative norms suitable for safe application to most individuals, none of the scales in this book do. Hence, the best course for users of these scales is to evaluate carefully the samples from which cutoff scores and means come. More reliance is reasonable on samples that (a) are similar to the client or research subject in question, (b) are based on community surveys, which are generally fairly representative of at least one community, (c) are large (in the hundreds), and (d) provide findings consistent with data from other studies. Scale users may also want to collect local sample data for use.

APPROPRIATE CLINICAL USE OF SCALES

As an extension of the philosophy underlying reliability and validity research, we suggest as a general clinical practice that clinicians consider client scale scores as findings to be tested against other data sources. For instance, a clinician can test the results of a self-report measure of depression against clinical observations of the client and direct questioning about what the client sees as his or her problem. A clinician finding a low mental status exam score can collect detailed information from the client and relevant others about the recent functioning of the client and then obtain results of a more specific neuropsychological testing.

By treating a scale score as a piece of evidence rather than as a conclusion in itself, clinicians can minimize assessment errors. This approach is especially important when a reason exists to suspect that a respondent is giving less than honest information. Wise test users realize that some clients, when they are the only source of information, can fake good or bad on almost any maladjustment measure and thereby make scale scores misleading or meaningless.

For further information on psychometrics or the professional, ethical use of scales, see the *Standards for Educational and Psychological Testing* (American Education Research Association, American Psychological Association, & National Council on Measurement in Education, 1985) and the other books in the reference list for this chapter.

REFERENCES

American Education Research Association, American Psychological Association, & National Council on Measurement in Education (1985). *Standards for educational and psychological testing*. Washington, D.C.: American Psychological Association.

Cicchetti, D. V. (1994). Guidelines, criteria, and rules of thumb for evaluating normed and standardized assessment instruments in psychology. *Psychological Assessment, 6*, 284–290.

Cohen, R. J., Montague, P., Nathanson, L. S., & Swerdlik, M. E. (1988). *Psychological testing: An introduction to tests and measurements*. Mountain View, CA: Mayfield.

Kline, P. (1993). *The handbook of psychological testing*. New York: Rutledge.

Nunnally, J. (1978). *Psychometric theory*. New York: McGraw-Hill.

CHAPTER 2

Delirium and Dementia

DELIRIUM RATING SCALE

Purpose and Development

The Delirium Rating Scale assess the severity of delirium (Trzepacz, Baker, & Greenhouse, 1988). It consists of 10 clinician-rated items, each of which reflects a different aspect of delirium.

Administration and Scoring

To rate the 10 items, the interviewer considers all available sources of information, which may include an interview with the patient, a mental status exam, medical tests, medical history, nurses' observations, and family reports. A rating scale with numeric values ranging from 0–2 to 0–4 is used for each item. The total score is the sum of all ratings; scores may range from 0 to 32 with higher scores indicating more severe delirium.

Sample Scores

Trzepacz et al. (1988) used the scale to assess 20 individuals diagnosed with delirium, nine diagnosed with dementia, nine diagnosed with schizophrenia, and nine with no diagnosis. Wada and Yamaguchi (1993) reported the intake scale scores of 28 elderly individuals with dementia, 12 of whom later improved within a week and 16 of whom did not. Rosen, Sweet, Mulsant, Rifai, Pasternak, & Zubenko (1994) gave the scale to 791 elderly patients, 70 of whom had delirium, 291 of whom had another organic disorder such as Alzheimer's-related dementia or multiinfarct dementia,

TABLE 1
Scores on the Delirium Rating Scale

Group	M	SD
Delirious*	23.0	4.8
Delirious***	14.4	3.8
Delirious**		
Improved within a week	14.0	1.9
Not improved within a week	18.4	2.7
Dementia*	4.6	2.1
Organic Disorder***	8.8	3.6
Schizophrenic*	3.3	1.6
Nonorganic Disorder***	5.6	2.8
No diagnosis*	.7	.5

*Trzepacz et al. (1988), **Wada and Yamaguchi (1993),
***Rosen et al. (1994).

and 430 of whom had a nonorganic disorder such as major depression or schizophrenia. Table 1 shows average scores for these groups.

Rosen et al. (1994) found that a cutoff score of 10 correctly identified 94% of delirious patients as having delirium and correctly identified 68% of patients with organic disorders and 91% of patients with nonorganic disorders as not having delirium.

Reliability

Interrater reliability of the scale has ranged from .86 to .97 (Trzepacz, 1988; Rockwood, 1993).

Validity

In samples of delirious patients both Trzepacz et al. (1988) and Rockwood (1993) found that those with higher scale scores had poorer mental status exam scores, and Trzepacz et al. (1988) found that those with higher scores performed worse on a trailmaking task.

Trzepacz et al. (1988) found that delirious patients had much higher scale scores than demented patients, schizophrenic patients, or normal individuals. Rosen et al. (1994) also reported that delirious patients had much higher scale scores than patients with other organic disorders and patients with nonorganic disorders. Wada and Yamaguchi (1993) found that delirious patients who had the highest scale scores when first tested showed the least improvement over time.

DELIRIUM RATING SCALE

Item 1: Temporal Onset of Symptoms

This item addresses the time course over which symptoms appear; the maximum rating is for the most abrupt onset of symptoms—a common pattern for delirium. Dementia is usually more gradual in onset. Other psychiatric disorders, such as affective disorders, might be scored with 1 or 2 points on this item. Sometimes delirium can be chronic (e.g., in geriatric nursing-home patients), and unfortunately only 1 or 2 points would be assessed in that situation.

0. No significant change from longstanding behavior, essentially a chronic or chronic-recurrent disorder
1. Gradual onset of symptoms, occurring within a 6-month period
2. Acute change in behavior or personality occurring over a month
3. Abrupt change in behavior, usually occurring over a 1- to 3-day period

Item 2: Perceptual Disturbances

This item rates most highly the extreme inability to perceive differences between internal and external reality, while intermittent misperceptions such as illusions are given 2 points. Depersonalization and derealization can be seen in other organic mental disorders like temporal lobe epilepsy, in severe depression, and in borderline personality disorder and thus are given only 1 point.

0. None evident by history or observation
1. Feelings of depersonalization or derealization
2. Visual illusions or misperceptions including macropsia, micropsia; e.g., may urinate in wastebasket or mistake bedclothes for something else
3. Evidence that the patient is markedly confused about external reality; e.g., not discriminating between dreams and reality

Item 3: Hallucination Type

The presence of any type of hallucination is rated. Auditory hallucinations alone are rated with less weight because of their common occurrence in primary psychiatric disorders. Visual hallucinations are generally associated with organic mental syndromes, although not exclusively, and are given 2 points. Tactile hallucinations are classically described in delirium, particularly due to anticholinergic toxicity, and are given the most points.

→

0. Hallucinations not present
1. Auditory hallucinations only
2. Visual hallucinations present by patient's history or inferred by observation, with or without auditory hallucinations
3. Tactile, olfactory, or gustatory hallucinations present with or without visual or auditory hallucinations

Item 4: Delusions

Delusions can be present in many different psychiatric disorders, but tend to be better organized and more fixed in nondelirious disorders and thus are given less weight. Chronic fixed delusions are probably most prevalent in schizophrenic disorders. New delusions may indicate affective and schizophrenic disorders, dementia, or substance intoxication but should also alert the clinician to possible delirium and are given 2 points. Poorly formed delusions, often of a paranoid nature, are typical of delirium.

0. Not present
1. Delusions are systematized, i.e., well-organized and persistent
2. Delusions are new and not part of a preexisting primary psychiatric disorder
3. Delusions are not well circumscribed; are transient, poorly organized, and mostly in response to misperceived environmental cues; e.g., are paranoid and involve persons who are in reality caregivers, loved ones, hospital staff, etc.

Item 5: Psychomotor Behavior

This item describes degrees of severity of altered psychomotor behavior. Maximum points can be given for severe agitation or severe withdrawal to reflect either the hyperactive or the hypoactive variant of delirium.

0. No significant retardation or agitation
1. Mild restlessness, tremulousness, or anxiety evident by observation and a change from patient's usual behavior
2. Moderate agitation with pacing, removing i.v.'s, etc.
3. Severe agitation, needs to be restrained, may be combative; or has significant withdrawal from the environment, but not due to major depression or schizophrenic catatonia

Item 6: Cognitive Status During Formal Testing

Information from the cognitive portion of a routine mental status examination is needed to rate this item. The maximum rating of 4 points is given for severe cognitive deficits while only 1 point is given for mild inattention, which could be attributed to pain and fatigue seen in medically ill persons. Two points are given for a relatively isolated cognitive deficit, such as memory impairment, which could be due to dementia or organic amnestic syndrome as well as to early delirium.

0. No cognitive deficits, or deficits which can be alternatively explained by lack of education or prior mental retardation
1. Very mild cognitive deficits which might be attributed to inattention due to acute pain, fatigue, depression, or anxiety associated with having a medical illness
2. Cognitive deficit largely in one major area tested, e.g., memory, but otherwise intact
3. Significant cognitive deficits which are diffuse, i.e., affecting many different areas tested; must include periods of disorientation to time or place at least once each 24-hr period; registration and/or recall are abnormal; concentration is reduced
4. Severe cognitive deficits, including motor or verbal perseverations, confabulations, disorientation to person, remote and recent memory deficits, and inability to cooperate with formal mental status testing

Item 7: Physical Disorder

Maximum points are given when a specific lesion or physiological disturbance can be temporally associated with the altered behavior. Dementias are often not found to have a specific underlying medical cause, while delirium usually has at least one identifiable physical cause.

0. None present or active
1. Presence of any physical disorder which might affect mental state
2. Specific drug, infection, metabolic, central nervous system lesion, or other medical problem which can be temporally implicated in causing the altered behavior or mental status

Item 8: Sleep–Wake Disturbance

Disruption of the sleep–wake cycle is typical in delirium, with demented persons generally having significant sleep disturbances much later in their course. Severe delirium is on a continuum with stupor and coma, and persons with a resolving coma are likely to be delirious temporarily.

0. Not present; awake and alert during the day, and sleeps without significant disruption at night

➤

1. Occasional drowsiness during day and mild sleep continuity disturbance at night; may have nightmares but can readily distinguish from reality
2. Frequent napping and unable to sleep at night, constituting a significant disruption of or a reversal of the usual sleep–wake cycle
3. Drowsiness prominent, difficulty staying alert during interview, loss of self-control over alertness and somnolence
4. Drifts into stuporous or comatose periods

Item 9: Lability of Mood

Rapid shifts in mood can occur in various organic mental syndromes, perhaps due to a disinhibition of one's normal control. The patient may be aware of this lack of emotional control and may behave inappropriately relative to the situation or to his or her thinking state, e.g., crying for no apparent reason. Delirious patients may score points on any of these items depending upon the severity of the delirium and upon how their underlying psychological state "colors" their delirious presentation. Patients with borderline personality disorder might score 1 or 2 points on this item.

0. Not present; mood stable
1. Affect/mood somewhat altered and changes over the course of hours; patient states that mood changes are not under self-control
2. Significant mood changes that are inappropriate to situation, including fear, anger, or tearfulness; rapid shifts of emotion, even over several minutes
3. Severe disinhibition of emotions, including temper outbursts, uncontrolled inappropriate laughter, or crying

Item 10: Variability of Symptoms

The hallmark of delirium is the waxing and waning of symptoms, which is given 4 points on this item. Demented as well as delirious patients, who become more confused at night when environmental cues are decreased, could score 2 points.

0. Symptoms stable and mostly present during daytime
2. Symptoms worsen at night
4. Fluctuating intensity of symptoms, such that they wax and wane during a 24-hr period

TOTAL SCORE _____

Mini-Mental State Exam

Purpose and Development

The Mini-Mental State Exam (Folstein, Folstein, & McHugh, 1975) is an 11-item test of cognitive ability used primarily to identify possible cases of dementia and to assess change in cognitive ability related to dementia. The test measures orientation to time and place, attention, short-term memory, and the ability to name objects, follow commands, write a sentence, and copy a design.

The scale appears to be the most commonly used mental status exam in the world (DesRosiers, 1992). It has been made a part of several batteries used to assess dementia and part of the Diagnostic Interview Schedule, which is commonly used in community surveys of psychiatric disorders (Tombaugh & McIntyre, 1992). Researchers have published over 500 journal articles involving the scale in the past several years, far more than all the similar measures combined. Researchers frequently use the scale as a standard against which to compare new measures (e.g., Jensen, Dehlin, & Gustafson, 1993).

Versions of the scale exist in many languages, including Castillian (Rodriquez-Alvarez, 1991), Chinese (Hill, Klauber, Salmon, Yu, Liv, Zhang, & Katzman, 1993), Dutch (Van der Cammen, Van Harskamp, Stronks, Passchier, & Schudel, 1992), German (Kummer, Gundel, Van Laak, & Hirche, 1992), Italian (Turrina, Dewey, Siani, Saviotti, Marchione, & Siciliani, 1993), Korean (Park & Ha, 1988), as well as languages that have a translation of the Diagnostic Interview Schedule.

Administration and Scoring

The instructions for administering the test are included with the scale items. Test users need to have with them a pencil and watch to show the respondent, a sheet of blank paper for the respondent to write on, and a blank piece of paper with the words "CLOSE YOUR EYES" on it in letters large enough for the respondent to see clearly.

Because various client characteristics might invalidate test results, it is wise for clinicians using the scale to inquire about the education of the respondent; note or ask about visual, hearing, and handwriting problems; and note whether the respondent better understands a language other than the one used by the clinician. Collecting this information will help the clinician modify the test in appropriate circumstances (e.g., by having someone administer it in another language) and interpret the test results.

The minimum possible score on each item is 0. Maximum possible scores vary from 1 to 5 depending on the item. Total scores, which are the sum of item scores, can range from 0 to 30, with higher scores indicating better cognitive ability.

Scale users have sometimes modified the scale items to suit their circumstances (Tombaugh & McIntyre, 1992). For instance, one multipart item asks what hospital the respondent is in. For a community survey, Folstein, Anthony, Parhead, Duffy, & Gruenberg (1985) asked instead for the names of two main nearby streets.

Another item asks the respondent to recall three words, with the choice of words left to the clinician. Commonly included words have included *apple, penny,* and *table,* as well as some combination of *flag, ball, tree, brown, ring, rose, dog,* and *elephant* (Tombaugh & McIntyre, 1992). Tombaugh and McIntyre (1992) mention *honesty* as an alternative sometimes used, but we suspect that such an abstract word might be substantially harder to remember than the others.

Generally, test users score the refusal to answer a question as 0 (Folstein et al., 1985). The rating of level of consciousness is not scored as part of the overall test, but it may provide useful information by itself.

We will provide the original version of the test (Folstein et al., 1971) with some additional directions from a later community survey version (Folstein et al., 1985), and our own intersecting pentagons. We suggest altering the phrasing of the serial 7's item from "can you subtract . . . ?" to "please subtract" in order to minimize refusals to try.

Cutoff and Sample Scores

In a comprehensive review of the scale, Tombaugh and McIntyre (1992) noted that clinicians and researchers generally consider a score of 23 or lower to indicate cognitive impairment, but that recently some test users have used a tripartite classification: 24–30 = no cognitive impairment, 18–23 = mild impairment, and 0–17 = severe impairment.

Tombaugh and McIntyre (1992) reviewed dozens of studies examining the value of using a score of 23 or less as a cutoff for a finding of dementia and concluded that most studies found that the scale correctly identified over 80% of persons diagnosed as demented and 80% of persons not diagnosed as demented on the basis of more in-depth assessments.

In a Baltimore community survey of over 3,000 individuals, Folstein et al. (1985) found a median score of 28.5 in individuals under 65 years old and a median of 26.5 in those over 65. As part of a community survey, Wiederholt, Cahn, Butters, Salmon, Kritz-Silverstein, and Barrett-Connor (1993) gave the test to 1,692 individuals over 54 years old in an upper-middle-class area of California and found mean scores of about 27.5, *SD* =

about 1.5, for individuals aged 55–74, and means scores of about 24–27, *SD* = about 3.0, for individuals aged 75–94. Lindal and Stephansson (1993) similarly found a mean score of about 28 (no SD) in 862 individuals aged 55–57 in an Iceland community survey.

Galasko, Abramson, Corey-Bloom, and Thal (1993) reported a mean score of about 17 (no SD) for 39 persons diagnosed as having probable Alzheimer's disease. Folstein et al. (1971) reported a much lower mean score of 9.6, *SD* = 5.8, for 29 demented individuals.

Reliability

Studies have found internal consistency for the scale as measured by Cronbach's alpha to be .96 in a sample of medical patients and to range from .54 to .77 in community surveys (Tombaugh & McIntyre, 1992). Test–retest reliability over periods ranging from one day to several weeks has ranged from .79 to .95 in groups that included demented individuals (Tombaugh & McIntyre, 1992).

Validity

Researchers have repeatedly found substantial correlations between Mini-Mental State scores and scores on other measures of mental status, memory, intelligence, neuropsychological functioning, and activities of daily living (Orrell, Howard, Payne, Bergmann, Woods, Everitt, & Levy, 1992; Tombaugh & McIntyre, 1992). Many other studies have consistently shown that lower scale scores are associated with various indicators of physical decay, including urinary incontinence, hearing loss, hospitalization, death, and signs of brain disease at autopsy (Tombaugh & McIntyre, 1992).

Although studies have shown that scale scores discriminate well between demented and normals, Tombaugh and McIntyre (1992) noted studies showing that scale scores were more accurate in assessing dementia with groups that contained a higher percentage of severely demented (vs. mildly demented) individuals, and that false identification of individuals as demented occurred more often when patients with other psychiatric disorders such as depression were included in the study. The most recent studies have confirmed that discriminations made by the test have lower validity with individuals who are depressed or have less education (Chaves & Izquierdo, 1992; Harper, Chacko, Kotik-Harper, & Kirby, 1992; Jagger, Clarke, & Anderson, 1992; Orrell et al., 1992; Tombaugh & McIntyre, 1992) or have a physical disability (Jagger et al., 1992). DesRosiers (1992) suggested that the education of the respondent be considered in making interpretations. Tombaugh and McIntyre (1992) recommended that the test not be used with individuals who have less than a ninth-grade education.

Other studies have found that scale scores significantly increase with appropriate treatment (Eagger, Levy, & Sahakian, 1992; Saletu, Moller, Grunberger, Deutsch, & Rossner, 1991).

MINI-MENTAL STATE EXAM

I would like to ask you some questions to check your concentration and your memory. Most of them will be easy.

Maximum Score	Actual Score	

ORIENTATION

5　　( )　What is the (year) (season) (date) (day of the week) (month)?

5　　( )　Where are we?: For instance, what (state) (county) (town) (hospital) (floor)?

REGISTRATION

3　　( )　I am going to name three objects. After I have said them, I want you to repeat them. Remember what they are because I am going to ask you to name them again in a few minutes. Please repeat the three items for me.

Say the names of three unrelated objects, clearly and slowly, about one second for each. For instance, "Apple" . . . "Table" . . . "Penny" . . . .

Score the first try. Give 1 point for each correct answer.

Repeat objects until all are learned, up to six trials. If he does not eventually learn all three, recall cannot be meaningfully tested.

ATTENTION AND CALCULATION

5　　( )　Can you subtract 7 from 100, and then subtract 7 from the answer you get and keep subtracting 7 until I tell you to stop?

Stop after five subtractions. Count as correct each time the difference between numbers is 7.

Alternatively, Now I am going to spell a word forward and I want you to spell it backward. The word is WORLD, W-O-R-L-D. Spell "world" backward.

Repeat if necessary, but not after spelling starts. The score is the number of letters in correct order. E.g. dlrow = 5, dlorw = 3.

RECALL

3　　( )　Now what were the three objects I asked you to remember? *Score 0–3.*

→

LANGUAGE

2   ( )   *Show wristwatch.* What is this called?
              Show pencil. What is this called?
1   ( )   I'd like you to repeat a phrase after me: "No ifs, ands, or
              buts."
              Allow only one trial.
1   ( )   Read the words on this page and then do what it says.
              Hand "CLOSE YOUR EYES" sheet. Score 1 if he closes eyes.
3   ( )   *Read full statement and **then** hand over paper.*
              I'm going to give you a piece of paper. When I do, take
              the paper in your right hand, fold the paper in half
              with both hands, and put the paper down on your lap.
              Score 1 point for each part correctly executed.
1   ( )   Write any complete sentence on that piece of paper for
              me.
              *Do not dictate a sentence; it is to be written spontaneously. It
              must contain a subject and a verb and be sensible. Correct
              grammar and punctuation are not necessary.*
1   ( )   Here is a drawing. Please copy the drawing on the
              same paper exactly as it is.
              *Use a drawing of intersecting pentagons, each side about 1
              in. All 10 angles must be present and 2 must intersect
              (form a 4-sided figure) to score 1 point. Tremor and rota-
              tion are ignored.*

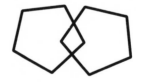

_____ TOTAL SCORE

ASSESS level of consciousness along a continuum

Alert	Drowsy	Stupor	Coma

Reprinted from *Journal of Psychiatric Research*, 12, M. F. Folstein, S. E. Folstein, & P. R. Folstein, "Mini-Mental State": A practical method for grading the cognitive state of patients for the clinician, pp. 196–198, Copyright 1975, with kind permission from Elsevier Science Ltd., The Boulevard, Langford Lane, Kidlington OX5 1GB, UK.

BLESSED–ROTH DEMENTIA SCALE

Purpose and Development

The Blessed–Roth Dementia Scale is a 22-item clinician-rated scale designed to assess severity of dementia (Blessed, Tomlinson, & Roth, 1968). The authors created items that tap competence in personal, domestic, and social activities, and changes in personality, interests, and drive. The scale is widely used by clinicians (Strang, Bradley, & Stockwell, 1989).

Administration and Scoring

The scale user obtains information from a relative or another individual in close contact with the patient. This individual responds to questions about the patient's functioning during the past six months. Disability is rated using a 0 to 1 scale for items 0 to 8, a 0 to 3 scale for items 9 to 11, and a 0 or 1 scale for items 12 to 22. The total score is the sum of all items. Scores can range from 0 to 28, with higher scores indicating more dementia.

Sample Scores

Blessed et al. (1968) reported that the mean scale score for 26 individuals with senile dementia was 13.92 (SD = 5.03), for 12 individuals with a functional psychosis it was 2.42 (SD = 1.44), for 14 individuals with delirium it was 2.00 (SD = 1.71), and for 8 control subjects who were physically ill it was 2.25 (SD = 1.75).

Reliability

Copeland and Wilson (1989) reported that an unpublished study by C. M. Lloyd found the scale had good test–retest reliability. Cole (1990) found that the scale had a rather low interrater reliability of .59.

Validity

The scale has been found to be associated with other measures of dementia (Eastwood, Lautenschlaeger, & Corbin, 1983). Blessed et al. (1968) found that individuals with higher scale scores later had higher post-mortem plaque counts and Perry, Tomlinson, Blessed, Bergman, Gibson, and Perry (1978) found a correlation between scale scores and a deficiency of brain choline acetyltransferase.

Blessed et al. (1968) reported that individuals who had been diagnosed with senile dementia had much higher scale scores than individuals with other diagnoses, including delirium. A study by Davis, Morris, and Grant (1990) confirmed that individuals diagnosed with dementia had much higher scores than others. Several studies have shown that the scale is sensitive to treatment interventions (e.g., Muratorio & 14 other authors, 1992; Spagnoli & 35 other authors, 1991).

BLESSED–ROTH DEMENTIA SCALE

Notes for General Guidance

Information should be obtained as far as possible from a relative in close and continual contact with the patient. Inquiries should be directed toward defining *changes* in capacity, habits, and personality. Allowance can be made in scoring for physical disabilities present that would of themselves restrict activities: e.g., you may ask "if your wife could walk normally, do you think she would be able to remember well enough to cope with shopping?"

Changes in Performance of Everyday Activities

Score 1 for significant and persisting disability; 1/2 for partial or intermittent disability; 0 for no change.

1. Inability to perform household tasks   1   1/2   0
2. Inability to cope with small sums of money   1   1/2   0
3. Inability to find way about indoors   1   1/2   0
4. Inability to find way about familiar streets   1   1/2   0
5. Inability to remember short lists of items, e.g., in shopping   1   1/2   0
6. Inability to recognize or interpret surroundings, e.g., whether at home or in another location such as a hospital, or to discriminate between relatives and medical/ nursing attendants, etc.   1   1/2   0
7. Inability to recall recent events of significance for the testee   1   1/2   0
8. Tendency to dwell in the past   1   1/2   0

Changes in Habits

Allocate the score most appropriate to the testee's usual capacity.

9. Eating:
   - Cleanly with proper utensils   0
   - Messily, e.g., with a spoon only   1
   - Can manage only simple solid foods, e.g., a biscuit   2
   - Has to be fed   3
10. Dressing:
    - Unaided and tidily   0
    - Slightly untidy, e.g., misplaced buttons   1

→

Wrong sequence, or omitting important items	2
Unable to dress	3

11. Sphincter control:

Complete	0
Occasional wet bed or pants	1
Frequent urinary incontinence	2
Incontinent of urine and feces	3

Changes in Personality, Interests, and Drive

Score 1 for each item reported provided this is a change, not a lifelong trait.

12. Increased rigidity	1
13. Increased egocentricity	1
14. Impaired regard for other people's feelings	1
15. Coarsening of affect (feelings)	1
16. Impaired emotional control, e.g., increased petulance, irritability or angry outbursts	1
17. Hilarity in inappropriate situations	1
18. Diminished emotional responsiveness	1
19. Sexual misdemeanor	1
20. Hobbies relinquished	1
21. Diminished initiative or drive	1
22. Purposeless overactivity	1

TOTAL SCORE _____

CORNELL SCALE FOR DEPRESSION IN DEMENTIA

Purpose and Uses

The 19-item clinician-rating Cornell Scale for Depression in Dementia (Alexopoulos, Abrams, Young, & Shamoian, 1988) was developed for use in assessing demented individuals, who as a group are more difficult to assess for depression than many other clients because of their intellectual deficits and tendency to experience rapidly shifting yet recurring moods. Alexopoulos and colleagues first reviewed the literature on depression in demented persons, collected information from geriatric psychiatrists and other experts, and then created items that can be rated primarily on the basis of observation.

Administration and Scoring

The clinician initially interviews the patient's caregiver and then briefly interviews the patient. The clinician chooses appropriate language to ask about each rating item. There are no set interview questions. The caregiver interview takes about 20 minutes and the patient interview about 10 minutes. If there is a large discrepancy between the information provided by the patient and the caregiver, the clinician interviews the caregiver again to try to find the basis for the differences (Alexopoulos et al., 1988).

The clinician uses a 0–2 scale to rate the client on 19 items. Scale scores are the sum of the ratings and can range from 0 to 38, with high scores indicating more depression. Scale users may decide that an item is unratable, but then the total scale score loses some meaning.

Sample Scores

Ott and Fogel (1992) found a mean score of 3.9 (SD = 2.8) for 25 outpatients evaluated at a memory disorders clinic for possible dementia. Alexopoulos et al. (1988) found a mean score of 4.7 (SD = 3.4) in 26 demented but nondepressed patients, and a mean score of 21.8 (SD = 4.0) for 12 demented patients diagnosed as having major depressive disorder.

Reliability

In a sample of demented patients, internal consistency as measured by Cronbach's alpha was .84 and interrater agreement as measured by weighted kappas was .62 and .63 (Alexopoulos et al., 1988).

Validity

Scale scores have been found to correlate .83 with levels of depression diagnosed on the basis of diagnostic criteria data collected by independent psychiatrists and to correlate significantly more highly with those depression levels than did Hamilton Depression Rating Scale scores, which did not even correlate significantly with depression levels in the most severely demented patients (Alexopoulos et al., 1988).

Ott and Fogel found that scale scores correlated .92 with the clinician-rated Hamilton Depression Rating Scale but only .40 with self-reported depression on the Geriatric Depression Scale in a group of outpatients being evaluated for dementia. The lower correlation with the self-report became even lower for clients who scored low on measures of either insight or mental status. Self-report scores were highly correlated with mental status and insight level, but the Cornell ratings were not, confirming the value of a clinician-rating with clients who have lower insight or mental status.

(Alexopoulos et al., 1988) also found that Cornell scores significantly decreased in demented patients after treatment for depression.

CORNELL SCALE FOR DEPRESSION IN DEMENTIA

SCORING SYSTEM

a = unable to evaluate
0 = absent
1 = mild or intermittent
2 = severe

Ratings should be based on symptoms and signs occurring during the week prior to interview. No score should be given if symptoms result from physical disability or illness.

A. MOOD-RELATED SIGNS

1. Anxiety	a	0	1	2
anxious expression, ruminations, worrying				
2. Sadness	a	0	1	2
sad expression, sad voice, tearfulness				
3. Lack of reactivity to pleasant events	a	0	1	2
4. Irritability	a	0	1	2
easily annoyed, short tempered				

B. BEHAVIORAL DISTURBANCE

5. Agitation	a	0	1	2
restlessness, handwringing, hair pulling				
6. Retardation	a	0	1	2
slow movements, slow speech, slow reactions				
7. Multiple physical complaints (score 0 if GI symptoms only)	a	0	1	2
8. Loss of interest	a	0	1	2
less involved in usual activities (score only if change occurred acutely, i.e., in less than 1 month)				

C. PHYSICAL SIGNS

9. Appetite loss	a	0	1	2
eating less than usual				
10. Weight loss	a	0	1	2
(score 2 if greater than 5 lb in 1 month)				

11. Lack of energy   a   0   1   2
    fatigues easily, unable to sustain activities
    (score only if change occurred acutely, i.e., in less than
    1 month)

D. CYCLIC FUNCTIONS

12. Diurnal variation of mood symptoms worse in the   a   0   1   2
    morning
13. Difficulty falling asleep   a   0   1   2
    later than usual for this individual
14. Multiple awakenings during sleep   a   0   1   2
15. Early morning awakening   a   0   1   2
    earlier than usual for this individual

E. IDEATIONAL DISTURBANCE

16. Suicide   a   0   1   2
    feels life is not worth living, has suicidal wishes, or
    makes suicide attempt
17. Poor self-esteem   a   0   1   2
    self-blame, self-depreciation, feelings of failure
18. Pessimism   a   0   1   2
    anticipation of the worst
19. Mood-congruent delusions   a   0   1   2
    delusions of poverty, illness, or loss

AGITATED BEHAVIOR SCALE

Purpose and Development

The Agitated Behavior Scale is a 14-item observer-based scale developed by Corrigan (1989) to assess agitation in individuals with brain trauma. It is intended mainly for use by staff members in inpatient settings. An initial pool of 39 items was generated on the basis of a literature review of previous descriptors for agitation and information provided by staff members working with head-trauma clients. The 14 items that had the best interrater reliability, contributed most to the total content realm of agitated behavior, and showed variance were selected for the scale. In a factor analytic study, Corrigan and Bogner (1994) found that a general construct of agitation underlies the scale, and that aggression, disinhibition, and lability were secondary underlying factors. In another factor analytic study, Fichera, Zielinski, Tremont, and Mittenberg (1994) found two main factors, psychomotor disinhibition and affective disinhibition.

Administration and Scoring

There is no fixed time interval for which the observer monitors the individual; however, Corrigan (1989) suggested a day or, in inpatient settings, a shift as an appropriate time interval for observation. The observer uses a 1 to 4 scale of frequency to rate the items. The 14 items are summed for a total score that may range from 1 to 56, with higher scores indicating more agitation.

Fichera et al. (1994) calculated subscale scores for Psychomotor Disinhibition by summing items 1, 6, 7, 8, 9, 10, and 11 and for Affective Disinhibition by summing items 2, 3, 4, 5, 12, 13, and 14. Scores on the subscales may range from 7 to 28, with higher scores indicating more disinhibition and agitation.

Sample Scores

In a sample of 150 head-injured patients with mild to severe injuries, Fichera et al. (1994) reported a mean total scale score of 17.6 (SD = 5.3). Another sample of 51 head-injured patients had a mean score of 18.73 (SD = 6.19) while a sample of orthopedic trauma patients with no neurological injury had a mean score of 15.31 (SD = 2.26) (Zielinski, Theroux-Fichera, Tremont, Rayls, & Mittenberg, 1994).

Reliability

Internal consistency as assessed by Cronbach's alpha ranged from .84 to .92 for four different observers in Corrigan's (1989) study and was .85 in Fichera et al.'s (1994) study. Corrigan (1989) reported interrater reliability ranged from .71 to .79.

Validity

Corrigan (1989) found that scale scores were associated with several other measures of agitation. Higher scale scores have also been found to be associated with poorer cognitive functioning (Corrigan & Mysiw, 1988; Corrigan, Mysiw, Gribble, & Chock, 1992), poorer attention (Corrigan et al., 1992), more severe coma, and more severe amnesia after a head injury (Fichera, Zielinski, & Mittenberg, 1993; Fichera et al., 1994).

Fichera et al. (1994) reported that patients with different types of head trauma showed different subscale profiles. Patients with frontal lesions were more likely to have high scores on the Psychomotor Disinhibition Scale while patients with diffuse trauma were more likely to have high scores on the Affective Disinhibition Scale.

Tracking the recovery of head trauma patients, Fichera et al. (1994) found that patients who had more severe injuries, subcortical lesions, or heavy preinjury alcohol use showed the most persistent agitation.

AGITATED BEHAVIOR SCALE

At the end of the observation period indicate whether each behavior was present and, if so, to what degree: slight, moderate, or extreme. The degree can be based on either the frequency of the behavior or the severity of a given incident. Use the following numerical values for every behavior listed. DO NOT LEAVE BLANKS.

1 = absent
2 = present to a slight degree
3 = present to a moderate degree
4 = present to an extreme degree

_____ 1. Short attention span, easy distractibility, inability to concentrate.
_____ 2. Impulsive, impatient, low tolerance for pain or frustration.
_____ 3. Uncooperative, resistant to care, demanding.
_____ 4. Violent and/or threatening violence toward people or property.
_____ 5. Explosive and/or unpredictable anger.
_____ 6. Rocking, rubbing, moaning, or other self-stimulating behavior.
_____ 7. Pulling at tubes, restraints, etc.
_____ 8. Wandering from treatment areas.
_____ 9. Restlessness, pacing, excessive movement.
_____ 10. Repetitive behaviors, motor and/or verbal.
_____ 11. Rapid, loud, or excessive talking.
_____ 12. Sudden changes of mood.
_____ 13. Easily initiated or excessive crying and/or laughter.
_____ 14. Self-abusiveness, physical and/or verbal.

_____ TOTAL SCORE

Reprinted with permission of Swets Publishing Service from Corrigan, J. D. (1989). Development of a scale for assessment of agitation following traumatic brain injury. *Journal of Clinical and Experimental Neuropsychology, 11,* 261–277.

REFERENCES

Alexopoulas, G., Abrams, R., Young, R., & Shamoian, C. (1988). Cornell Scale for Depression in Dementia. *Biological Psychiatry, 23,* 271–284.
Blessed, G., Tomlinson, B. E., & Roth, M. (1968). The association between quantitative measures of dementia and of senile change in the cerebral grey matter of elderly subjects. *British Journal of Psychiatry, 114,* 797–811.
Chaves, M. L., & Izquierdo, I. (1992). Differential diagnosis between dementia and depression: A study of efficiency increment. *Acta Neurologica Scandinavica, 85,* 378–382.
Cole, M. G. (1990). Interrater reliability of the Blessed Dementia Scale. *Canadian Journal of Psychiatry, 35,* 328–330.
Copeland, J. R. M., & Wilson, K. C. M. (1989). Rating scales in old age psychiatry. In C. Thompson (Ed.), *The instruments of psychiatric research* (pp. 305–335). New York: Wiley.
Davis, P. B., Morris, J. C., & Grant, E. G. (1990). Brief screening tests versus clinical staging in senile dementia of the Alzheimer type. *Journal of the American Geriatrics Society, 38,* 129–135.
Corrigan, J. D. (1989). Development of a scale for assessment of agitation following traumatic brain injury. *Journal of Clinical and Experimental Neuropsychology, 11,* 261–277.
Corrigan, J. D., & Bogner, J. A. (1994). Factor structure of the Agitated Behavior Scale. *Journal of Clinical and Experimental Neuropsychology, 16,* 386–392.
Corrigan, J. D., & Mysiw, W. J. (1988). Agitation following traumatic head injury: Equivocal evidence for a discrete stage of cognitive recovery. *Archives of Physical Medicine and Rehabilitation, 69,* 487–492.
Corrigan, J. D., Mysiw, W. J., Gribble, M. W., & Chock, S. K. (1992). Agitation, cognition and attention during post-traumatic amnesia. *Brain Injury, 6,* 155–160.
DesRosiers, G. (1992). Primary or depressive dementia: Mental status screening. *International Journal of Neuroscience, 64,* 33–67.
Eagger, S. A., Levy, R., & Sahakian, B. J. (1992). Tacrine in Alzheimer's disease. *Acta Neurologica Scandinavica, 85,* 75–80.
Eastwood, M. R., Lautenschlaeger, E., & Corbin, S. (1983). A comparison of clinical methods for assessing dementia. *Journal of the American Geriatric Society, 31,* 342–347.
Fichera, S., Zielinski, R., & Mittenberg, W. (1993). Neuropsychological correlates of post-traumatic agitation. *Journal of Clinical and Experimental Neuropsychology, 15,* 105–106.
Fichera, S., Zielinski, R., Tremont, G., & Mittenberg, W. (1994). Psychometric properties of the Agitated Behavior Scale. *Archives of Clinical Neuropsychology, 9,* 127–129.
Folstein, M., Anthony, J., Parhead, J., Duffy, B., & Gruenberg, E. (1985). The meaning of cognitive impairment in the elderly. *Journal of the American Geriatrics Society, 33,* 228–235.
Folstein, M., Folstein, S., & McHugh, P. R. (1971). "Mini-Mental State": A practical method for grading the cognitive state of patients for the clinician. *Journal of Psychiatric Research, 12,* 189–198.
Galasko, D., Abramson, I., Corey-Bloom, J., & Thal, L. J. (1993). Repeated exposure to the Mini-Mental State Examination and the Information-Memory-Concentration Test results in a practice effect in Alzheimer's disease. *Neurology, 43,* 1559–1563.
Harper, R. G., Chacko, R. C., Kotik-Harper, D., & Kirby, H. B. (1992). Comparison of two cognitive screening measures for efficacy in differentiating dementia from depression in a geriatric inpatient population. *Journal of Neuropsychiatry and Clinical Neurosciences, 4,* 179–184.
Hill, L. R., Klauber, M. R., Salmon, D. P., Yu, E. S., Liv, W. T., Zhang, M., & Katzman, R. (1993). Functional status, education, and the diagnosis of dementia in the Shanghai survey. *Neurology, 43,* 138–145.

Jagger, C., Clarke, M., & Anderson, J. (1992). Screening for dementia: A comparison of two tests using receiver operating characteristics (ROC) analysis. *International Journal of Geriatric Psychiatry, 7,* 659–665.

Jensen, E., Dehlin, O., & Gustafson, L. (1993). A comparison between three psychogeriatric rating scales. *International Journal of Geriatric Psychiatry, 8,* 215–229.

Kummer, J., Gundel, L., Van Laak, H. H., & Hirche, H. (1992). Efficacy and tolerance of naftidrofuryl in multi-infarct dementia: A placebo-controlled double-blind study. *Zeitschrift fur Gerontopsychologie and Psychiatrie, 5,* 25–41.

Lindal, E., & Stephansson, J. G. (1993). Mini-Mental State Examination scores: Gender and lifetime psychiatric disorders. *Psychological Reports, 72,* 631–641.

Muratorio, A., & 14 other authors (1992). A neurotropic approach to the treatment of multi-infarct dementia using 1-alpha-glycerylphosphorylcholine. *Current Therapeutic Research, 52,* 741–752.

Orrell, M. W., Howard, R., Payne, A., Bergmann, K., Woods, R., Everitt, B., & Levy, R. (1992). Differentiation between organic and functional psychiatric illness in the elderly: An evaluation of four cognitive tests. *International Journal of Geriatric Psychiatry, 7,* 263–275.

Ott, B., & Fogel, B. (1992). Measurement of depression in dementia: Self vs. clinician rating. *International Journal of Geriatric Psychiatry, 7,* 899–904.

Park, J. H., & Ha, J. C. (1988). Cognitive impairment among the elderly in a Korean rural community. *Acta Psychiatrica Scandanavica, 77,* 52–57.

Perry, E. K., Tomlinson, B. E., Blessed, G., Bergman, K., Gibson, P. H., & Perry, R. H. (1978). Correlation of cholinergic abnormalities with senile plaques and mental test scores in senile dementia. *British Medical Journal, 2,* 1457–1459.

Rockwood, K. (1993). The occurrence and duration of symptoms in elderly patients with delirium. *Journal of Gerontology, 48,* 162–166.

Rodriquez-Alvarez, M. (1991). The presence of a temporal orientation impairment in heroin users. *Revista de Psicologia Universitas Tarragonensis, 13,* 59–64.

Rosen, J., Sweet, R. A., Mulsant, B. H., Rifai, A. H., Pasternak, R., & Zubenko, G. S. (1994). The Delirium Rating Scale in a psychogeriatric inpatient setting. *Journal of Neuropsychiatry and Clinical Neuroscience, 6,* 30–35.

Saletu, B, Moller, H. F., Grunberger, J., Deutsch, H., & Rossner, M. (1990–91). Propentofylline in adult-onset cognitive disorders: Double-blind, placebo-controlled, clinical, psychometric and brain mapping studies. *Neuropsychobiology, 24,* 173–184.

Spagnoli, A., & 35 other authors (1991). Long-term acetyl-1-carnitine treatment in Alzheimer's disease. *Neurology, 41,* 1726–1732.

Strang, J., Bradley, B., & Stockwell, T. (1989). Assessment of drug and alcohol use. In C. Thompson (Ed.), *The instruments of psychiatric research* (pp. 211–235). New York: Wiley.

Tombaugh, T. N., & McIntyre, N. J. (1992). The Mini-Mental State Examination: A comprehensive review. *Journal of the American Geriatrics Society, 40,* 922–935.

Trzepacz, P. T., Baker, R. W., & Greenhouse, J. (1988). A symptom rating scale for delirium. *Psychiatry Research, 23,* 89–97.

Turrina, D. C., Dewey, M. E., Siani, R., Saviotti, F., Marchione, N., & Siciliani, O. (1993). Performance of the Italian version of the Mini-Mental State Examination in day hospital geriatric medical patients. *International Journal of Geriatric Psychiatry, 8,* 649–654.

Van der Cammen, J. J., Van Harskamp, F., Stronks, D. L., Passchier, J., & Schudel, W. J. Value of the Mini-Mental State Examination and informants' data for the detection of dementia in geriatric outpatients. *Psychological Reports, 71,* 1003–1009.

Wada, Y., & Yamaguchi, N. (1993). Delirium in the elderly: Relationship of clinical symptoms to outcome. *Dementia, 4,* 113–116.

Wiederholt, W. C., Cahn, D., Butters, N. M., Salmon, D. P., Kritz-Silverstein, D., & Barrett-Connor, E. (1993). Effects of age, gender and education on selected neuropsychological tests in an elderly community cohort. *Journal of the American Geriatrics Society, 41*, 639–647.

Zielinski, R. E., Theroux-Fichera, S., Tremont, G., Rayls, K. R., & Mittenberg, W. (1994). Normative data for the agitated behavior scale. *The Clinical Neuropsychologist, 8*, 348–350.

Substance-Related Disorders

CAGE ALCOHOL INTERVIEW SCHEDULE

Purpose and Development

The CAGE, developed by J.A. Ewing and B.A. Rouse, is a 4-item interview schedule that assesses alcohol abuse. The name "CAGE" comes from letters in the four questions: *cut, annoyed, guilty, eye*-opener (Mayfield, McLeod, & Hall, 1974). The CAGE is much briefer than most alcohol screening measures and can therefore serve as a way for health and mental health professionals to quickly screen clients for alcohol abuse as a supplement to assessment for other problems. The CAGE is very widely used in applied settings (Strang, Bradley, & Stockwell, 1989).

Administration and Scoring

Before asking the CAGE questions, one might want to ask the client whether he or she ever drinks, as Mayfield et al. (1974) did. A negative answer might be reason to forgo asking the CAGE questions.

The scale does not limit responses to any time frame, so the interviewer should inquire about the time frame of all affirmative responses in order to determine whether drinking is a current problem (Jacobson, 1989). Clients can easily fake good or bad on this obvious interview schedule, so when a scale user has reason to suspect that responses are not accurate, it is best to collect related information from other sources (Jacobson, 1989), such as family members and treatment records.

It is easy to convert the CAGE into a questionnaire, as Werner & Greene (1992) did to assess hundreds of college students. No evidence appears to exist about whether scores differ between questionnaire and interview formats.

Affirmative responses are summed for a total score. Scores can range from 0 to 4, with higher scores indicating more alcohol problems.

Cut-Off and Sample Scores

Mayfield et al. (1974) recommend that two or more affirmative responses to the questions be viewed as suggesting an alcohol problem and justifying an in-depth examination of drinking patterns, causes, and results. Several studies have examined the classification value of this cut-off. With psychiatric inpatients who were diagnosed as alcoholic or not alcoholic, Mayfield et al. (1974) found 81% accuracy in identifying alcoholics and 89% accuracy in identifying nonalcoholics. Mischke and Venneri (1987) evaluated the cut-off against alcohol counselor conclusions about whether convicted drunk drivers were alcoholics and found 86% correct classification of alcoholics and 60% correct classification of nonalcoholics.

With regard to medical patients, Moore, Bone, Geller, Mamon, Stokes, & Levine (1989) concluded that on the basis of prior studies that the CAGE has about 80% accuracy. Later studies have confirmed this. For instance, in a group of elderly medicine outpatients, Buschbaum, Buchanan, Welsh, Centor, & Schnoll (1992) used Diagnostic Interview Schedule alcohol abuse or dependence diagnoses as a standard and found 70% accuracy in identifying alcoholics and 91% accuracy in identifying nonalcoholics. Bauschbaum et al. (1992) noted accuracy rates of 80–85% with regard to two other recently published studies of primary care patients. However, studies of college students using questionnaire forms of the scale have found lower classification accuracy with regard to groups defined by quantity of alcohol consumed (Heck & Lichtenberg, 1990; Smith, Collins, Kreisberg, Volpicelli, & Alterman, 1987). See Smart et al. (1992) for descriptions of other cut-off studies.

In an Ontario community survey of 703 adults, Smart, Adlaf, & Knoke (1991) found a mean score of .44, $SD = .84$.

Reliability

Mischke and Venneri (1987) found internal consistency, as measured by Cronbach's alpha, to be .71 for the CAGE. Smart et al. (1991) found an average interitem correlation of .58.

Validity

Studies have shown that scale scores are correlated with scores on other measures of alcohol abuse and a diagnosis of alcohol abuse or dependence (Lee & DeFrank, 1988; Susman, Sitorius, Schneider, & Gilbert, 1992) and with level of alcohol use (Heck, 1991; Lee & DeFrank, 1988; Nystrom, Perasalo, & Salapuro, 1993; Werner & Greene, 1992).

Bernadt, Mumford, and Murray (1984) found that scale scores discriminated significantly between diagnosed alcoholics and other psychiatric inpatients. Similarly, the studies mentioned above that tested the classification accuracy of the scale also serve as strong evidence of validity.

Finally, studies have shown that the scale identifies alcoholics more accurately than blood tests (Bell & Steensland, 1987; Lairson, Harlow, Cobb, Harrist, Martin, Ramby, Rustin, & Swint, 1992) and better than physicians not using a scale (Moore et al., 1989).

CAGE ALCOHOL INTERVIEW SCHEDULE

1. Have you ever felt you should cut down on your drinking?
2. Have people annoyed you by criticizing your drinking?
3. Have you ever felt bad or guilty about your drinking?
4. Have you ever had a drink first thing in the morning to steady your nerves or get rid of a hang-over (eye-opener)?

SELF-ADMINISTERED ALCOHOLISM SCREENING TEST (SAAST)

Purpose and Development

The SAAST, developed by Swenson & Morse (1975), is a self-administered version of the popular Michigan Alcoholism Screening Test (MAST;
Selzer, 1971). When the many versions of the MAST are considered together, the MAST is the most widely used scale in the substance abuse field
(Jacobson, 1989; Strang, Bradley, & Stockwell, 1989). The SAAST includes
modified wordings of 24 of the 25 MAST items.

The original SAAST included 34 items (Swenson & Morse, 1975), but
later modifications included one or more additional items (Davis, de la
Fuente, Morse, Landa, & O'Brien, 1989). We will provide a 35-item version
which includes the original 34 items plus one more item (our #29) described by Hurt, Morse, & Swenson (1980). This version has been the most
used one in recently published articles.

Generally the client completes the scale. Alternatively, a close friend
or relative of the client can do so (Swenson & Morse, 1975; Loethen &
Khavari, 1990) or the client's counselor can complete the scale (Swenson &
Morse, 1975).

Administration and Scoring

The scale score is the sum of "no" responses to questions 2, 5, 7, and 8,
and "yes" responses to the other questions. Scores can range from 0 to 35,
with higher scores indicating more alcohol problems.

Although it is not completely clear to what extent nonroutine administration methods might affect scale scores, in a group of inpatient alcoholics, Swenson and Morse (1975) found similar scores for self-completion
and completion by a spouse regarding the inpatient, and scores about a
standard deviation (5 points) higher when alcohol counselors completed
the ratings regarding the inpatient. Loethen and Khavari (1990) also found
similar scores between SAAST's completed by alcoholics and SAAST's
completed by friends and relatives regarding the alcoholics.

Cut-off and Sample Scores

Swenson and Morse (1975) recommended interpreting a score of 6 or
less as indicating no alcoholism, 7–9 as indicating a strong possibility of
alcoholism, and 10 or more as indicating probable alcoholism. Using the
recommended cutoff of 10, Swenson and Morse (1975) correctly identified
84% of 100 alcoholic patients as alcoholics and 97% of medical patients as

nonalcoholics. Davis and Morse (1987) found 88–89% accuracy in classifying 583 alcoholic inpatients.

Davis, Hurt, Morse, & O'Brien (1987) reported a mean of 2.69 (SD = 1.74) for 636 nonalcoholic medical patients and 15.87 (SD = 5.92) for 473 alcoholics.

Reliability

Davis et al. (1987) found Kudor–Richardson formula 20 (internal consistency) to be .81. In a review of alcohol-abuse measures, Jacobson (1989) concluded that the scale has reasonably good reliability.

Validity

Scale scores have been found to correlate with biochemical indicators of alcohol use (Peterson, Scott, & Jovanovic-Peterson, 1991) and with other psychological measures of alcoholism (Loethen & Khavari, 1990). Several studies have found evidence that scale scores distinguish between normals and individuals otherwise found to have alcohol-use problems (Davis et al., 1987; Russell & Bigler, 1979; Smith & Pristach, 1990; Swenson & Morse, 1975). Further, the acceptable validity of the MAST as documented by many studies (Lee, 1992) can to some extent be extended to the SAAST because of the great overlap in items. Jacobson (1989), after reviewing the validity research on the SAAST, concluded that the scale has reasonably good validity.

SELF-ADMINISTERED ALCOHOL SCREENING TEST

Please write "Y" for yes or "N" for no to the left of each question.

_____ 1. Do you enjoy a drink now and then? (If you never drink alcoholic beverages, and have no previous experience with drinking, do not continue with questionnaire.)

_____ 2. Do you feel you are a normal drinker (that is, drink no *more* than average)?

_____ 3. Have you ever awakened the morning after some drinking the night before and found you could not remember a part of the evening?

_____ 4. Do close relatives ever worry about your drinking?

_____ 5. Can you stop drinking without a struggle after one or two drinks?

_____ 6. Do you ever feel guilty about your drinking?

_____ 7. Do friends or relatives think you are a normal drinker?

_____ 8. Are you always able to stop drinking when you want to?

_____ 9. Have your ever attended a meeting of Alcoholics Anonymous (AA) because of your drinking?

_____ 10. Have you gotten into physical fights when drinking?

_____ 11. Has your drinking ever created problems between you and your wife, husband, parent, or near relative?

_____ 12. Has your wife, husband, or other family member ever gone to anyone for help about your drinking?

_____ 13. Have you ever lost friendships because of your drinking?

_____ 14. Have you ever gotten into trouble at work because of drinking?

_____ 15. Have you ever lost a job because of drinking?

_____ 16. Have you ever neglected your obligations, your family, or your work for two or more days in a row because you were drinking?

_____ 17. Do you ever drink in the morning?

_____ 18. Have you ever felt the need to cut down on your drinking?

_____ 19. Have there been times in your adult life when you have found it necessary to completely avoid alcohol?

_____ 20. Have you ever been told you have liver trouble? Cirrhosis?

_____ 21. Have you ever had delirium tremens (DTs)?

_____ 22. Have you ever had severe shaking, heard voices, or seen things that weren't there after heavy drinking?

_____ 23. Have you ever gone to anyone for help about your drinking?

_____ 24. Have you ever been in a hospital because of drinking?

_____ 25. Have you been told by a doctor to stop drinking?

➤

_____ 26. Have you ever been a patient in a psychiatric hospital or on a psychiatric ward of a general hospital?

_____ 27. Was your drinking part of the problem that resulted in that hospitalization?

_____ 28. Have you ever been a patient at a psychiatric or mental health clinic or gone to any doctor, social worker, or clergyman for help with any emotional problem?

_____ 29. Was your drinking part of the problem?

_____ 30. Have you ever been arrested, even for a few hours, because of drunken behavior (not driving)? How many times? _____

_____ 31. Have you ever been arrested, even for a few hours, because of driving while intoxicated? How many times? _____

_____ 32–35. Have any of the following relatives ever had problems with alcohol?

_____ 32. (A) Parents

_____ 33. (B) Brothers or sisters

_____ 34. (C) Husband or wife

_____ 35. (D) Children

Reprinted from Swenson et al. (1975, pp. 207–208), with permission of the Mayo Clinic Proceedings.

Drug Abuse Screening Test

Purpose and Uses

The 28-item self-report Drug Abuse Screening Test (Skinner, 1982), often called the DAST, is the Michigan Alcoholism Screening Test (MAST) with the wording changed to ask about "drugs" rather than alcohol. The Drug Abuse Screening Test provides a total score based on information about the negative psychological, social, job, medical, and legal effects of drug use. Two factor analyses have indicated that the scale is unidimensional (Langevin & Lang,1990; Skinner, 1982), but a factor analysis by Skinner and Goldberg (1986) found four to six factors, including factors best described as dependence, social problems, medical problems, and previous treatment.

Administration and Scoring

Respondents answer yes or no to questions. Summing "no" responses to items 4, 5, and 7, and "yes" responses to the other items leads to a scale score which can range from 0 to 28, with higher scores indicating more substance abuse.

We will provide the scale items with Skinner's (1982) instructions, which do not substantially define the term "drugs." When Skinner created the scale virtually everyone would interpret drugs to exclude alcohol and tobacco. More recently, many substance abuse professionals have begun characterizing alcohol and tobacco as drugs, and as a result some clients may be unsure about the meaning of the term "drug" in the items. Scale users therefore may want to make explicit that the scale is not asking about alcohol or tobacco use.

Cutoff and Sample Scores

In a group of substance abuse and psychiatric patients, Staley and El-Guebaly (1990) found that using 8 as the minimum score (cutoff) for categorizing someone as a substance abuser led to correctly identifying 93% of substance abusers and 88% of nonabusers. Cut-offs of 6 to 11 worked about as well as 8.

For a group of 105 narcotic users seeking help at an addiction treatment center, Skinner and Goldberg (1986) found a mean score of 12.8 (*SD* = 3.6).

Reliability

Langevin and Lang (1990), Skinner (1982), and Skinner and Goldberg (1986) found internal consistency as measured by Cronbach's alpha to range from .74 to .92.

Validity

Skinner (1982) found that scales scores correlated significantly with frequency of self-reported use of several types of drugs (such as heroin). Skinner and Goldberg (1986) found that scale scores correlated with the number of drugs currently being used. Bilal, Khatter, Hassan, and Berry (1992) found that responses on several of the scale items correlated significantly with findings of amphetamines in the urine of conscripts. Skinner (1982) found that individuals seeking help for drug problems had significantly higher scale scores than individuals seeking help for alcohol problems only, and Staley and El-Guebaly (1990) found significantly higher scale scores for individuals in a substance treatment program than for psychiatric patients.

On the negative side, Skinner (1982) found that higher scale scores were associated with higher scores on a measure of carelessness and with lower scores on measures of denial and social desirability responding.

DRUG ABUSE SCREENING TEST

The following questions concern information about your involvement with and abuse of drugs. Drug abuse refers to (1) the use of prescribed or "over-the-counter" drugs in excess of the directions and (2) any nonmedical use of drugs. Carefully read each statement and decide whether your answer is yes or no. Then circle the appropriate response.

Yes No 1. Have you used drugs other than those required for medical reasons?

Yes No 2. Have you abused prescription drugs?

Yes No 3. Do you abuse more than one drug at a time?

Yes No 4. Can you get through the week without using drugs (other than those required for medical reasons)?

Yes No 5. Are you always able to stop using drugs when you want to?

Yes No 6. Do you abuse drugs on a continuous basis?

Yes No 7. Do you try to limit your drug use to certain situations?

Yes No 8. Have you had "blackouts" or "flashbacks" as a result of drug use?

Yes No 9. Do you ever feel bad about your drug abuse?

Yes No 10. Does your spouse (or parents) ever complain about your involvement with drugs?

Yes No 11. Do your friends or relatives know or suspect you abuse drugs?

Yes No 12. Has drug abuse ever created problems between you and your spouse?

Yes No 13. Has any family member ever sought help for problems related to your drug use?

Yes No 14. Have you ever lost friends because of your use of drugs?

Yes No 15. Have you ever neglected your family or missed work because of your use of drugs?

Yes No 16. Have you ever been in trouble at work because of drug abuse?

Yes No 17. Have you ever lost a job because of drug abuse?

Yes No 18. Have you gotten into fights when under the influence of drugs?

Yes No 19. Have you ever been arrested because of unusual behavior while under the influence of drugs?

Yes No 20. Have you ever been arrested for driving while under the influence of drugs?

➤

Yes   No   21. Have you engaged in illegal activities in order to obtain drugs?

Yes   No   22. Have you ever been arrested for possession of illegal drugs?

Yes   No   23. Have you ever experienced withdrawal symptoms as a result of heavy drug intake?

Yes   No   24. Have you had medical problems as a result of your drug use (e.g., memory loss, hepatitis, convulsions, bleeding, etc.)?

Yes   No   25. Have you ever gone to anyone for help for a drug problem?

Yes   No   26. Have you ever been in hospital for medical problems related to your drug use?

Yes   No   27. Have you ever been involved in a treatment program specifically related to drug use?

Yes   No   28. Have you been treated as an out-patient for problems related to drug abuse?

Reprinted from Skinner, H. A. (1982). The Drug Abuse Screening Test. *Addictive Behaviors, 7,* 363–371. Elsevier Science Ltd, Pergamon Imprint, Oxford, England.

FAGERSTROM TEST FOR NICOTINE DEPENDENCE

Nature and Uses

The 6-item self-report Fagerstrom Test for Nicotine Dependence (Heatherton, Kozlowski, Frecker, & Fagerstrom (1991) is a revision of the 8-item Fagerstrom Tolerance Questionnaire (Fagerstrom, 1978), which has been very popular for years. The revision was prompted by evidence that the earlier scale was not homogeneous, had low internal consistency (under .60), contained items that added little but error variance, one item (whether the respondent inhales) had virtually no variance, another item (nicotine yield) tended to provide inaccurate information, and two items (time to first cigarette of day and number of cigarettes per day) had scoring levels that tended to obscure important differences (Heatherton et al., 1991). The revision involved eliminating the inhalation and nicotine yield items and modifying the rating levels for time to first cigarette and number of cigarettes per day.

A factor analysis of the modified scale found that it was reasonably homogeneous and much more so than the earlier version of the scale (Heatherton et al., 1991).

Administration and Scoring

For each question, respondents choose from a selection of two to four possible answers. For item 1, score "within 5 minutes" as 3, "6–30 minutes" as 2, "31–60 minutes" as 1, and "after 90 minutes" as 0. For items 2, 5, and 6, score "yes" responses as 1 and "no" responses as 0. For item 3, score "first one in the morning" as 1 and "all others" as 0. For item 4, score the four responses in order 0 to 3.

The scale score is the sum of all responses. Scores can range from 0 to 10, with higher scores indicating more dependence.

Reliability

Cronbach's alpha for the Dependence scale has varied from .61 (Heatherton et al., 1991) to .64 (Pomerleau, Carton, Lutzke, Flessland, & Pomerleau, 1994), always higher than found for the prior version of the scale. Pomerleau et al. (1994) found a test–retest reliability of .88 for periods of about two to six weeks.

Validity

Scale scores have been found to correlate with carbon monoxide levels in breath samples (Heatherton et al., 1991), levels of cotinine (a metabolite of nicotine) in salivary samples (Heatherton et al., 1991; Pomerleau et al., 1994), scores on a measure of addictive reasons for smoking, and number of years smoked (Pomerleau et al., 1994). Heatherton et al. (1994) and Pomerleau et al. (1994) found that the correlations between the scale and other variables studied were similar to the correlations between the prior version of the scale and these variables.

With the overlap in items between the scale and its earlier version, we believe that the many studies supporting the validity of the earlier version also serve to some extent to support the validity of the modified scale. After reviewing research on the earlier version of the scale, Shiffman (1988) concluded that studies have consistently found that scale scores predict severity of craving, withdrawal symptoms, and relapse. Perhaps most important as a practical matter, studies have consistently found that among individuals who are trying to quit, those who have high scores on the earlier version tend to benefit the most from prescribed nicotine supplements (Shiffman, 1988).

Fagerstrom Test for Nicotine Dependence

For each question, circle one answer.

1. How soon after you wake up do you smoke your first cigarette?

   Within 5 minutes   6–30 minutes   31–60 minutes   After 60 minutes

2. Do you find it difficult to refrain from smoking in places where it is forbidden e.g. in church, at the library, in cinema, etc.?

   Yes   No

3. Which cigarette would you hate most to give up?

   The first one in the morning   All others

4. How many cigarettes/day to you smoke?

   10 or less   11–20   21–30   31 or more

5. Do you smoke more frequently during the first hours after waking than during the rest of the day?

   Yes   No

6. Do you smoke if you are so ill that you are in bed most of the day?

   Yes   No

Reprinted with permission of Dr. Karl-Olav Fagerstrom.

HORN–WAINGROW REASONS FOR SMOKING SCALE

Nature and Uses

The Reasons for Smoking Scale (Ikard, Green, & Horn, 1969) is a 23-item self-report measure of reasons the respondent smokes. The scale is based on a theory of Tomkins (1966) that postulated four explanations for smoking: smoking to reduce negative feelings, smoking to increase positive feelings, habitual smoking (no emotional effect), and addictive smoking (smoking to end negative feelings caused by the lack of smoking and to obtain the positive feelings that occur when the withdrawal ends).

Horn and Waingrow created the scale by revising a scale developed by Schwartz and Little to measure these reasons for smoking (see Ikard et al., 1969). The Horn–Waingrow scale has been used in dozens of published studies (Tate, Schmitz, & Stanton, 1991). An 18-item version of the scale is sometimes used (e.g., Niura, Goldstein, Ward, & Abrams 1989), but we prefer the original 23-item scale because more psychometric evaluations have been reported on it.

The scale can be used to study smoking motivations in groups or individuals and to help devise treatment plans (Shiffman, 1988). Theoretically, smokers high on a particular motivation (e.g., negative affect reduction) might benefit the most from treatment focused on that motivation (e.g., stress management training).

Administration and Scoring

For each item, respondents indicate how often a statement is true for them on a 5-point scale (1 = never, 2 = seldom, 3 = occasionally, 4 = frequently, 5 = always).

The 23-item Horn–Waingrow scale has six subscales that measure motivations for smoking. A factor analysis identified the items that make up each subscale (Ikard et al., 1969): negative affect reduction (items 3, 7, 11, 14, 17, 19), pleasurable relaxation (items 16, 21), stimulation (items 1, 9, 23), addiction (craving after a period of not smoking; items 5, 10, 13, 18, 22), habituation (automatic; items 2, 8, 15, 20), and sensorimotor stimulation (items 4, 6, 12). Many studies (e.g., Livson & Leino, 1988) have substantiated the 6-factor structure originally reported by Ikard et al. (1969).

Sample Scores

Tate, Schmitz, & Stanton (1991) reported mean scores for 61 college student smokers. See Table 1. The scale developers (Ikard et al., 1969) recommend considering mean subscale scores to be "high" if they are over 3.

TABLE 1
Reasons for Smoking Subscale Means and Reliability

| | | | | Reliability | |
| | | | | Test–Retest | |
Subscale	*Mean*	*SD*	Alpha	Several days	Three years
Negative affect reduction	3.5	0.7	.83	.73	.64
Pleasurable relaxation	3.9	0.6	.76	.43	.62
Stimulation	2.7	0.8	.75	.61	.51
Addictive	2.9	0.8	.78	.75	.48
Habitual	2.1	0.6	.60	.74	.53
Sensorimotor manipulation	2.4	0.8	.64	.89	.67

Reliability and Stability

Table 1 provides reported subscale alpha coefficients (Tate et al., 1991), test–retest reliability coefficients for several days (Mausner and Platt 1971), and test-retest stability coefficients for three years (Costa, McCrae, & Bosse, 1980), all for current smokers.

Validity

Studies have found that various Reasons for Smoking subscale scores correlated with number of cigarettes smoked (Ikard et al., 1969), tar and nicotine consumption (Bosse, Garvey, & Glynn, 1980), and daily self-monitoring of reasons for smoking using a format similar to the Reasons for Smoking Scale (Tate et al., 1991). There was no clear pattern of which subscales correlated with other variables.

In treatment studies, some subscales predicted withdrawal signs, urge to smoke, number of cigarettes smoked (Niura et al., 1989; 18-item scale) and maintained abstinence (Mothersill, McDowell, & Rosser 1988). O'Connell and Shiffman (1988) found that individuals with high pretreatment Negative Affect Reduction subscale scores were more likely than others to relapse in situations involving negative emotions.

In a recent review of research on the Reasons for Smoking Scale, Tate et al. (1991) rated the validity data weak and inconsistent. The reviewers based their negative conclusion about validity in large part on a number of studies that were not designed to test the validity of the scale and that provide ambiguous information at best. We do agree, however, that validity results for the subscales have not been consistent.

HORN-WAINGROW REASONS FOR SMOKING SCALE

Please use the scale below to indicate the extent to which each statement is true for you. Mark your response to the left of the item.

1 = never
2 = seldom
3 = occasionally
4 = frequently
5 = always

_____ 1. I smoke cigarettes to stimulate me, to perk myself up.
_____ 2. I've found a cigarette in my mouth and didn't remember putting it there.
_____ 3. When I smoke a cigarette, part of the enjoyment is watching the smoke as I exhale it.
_____ 4. When I am trying to solve a problem, I light up a cigarette.
_____ 5. I am very much aware of the fact when I am not smoking a cigarette.
_____ 6. Part of the enjoyment of smoking a cigarette comes from the steps I take to light up.
_____ 7. When I feel "blue" or want to take my mind off cares and worries, I smoke cigarettes.
_____ 8. I smoke cigarettes automatically without even being aware of it.
_____ 9. I smoke cigarettes in order to keep myself from slowing down.
_____ 10. I get a real gnawing hunger for a cigarette when I haven't smoked for a while.
_____ 11. When I feel uncomfortable or upset about something, I light up a cigarette.
_____ 12. Handling a cigarette is part of the enjoyment of smoking it.
_____ 13. Between cigarettes, I get a craving that *only* a cigarette can satisfy.
_____ 14. I light up a cigarette when I feel angry about something.
_____ 15. I light up a cigarette without realizing I still have one burning in the ashtray.
_____ 16. I find cigarettes pleasurable.
_____ 17. When I feel ashamed or embarrassed about something, I light up a cigarette.
_____ 18. When I have run out of cigarettes, I find it almost unbearable until I can get them.
_____ 19. Few things help better than cigarettes when I'm feeling upset.

_____ 20. I smoke cigarettes just from habit, without even really wanting the one I'm smoking.

_____ 21. Smoking cigarettes is pleasant and relaxing.

_____ 22. I do not feel contented for long unless I am smoking a cigarette.

_____ 23. I smoke cigarettes to give me a "lift."

Reprinted from Ikard et al. (1969, pp. 652–653) by courtesy of Marcel Dekker, Inc.

SUBJECTIVE OPIATE WITHDRAWAL SCALE AND OBJECTIVE
OPIATE WITHDRAWAL SCALE

Nature and Uses

Handelsman, Cochrane, Aronson, Ness, Rubinstein, and Kanof (1987)
developed the Subjective Opiate Withdrawal Scale as a self-report measure of 16 common opiate withdrawal characteristics and the Objective
Opiate Withdrawal Scale as a measure of 13 common characteristics of
opiate withdrawal that others can observe.

Administration and Scoring

For the Subjective scale, respondents use a 0–4 rating scale to rate to
what extent they are currently experiencing each of 16 characteristics.
Scores can range from 0 to 64, with higher scores indicating more withdrawal.

For the Objective scale, the rater observes the subject for about 10
minutes. No interaction between the rater and the subject is required. The
observer rates each characteristic as either present (1) or not present (0).
Scores can range from 0 to 13, with higher scores indicating more withdrawal.

Sample Scores

Handelsman et al. (1987) provided the scores listed in Table 1 for 11
patients on admission to a opiate detoxification ward and again after they
were stabilized on methadone. Twenty-one patients who were abusing
opiates as well as other drugs are listed separately.

Reliability

Handelsman et al. (1987) administered the Subjective scale on two
occasions one week apart to 72 individuals they expected to maintain
stable levels of methadone use or nonuse. The correlation was .60. We were
unable to find any internal consistency data on the scale.

Handelsman et al. (1987) determined interrater reliability for the 13
Objective scale items to range from .50 for anxiety to .99 for abdominal
cramps, with most kappas over .80 but no correlation for vomiting because
this behavior was never observed. No interrater correlations were reported for total scale scores.

TABLE 1
Opiate Withdrawal Scale Scores (Handelsman et al., 1987)

Group	Scale	Score on admission		Score after methadone	
		Mean	*SD*	*Mean*	*SD*
Opiate abuse	Subjective	24.3	2.2	5.6	1.5
	Objective	2.5	0.4	0.3	0.4
Opiate and other drug abuse	Subjective	23.1	2.8	14.4	2.4
	Objective	2.0	0.4	0.9	0.2

As the studies above indicate, only meager evidence of reliability exists for the two scales. Hence, it is best to be cautious in comparing small differences or changes in scale scores.

Validity

Two types of validity data exist for the two scales. First, for each scale, studies found that scores decreased significantly in opiate abusers after they received methadone (Handelsman et al., 1987; Loimer, Linzmayer, and Grunberger, 1991). Second, opiate abusers given naloxone (which causes opiate withdrawal) showed significantly increased scores compared to opiate abusers given a placebo (Handelsman et al., 1987). However, Loimer et al. (1991) found that the Subjective and Objective scale scores did not correlate significantly with each other in 20 opiate addicts.

THE SUBJECTIVE OPIATE WITHDRAWAL SCALE

Using the scale below, put a number to the left of each statement to indicate how you are feeling now.

0 = not at all
1 = a little
2 = moderately
3 = quite a bit
4 = extremely

_____ 1. I feel anxious.
_____ 2. I feel like yawning.
_____ 3. I'm perspiring.
_____ 4. My eyes are tearing.
_____ 5. My nose is running.
_____ 6. I have goose flesh.
_____ 7. I am shaking.
_____ 8. I have hot flashes.
_____ 9. I have cold flashes.
_____ 10. My bones and muscles ache.
_____ 11. I feel restless.
_____ 12. I feel nauseous.
_____ 13. I feel like vomiting.
_____ 14. My muscles twitch.
_____ 15. I have cramps in my stomach.
_____ 16. I feel like shooting up now.

THE OBJECTIVE OPIATE WITHDRAWAL SCALE

Observer: Score one point for each of the 13 items observed.

1. Yawning (One or more)
2. Rhinorrhea (three or more sniffs per observation period)
3. Pilorection (gooseflesh—observe patient's arm)
4. Perspiration
5. Lacrimation
6. Mydriasis
7. Tremors (hands)
8. Hot and cold flashes (shivering or huddling for warmth)
9. Restlessness (frequent shifts of position)

10. Vomiting
11. Muscle twitches
12. Abdominal cramps (holding stomach)
13. Anxiety
    (Score if any of below symptoms present; range: mild to severe.)
    Mild: observable manifestations—foot shaking, fidgeting, finger tapping
    Moderate to severe: agitation, unable to sit, trembling, panicky; complains of difficulty in breathing, choking sensations, palpitations

Reprinted from Handelsman et al. (1987; pp. 296–297), by courtesy of Marcel Dekker, Inc.

REFERENCES

Bell, H., & Steensland, H. (1987). Serum activity of gamma-glutamyltranspeptidase (GGT) in relation to estimated alcohol consumption and questionnaires in alcohol dependence syndrome. *British Journal of Addiction, 82*, 1021–1026.

Bernadt, M., Mumford, J., & Murray, R. (1984). A discriminant-function analysis of screening tests for excessive drinking and alcoholism. *Journal of Studies on Alcohol, 45*, 81–86.

Bilal, A. M., Khattar, M. A., Hassan, K. I., & Berry, D. (1992). Psychosocial and toxicological profile of drug misuse in male army conscripts in Kuwait. *Acta Psychiatrica Scandinavica, 86*, 104–107.

Bosse, R., Garvey, A.J., & Glynn, R.J. (1980). Age and addiction to smoking. *Addictive Behaviors, 3*, 35–38.

Buchsbaum, D. G., Buchanan, R. G., Welsh, J., Centor, R. M., & Schnoll, S. H. (1992). Screening for drinking disorders in the elderly using the CAGE Questionnaire. *Journal of the American Geriatrics Society, 40*, 662–665.

Costa, P. O., McCrae, R. R., & Bosse, R. (1980). Smoking motive factors: a review and replication. *International Journal of the Addictions, 15*, 537–549.

Davis, L., de la Fuente, J., Morse, R., Landa, E., & O'Brien, P. (1989). Self-administered alcoholism screening test (SAAST): Comparison of classificatory accuracy in two cultures. *Alcoholism: Clinical and Experimental Research, 13*, 224–228.

Davis, L., & Morse, R. (1987). Age and sex differences in the responses of alcoholics to the Self-Administered Alcoholism Screening Test. *Journal of Clinical Psychology, 43*, 423–430.

Davis, L., Hurt, R., Morse, R., & O'Brien, P. (1987). Discriminant analysis of the Self-Administered Alcoholism Screening Test. *Alcoholism: Clinical and Experimental Research, 11*, 269–273.

Handelsman, L., Cochrane, K. J., Aronson, M. J., Ness, R., Rubinstein, K. J., & Kanof, P. D. (1987). Two rating scales for opiate withdrawal. *American Journal of Drug and Alcohol Abuse, 13*, 293–308.

Heatherton, T., Kozlowski, L., Frecker, R., & Fagerstrom, K. (1991). The Fagerstrom Test for Nicotine Dependence: A revision of the Fagerstrom Tolerance Questionnaire. *British Journal of Addiction, 86*, 1119–1127.

Heck, E. J. (1991). Developing a screening questionnaire for problem drinking in college students. *Journal of American College Health, 39*, 227–231.

Heck, E. J., & Lichtenberg, J. W. (1990). Validity of the CAGE in screening for problem drinking in college students. *Journal of College Student Development, 31*, 359–364.

Hurt, R. D., Morse, R. M., & Swenson, W. M. (1980). Diagnosis of alcoholism with a self-screening alcoholism screening test. *Mayo Clinic Proceedings, 55*, 365–370.

Ikard, F. F., Green, D. E., & Horn, D. H. (1969). A scale to differentiate between types of smoking as related to the management of affect. *International Journal of the Addictions, 4*, 649–659.

Jacobson, G. (1989). A comprehensive approach to pretreatment evaluation: Detection, assessment, and diagnosis of alcoholism. In R. Hester & W. Miller (Eds.), *Handbook of Alcoholism Treatment Approaches* (pp. 17–53). New York: Pergamon.

Lairson, D. R., Harlow, K., Cobb, J., Harrist, R., Martin, D., Ramby, R., Rustin, T., & Swint, J. (1992). Screening for patients with alcohol problems: severity of patients identified by the CAGE. *Journal of Drug Education, 22*, 337–352.

Langevin, R., & Lang, R. A. (1990). Substance abuse among sex offenders. *Annals of Sex Research, 3*, 397–424.

Lee, A. (1992). Diagnosing alcoholism: Toward a multisource approach. In C. Stout, J. Levitt, & D. Ruben (Eds.), *Handbook for Assessing and Treating Addictive Disorders* (pp. 83–96). New York: Greenwood.

Lee, D. J., & DeFrank, R. S. (1988). Interrelationships among self-reported alcohol intake, physiological indices and alcoholism screening measures. *Journal of Studies on Alcohol, 49*, 532–537.

Loethen, G., & Khavari, K. (1990). Comparison of the Self-Administered Alcohol Screening Test (SAAST) and the Khavari Alcohol Test (KAT): Results from an alcoholic population and their collaterals. *Alcoholism: Clinical and Experimental Research, 14*, 756–760.

Loimer, N., Linzmayer, L., & Grunberger, J. (1991). Comparison between observer assessment and self-rating of withdrawal distress during opiate detoxification. *Drug and Alcohol Dependence, 28*, 265–268.

Mayfield, D, McLeod, G., & Hall, P. (1974). The CAGE Questionnaire: Validation of a new alcoholism instrument. *American Journal of Psychiatry, 131*, 1121–1123.

Mischke, H., & Venneri, R. (1987). Reliability and validity of the MAST, Mortimer-Filkins Questionnaire and CAGE in DWI assessment. *Journal of Studies on Alcohol, 48*, 492–501.

Moore, R. D., Bone, L. R., Geller, G., Mamon, J. A., Stokes, E. J., & Levine, D. M. (1989). Prevalence, detection, and treatment of alcoholism in hospitalized patients. *Journal of the American Medical Association, 261*, 403–407.

Mothersill, K. J., McDowell, I., & Rosser, W. (1988). Subject characteristics and long-term post-program smoking cessation. *Addictive Behaviors, 13*, 29–36.

Niura, R., Goldstein, M. G., Ward, K. D., & Abrams, D. B. (1989). Reasons for smoking and severity of residual nicotine withdrawal symptoms when using nicotine chewing gum. *British Journal of Addiction, 84*, 681–687.

Nystrom, M., Perasalo, J., & Salaspuro, M. (1993). Screening for heavy drinking and alcohol-related problems in young university students: The CAGE, the Mm-MAST and the trauma score questionnaires. *Journal of Studies on Alcohol, 54*, 528–533.

O'Connell, K. A., & Shiffman, S. (1988). Negative affect smoking and smoking relapse. *Journal of Substance Abuse, 1*, 25–33.

Peterson, C., Scott, B., & Jovanovic-Peterson, L. (1991). Hemoglobin associated acetaldehyde correlates with the self- administered Alcohol Screening Test but not glycated hemoglobin in Type II diabetes mellitus. *Alcohol, 8*, 183–185.

Pomerleau, C., Carton, S., Lutzke, M., Flessland, K., & Pomerleau, O. (1994). Reliability of the Fagerstrom Tolerance Questionnaire and the Fagerstrom Test for Nicotine Dependence. *Addictive Behaviors, 19*, 33–39.

Russell, M., & Bigler, L. (1979). Screening for alcohol-related problems in an outpatient obstetric–gynecologic clinic. *American Journal of Obstetrics and Gynecology, 134*, 4–12.

Selzer, M. (1971). The Michigan Alcohol Screening Test: The quest for a new diagnostic instrument. *American Journal of Psychiatry, 127*, 1653–1658.

Shiffman, S. (1988). Behavioral Assessment. In D. Donovan & G. Marlatt (Eds.), *Assessment of Addictive Behaviors*, pp. 139–188. New York: Guilford.

Skinner, H. A. (1982). The Drug Abuse Screening Test. *Addictive Behaviors, 7*, 363–371.

Skinner, H. A., & Goldberg, A. E. (1986). Evidence for a drug dependent syndrome among narcotic users. *British Journal of Addiction, 81*, 479–484.

Smart, R. G., Adlaf, E. M. & Knoke, D. (1991). Use of the CAGE scale in a population survey of drinking. *Journal of Studies on Alcohol, 52*, 593–596.

Smith, C., & Pristach, C. (1990). Utility of the Self-Administered Alcoholism Screening Test (SAAST) in schizophrenic patients. *Alcoholism: Clinical and Experimental Research, 14*, 690–694.

Smith, D. S., Collins, M. Kreisbert, J. P., Volpicelli, J. R., & Alterman, A. I. (1987). Screening for problem drinking in college freshmen. Special Issue: Students, alcohol, and college health. *Journal of American College Health, 36*, 89–94.

Staley, D., & El-Guebaly, N. (1990). Psychometric properties of the Drug Abuse Screening Test in a psychiatric patient population. *Addictive Behaviors, 15*, 257–264.

Strang, J., Bradley, B., & Stockwell, T. (1989). Assessment of drug and alcohol use. In C. Thompson (Ed.), *The Instruments of Psychiatric Research* (pp. 211–237). New York: Wiley.

Susman, J., Sitorius, M., Schneider, M., & Gilbert, C. (1992). Effect of a substance abuse curriculum on the recognition of alcoholism by family medicine residents. *Journal of Alcohol and Drug Education, 38*, 98–105.

Swenson, W., & Morse, R. (1975). The use of a self-administered alcoholism screening test (SAAST) in a medical center. *Mayo Clinic Proceedings, 50*, 204–208.

Tate, J. C., Schmitz, J. M., & Stanton, A. L. (1991). A critical review of the Reasons for Smoking Scale. *Journal of Substance Abuse, 3*, 441–455.

Tomkins, S. S. (1966). Psychological model for smoking behavior. *American Journal of Public Health, 56*, 17–20.

Werner, M. J., & Greene, J. W. (1992). Problem drinking among college freshmen. *Journal of Adolescent Health, 13*, 487–492.

Schizophrenia and Related Disorders

Scale for the Assessment of Negative Symptoms and
Scale for the Assessment of Positive Symptoms

Purpose and Uses

Andreasen (1982) developed the Scale for the Assessment of Negative Symptoms (SANS) to measure negative schizophrenic symptoms, including affective blunting, alogia (impoverished thinking and speaking), avolition, anhedonia, and attentional impairment. She developed the Scale for the Assessment of Positive Symptoms (SAPS) to measure positive schizophrenic symptoms, including hallucinations, delusions, formal positive thought disorder, bizarre behavior, and inappropriate affect (Andreasen, 1984; Andreasen, 1990). Together the scales provide a fairly comprehensive set of schizophrenia-symptom ratings.

Andreasen (1989) created the two scales because of prior theorizing and research findings suggesting that at least two types of schizophrenia exist, each with separate effects, outcomes, and causes. (See, for example, Strauss, Carpenter, and Bartko, 1974.) The ultimate hope of researchers is that more effective treatments and preventive methods will result from this line of inquiry.

Both scales consist of clinician ratings of symptoms Andreasen (1989) considered important on the basis of her clinical experience. The symptoms are quite similar to those mentioned in the DSM-IV description of schizophrenia. Andreasen created the scales on the foundation of two scales she had previously created—the Scale for the Assessment of

Thought, Language, and Communication and the Affect Rating Scale—as well as the Schedule for Affective Disorders and Schizophrenia (Andreasen & Olsen, 1982; Andreasen, 1989). Over the years Andreasen modified the scales, deleting a clinician catatonia rating, deleting patient self-ratings for the symptom clusters, and moving the inappropriate affect item from the Affective Flattening subscale of the Negative Symptoms Scale to be a one-item subscale of the Positive Symptoms Scale (Andreasen, 1990). We will give the versions of the scales Andreasen provided us in 1994.

The Negative Symptoms measure is the measure of negative symptoms most used in published research. The Positive Symptoms measure is often, but not always, used in conjunction with the Negative Symptoms measure. Researchers have translated the scales into Dutch, French, German, Japanese, Korean, and Spanish (Andreasen, 1990).

Because of the importance of discovering the true structure of types of schizophrenia, many researchers have factor-analyzed subscale scores on Negative and Positive Symptoms measures. The results have varied, but most researchers have concluded that the nine subscales fit a 3- or 4-factor model better than Andreasen's original 2-factor concept of positive and negative. The studies generally have found support for (a) a negative factor, made up of alogia, affective blunting, avolition, anhedonia, and attentional impairment, (b) a delusion/hallucination factor, and (c) a disorganization factor, including positive formal thought disorder and bizarre behavior (Andreasen, Swayze, Flaum, O'Leary, & Alliger, 1994; Klimidis, Stuart, Minas, Copolov & Singh, 1993; Peralta, de Leon, & Cuesta, 1992). Occasionally, studies find that bizarre behavior loads by itself on a fourth factor (Peralta et al., 1992). Also, some studies find that attentional impairment loads on the disorganization factor (Peralta et al., 1992).

Interpretation of the results is difficult, however, because different language versions of the measures have been used in studies along with different rotation techniques, and usually far too few subjects to allow the conclusion that an identified factor structure is generalizable (Peralta et al., 1992).

Administration and Scoring

For the Negative Symptoms Scale, clinicians use a 0–5 scale to rate the patient on each of 19 symptoms. Clinicians base the ratings on hospital records, a clinical interview, direct observations, family reports, and consultation with staff members (Andreasen, 1984). Andreasen (1984) recommended that the interviewer initially ask the patient about neutral topics to allow five to ten minutes in which to observe how the patient speaks and then go on to ask about relevant symptoms. The rating form includes suggested interview questions. For each of the five subscales, the clinician also uses the 0–5 scale to provide a global rating for that symptom. Andreasen (1984) noted that a single extremely severe symptom can lead to a very high global rating, even if other symptoms of this type are not present. Ratings are usually made for the prior month, although the prior week may be used instead (Andreasen, 1984).

For the Negative Symptoms Scale, summing the five global ratings leads to a "summary score," which can range from 0 to 25, with higher scores indicating more severe symptoms. Summing the individual items in each subscale leads to a "symptom complex" score, which can range from 0 to as high as 30 (depending on the number of items in the subscale), with higher scores indicating more severe symptoms. Summing the symptom complex scores leads to a "composite score," which can range from 0 to 95, with higher scores indicating more severe symptoms (Silk & Tandon, 1991).

The 31-item Positive Symptoms Scale, with its six subscales, operates the same way. Summary scores can range from 0 to 25, and scale composite scores can range from 0 to 155, with higher scores indicating more severe symptoms.

Cutoff and Sample Scores

Andreasen and her colleagues have created two sets of criteria for classifying schizophrenics. Andreasen, Flaum, Swayze, Tyrrell, and Arndt (1990) initially suggested relatively exclusive criteria such that schizophrenics be classified as *negative* if they have at least 2 of the 5 Negative Symptom global ratings at marked or severe (4 or 5) and none of the global Positive Symptoms at that level; *positive* if they have at least one of the global Positive Symptoms at marked or severe and none of the global Negative Symptoms; and *mixed* if they do not meet the criteria for either positive or negative or if they meet the criteria for both.

Andreasen et al. (1990) also tested more inclusive criteria in which schizophrenics are classified as *negative* if they have 2 of 5 Negative Symptom global ratings at marked or severe, regardless of whether they have any global Positive Symptoms at that level. Andreasen et al. (1990) and Fenton and McGlashan (1992) found that the more inclusive criteria led to four to five times as many schizophrenics being classified as negative. Fenton and McGlashan (1992) reported evidence that the more inclusive criteria are superior in creating a group of negative schizophrenics who differ from other schizophrenics in chronicity. Andreasen et al. (1990) found no difference in this regard.

Reliability

Internal consistency as measured by Cronbach's alpha for the global ratings has ranged in various studies from .78 to .85 for the Negative Symptoms Scale and .30 to .48 for the Positive Symptoms Scale (Peralta et al., 1992). The low internal consistency for the Positive Symptoms Scale is consistent with the common finding that it is multifactorial.

Subscale internal consistency as measured by Cronbach's alpha for the individual items of the Negative subscales has ranged from .63 to .86 (Andreasen, 1990; Peralta et al., 1992).

In a review of studies on the Negative Symptoms Scale, Andreasen (1989) found interrater reliability for the summary score of global ratings to range from .70 to .88 for the English version, with similar levels for versions in other languages. In another review of studies, Silk and Tandon (1992) reported that the individual negative items had interrater correlations ranging from .70 to .92.

For the Positive Symptoms Scale global ratings, Fenton and McGlashan (1991) found interrater reliability was .85 when raters used highly detailed admissions records.

Validity

Kay (1991, pp. 70–71) summarized two studies that found high correlations (a) between the Negative Symptoms total global scores and another negative-schizophrenia scale, and (b) between the Positive Symptoms total global scores and another positive-schizophrenia scale. Fenton and McGlashan (1992) compared several different measures of negative symptoms and found that the Andreasen's Negative Symptoms Scale correlated .80 to .90 with the other measures and had the highest correlation with a composite measure of future long-term outcome, which included hospitalizations, symptoms, work functioning, and social functioning.

Andreasen (1982) used the ratings that now make up the Positive and Negative Symptoms scales, along with historical data about the patients, to classify patients into groups of positive, negative, and mixed schizophrenia. The negative schizophrenia group (a) had lower education levels, (b) had poorer premorbid adjustment, (c) were less likely to have a job, (d) had larger ventricular-brain ratios, (e) had lower scores on the Mini Mental Status Exam, and (f) had lower globally rated functioning. Andreasen et al. (1990) later replicated these findings, except for the association with ventricular-brain ratios, and also found that the negative schizophrenics had lower scores on several intelligence measures.

In a group of soldiers who became overtly schizophrenic, Rosse and Kleinberg (1993) found those with high Negative Symptom scores when diagnosed had become schizophrenic sooner after joining the military than the other schizophrenics. The study found no association between Positive Symptom scores and how soon the soldiers became schizophrenic.

SCALE FOR THE ASSESSMENT OF NEGATIVE SYMPTOMS

AFFECTIVE FLATTENING OR BLUNTING

Affective flattening or blunting manifests itself as a characteristic impoverishment of emotional expression, reactivity, and feeling. Affective flattening can be evaluated by observation of the subject's behavior and responsiveness during a routine interview. The rating of some items may be affected by drugs, since the Parkinsonian side-effect of phenothiazines may lead to mask-like faces and diminished associated movements. Other aspects of affect, such as responsivity or appropriateness, will not be affected, however.

Unchanging Facial Expression

The subject's face appears wooden, mechanical, frozen. It does not change expression, or changes less than normally expected, as the emotional content of discourse changes. Since phenothiazines may partially mimic this effect, the interviewer should be careful to note whether or not the subject is on medication, but should not try to "correct" the rating accordingly.

Not at all: Subject is normal or labile	0
Questionable decrease	1
Mild: Occasionally the subject's expression is not as full as expected	2
Moderate: Subject's expressions are dulled overall, but not absent	3
Marked: Subject's face has a flat "set" look, but flickers of affect arise occasionally	4
Severe: Subject's face looks "wooden" and changes little, if at all throughout the interview	5

Decreased Spontaneous Movements

The subject sits quietly throughout the interview and shows few or no spontaneous movements. He does not shift position, move his legs, move his hands, etc., or does so less than normally expected.

Not at all: Subject moves normally or is overactive	0
Questionable decrease	1
Mild: Some decrease in spontaneous movements	2
Moderate: Subject moves three or four times during the interview	3

Marked: Subject moves once or twice during the interview   4
Severe: Subject sits immobile throughout the interview   5

Paucity of Expressive Gestures

The subject does not use his body as an aid in expressing his ideas, through such means as hand gestures, sitting forward in his chair when intent on a subject, leaning back when relaxed, etc. This may occur in addition to decreased spontaneous movements.

Not at all: Subject uses expressive gestures normally or exces-   0
   sively
Questionable decrease   1
Mild: Some decrease in expressive gestures   2
Moderate: Subject uses body as an aid in expression at least   3
   three or four times
Marked: Subject uses body as an aid in expression only once or   4
   twice
Severe: Subject never uses body as an aid in expression   5

Poor Eye Contact

The subject avoids looking at others or using his eyes as an aid in expression. He appears to be staring into space even when he is talking.

Not at all: Good eye contact and expression   0
Questionable decrease   1
Mild: Some decrease in eye contact and eye expression   2
Moderate: Subject's eye contact is decreased by at least half of   3
   normal
Marked: Subject's eye contact is very infrequent   4
Severe: Subject almost never looks at interviewer   5

Affective Nonresponsivity

Failure to smile or laugh when prompted may be tested by smiling or joking in a way which would usually elicit a smile from a normal individual. The examiner may also ask, "Have you forgotten how to smile?" while smiling himself.

Not at all   0
Questionable decrease   1
Mild: Slight but definite lack in responsivity   2
Moderate: Subject occasionally seems to miss the cues to respond   3

→

Marked: Subject seems to miss the cues to respond most of the   4
    time
Severe: Subject is essentially unresponsive, even on prompting   5

Lack of Vocal Inflections

While speaking, the subject fails to show normal vocal emphasis patterns. Speech has a monotonic quality, and important words are not emphasized through changes in pitch or volume. Subject also may fail to change volume with changes of subject so that he does not drop his voice when discussing private topics nor raise it as he discusses things which are exciting or for which louder speech might be appropriate.

Not at all: Normal vocal inflections   0
Questionable decrease   1
Mild: Slight decrease in vocal inflections   2
Moderate: Interviewer notices several instances of flattened vo-   3
    cal inflections
Marked: Obvious decrease in vocal inflection   4
Severe: Subject's speech is a continuous monotone   5

Global Rating of Affective Flattening

The global rating should focus on overall severity of affective flattening or blunting. Special emphasis should be given to such core features as unresponsiveness, inappropriateness, and an overall decrease in emotional intensity.

No flattening: Normal affect   0
Questionable affective flattening   1
Mild affective flattening   2
Moderate affective flattening   3
Marked affective flattening   4
Severe affective flattening   5

ALOGIA

Alogia is a general term coined to refer to the impoverished thinking and cognition that often occur in subjects with schizophrenia (Greek *a* = no, none; *logos* = mind, thought). Subjects with alogia have thinking processes that seem empty, turgid, or slow. Since thinking cannot be observed directly, it is inferred from the subject's speech. The two major manifestations of alogia are nonfluent empty speech (poverty of speech) and fluent empty speech (poverty of content of speech). Blocking and increased latency of response may also reflect alogia.

Poverty of Speech

There is restriction in the *amount* of spontaneous speech, so that replies to questions tend to be brief, concrete, and unelaborated. Unprompted additional information is rarely provided. Replies may be monosyllabic, and some questions may be left unanswered altogether. When confronted with this speech pattern, the interviewer may find himself frequently prompting the subject in order to encourage elaboration of replies. To elicit this finding, the examiner must allow the subject adequate time to answer and to elaborate his answer.

No poverty of speech: A substantial and appropriate number of replies to questions include additional information   0

Questionable poverty of speech   1

Mild: Occasional replies do not include elaborated information even though this is appropriate   2

Moderate: Some replies do not include appropriately elaborated information, and some replies are monosyllabic or very brief ("Yes." "No." "Maybe." "I don't know." "Last week.")   3

Marked: Answers are rarely more than a sentence or a few words in length   4

Severe: Subject says almost nothing and occasionally fails to answer questions   5

Poverty of Content of Speech

Although replies are long enough so that speech is adequate in amount, it conveys little information. Language tends to be vague, often over-abstract or over-concrete, repetitive, and stereotyped. The interviewer may recognize this finding by observing that the subject has spoken at some length but has not given adequate information to answer the question. Alternatively, the subject may provide enough information, but require many words to do so, so that a lengthy reply can be summarized in a sentence or two. Sometimes the interviewer may characterize the speech as "empty philosophizing."

EXCLUSIONS: This finding differs from circumstantiality in that the circumstantial subject tends to provide a *wealth of detail*.

EXAMPLE: *Interviewer*: "Why is it, do you think, that people believe in God?" *Subject*: "Well, first of all because he, uh, he are the person that is their personal savior. He walks with me and talks with me. And, uh, the understanding that I have, um, a lot of peoples, they don't really, uh, know they own personal self. Because, uh, they ain't, they all, just don't know they personal self. They don't know that he, uh, seemed like to me, a lot of 'em don't understand that he walks and talks with them."

No poverty of content	0
Questionable	1
Mild: Occasional replies are too vague to be comprehensible or can be markedly condensed	2
Moderate: Frequent replies which are vague or can be markedly condensed to make up at least a quarter of the interview	3
Marked: At least half of the subject's speech is composed of vague or incomprehensible replies	4
Severe: Nearly all the speech is vague, incomprehensible, or can be markedly condensed	5

Blocking

Interruption of a train of speech before a thought or idea has been completed. After a period of silence which may last from a few seconds to minutes, the person indicates that he cannot recall what he had been saying or meant to say. Blocking should only be judged to be present if a person voluntarily describes losing his thought or if, upon questioning by the interviewer, the person indicates that that was the reason for pausing.

No blocking	0
Questionable	1
Mild: A single instance noted during a forty-five minute period	2
Moderate: Occurs twice during forty-five minutes	3
Marked: Occurs three or four times during forty-five minutes	4
Severe: Occurs more than four times in forty-five minutes	5

Increased Latency of Response

The subject takes a longer time to reply to questions than is usually considered normal. He may seem "distant" and sometimes the examiner may wonder if he has even heard the question. Prompting usually indicates that the subject is aware of the question, but has been having difficulty in formulating his thoughts in order to make an appropriate reply.

Not at all	0
Questionable	1
Mild: Occasional brief pauses before replying	2

Moderate: Often pauses several seconds before replying   3
Marked: Usually pauses at least ten to fifteen seconds before   4
  replying
Severe: Long pauses prior to nearly all replies   5

Global Rating of Alogia

Since the core features of alogia are poverty of speech and poverty of content of speech, the global rating should place particular emphasis on them.

No alogia   0
Questionable   1
Mild: Mild but definite impoverishment in thinking   2
Moderate: Significant evidence for impoverished thinking   3
Marked: Subject's thinking seems impoverished much of the   4
  time
Severe: Subject's thinking seems impoverished nearly all of the   5
  time

AVOLITION–APATHY

Avolition manifests itself as a characteristic lack of energy, drive, and interest. Subjects are unable to mobilize themselves to initiate or persist in completing many different kinds of tasks. Unlike the diminished energy or interest of depression, the avolitional symptom complex in schizophrenia is usually not accompanied by saddened or depressed affect. The avolitional symptom complex often leads to severe social and economic impairment.

Grooming and Hygiene

The subject displays less attention to grooming and hygiene than normal. Clothing may appear sloppy, outdated, or soiled. The subject may bathe infrequently and not care for hair, nails, or teeth—leading to such manifestations as greasy or uncombed hair, dirty hands, body odor, or unclean teeth and bad breath. Overall, the appearance is dilapidated and disheveled. In extreme cases, the subject may even have poor toilet habits.

How often do you bathe or shower?
Do you change your clothes every day?
How often do you do laundry?

No evidence of poor grooming and hygiene   0

→

Questionable   1

Mild: Some slight but definite indication of inattention to ap-   2
pearance, i.e., messy hair or disheveled clothes

Moderate: Appearance is somewhat disheveled, i.e., greasy hair,   3
dirty clothes

Marked: Subject's attempts to keep up grooming or hygiene are   4
minimal

Severe: Subject's clothes, body, and environment are dirty and   5
smelly

Impersistence at Work or School

The subject has had difficulty in seeking or maintaining employment (or schoolwork) as appropriate for his age and sex. If a student, he does not do homework and may even fail to attend class. Grades will tend to reflect this. If a college student, there may be a pattern of registering for courses, but having to drop several or all of them before the semester is completed. If of working age, the subject may have found it difficult to work at a job because of inability to persist in completing tasks and apparent irresponsibility. He may go to work irregularly, wander away early, complete them in a disorganized manner. He may simply sit around the house and not seek any employment or seek it only in an infrequent and desultory manner. If a housewife or retired person, the subject may fail to complete chores, such as shopping or cleaning, or complete them in an apparently careless and half-hearted way.

Have you been having any problems at (work, school)?
Do you ever start some project and just never get around to finishing it?

No evidence of impersistence at work or school   0

Questionable   1

Mild: Slight indications of impersistence, i.e., missing a couple   2
days of school or work

Moderate: Subject often has poor performance at work or school   3

Marked: Subject has much difficulty maintaining even a below   4
normal level of work or school

Severe: Subject consistently fails to maintain a record at work or   5
school

Physical Anergia

The subject tends to be physically inert. He may sit in a chair for hours at a time and not initiate any spontaneous activity. If encouraged to become involved in an activity, he may participate only briefly and then wander away or disengage himself and return to sitting alone. He may spend large amounts of time in some relatively mindless and physically inactive task such as watching TV or playing solitaire. His family may report that he spends most of his time at home "doing nothing except sitting around." Either at home or in an inpatient setting he may spend much of time sitting in his room.

Are there times when you lie or sit around most of the day?
(Does this ever last longer than one day?)

No evidence of physical anergia	0
Questionable	1
Mild anergia	2
Moderate: Subject lies in bed or sits immobile at least quarter of normal waking hours	3
Marked: Subject lies in bed or sits immobile at least half of normal waking hours	4
Severe: Subject lies in bed or sits immobile for most of the day	5

Global Rating of Avolition–Apathy

The global rating should reflect the overall severity of the avolition symptoms, given expectational norms for the subject's age and social status or origin. In making the global rating, strong weight may be given to only one or two prominent symptoms if they are particularly striking.

No avolition	0
Questionable	1
Mild, but definitely present	2
Moderate avolition	3
Marked avolition	4
Severe avolition	5

ANHEDONIA–ASOCIALITY

This symptom complex encompasses the schizophrenic subject's difficulties in experiencing interest or pleasure. It may express itself as a loss of interest in pleasurable activities, an inability to experience pleasure when participating in activities normally considered pleasurable, or a lack of involvement in social relationships of various kinds.

➤

Recreational Interests and Activities

The subject may have few or no interests, activities, or hobbies. Although this symptom may begin insidiously or slowly, there will usually be some obvious decline from an earlier level of interest and activity. Subjects with relatively milder loss of interest will engage in some activities which are passive or nondemanding, such as watching TV, or will show only occasional or sporadic interest. Subjects with the most extreme loss will appear to have a complete and intractable inability to become involved in or enjoy activities. The rating in this area should take both the quality and quantity of recreational interests into account.

Have you felt interested in the things you usually enjoy?
(Have they been as fun as usual?)
Have you been watching TV or listening to the radio?

No inability to enjoy recreational interests or activities	0
Questionable	1
Mild inability to enjoy recreational activities	2
Moderate: Subject often is not "up" for recreational activities	3
Marked: Subject has little interest in and derives only mild pleasure from recreational activities	4
Severe: Subject has no interest in and derives no pleasure from recreational activities	5

Sexual Interest and Activity

The subject may show a decrement in sexual interest and activity, as judged by what would be normal for the subject's age and marital status. Individuals who are married may manifest disinterest in sex or may engage in intercourse only at the partner's request. In extreme cases, the subject may not engage in any sex at all. Single subjects may go for long periods of time without sexual involvement and make no effort to satisfy this drive. Whether married or single, they may report that they subjectively feel only minimal sex drive or that they take little enjoyment in sexual intercourse or in masturbatory activity even when they engage in it.

Have you noticed any changes in your sex drive?

No inability to enjoy sexual activities	0
Questionable decrement in sexual interest and activity	1
Mild decrement in sexual interest and activity	2
Moderate: Subject occasionally has noticed decreased interests in and/or enjoyment from sexual activities	3

Marked: Subject has little interest in and/or derives little plea- 4
sure from sexual activities
Severe: Subject has no interest in and/or derives no pleasure 5
from sexual activities

Ability to Feel Intimacy and Closeness

The subject may display an inability to form close and intimate relationships of a type appropriate for age, sex, and family status. In the case of
a younger person, this area should be rated in terms of relationships with
the opposite sex and with parents and siblings. In the case of an older
person who is married, the relationship with spouse and with children
should be evaluated, while older unmarried individuals should be judged
in terms of relationships with the opposite sex and family members who
live nearby. Subjects may display few or no feelings of affection to available family members. Or they may have arranged their lives so that they
are completely isolated from any intimate relationships, living alone and
making no effort to initiate contacts with family or members of the opposite sex.

Have you been having any problems with your (family, spouse)?
How would you feel about visiting with your (family, parents, spouse, etc.)?

No inability to feel intimacy and closeness 0
Questionable inability 1
Mild, but definite inability to feel intimacy and closeness 2
Moderate: Subject appears to enjoy family or significant others 3
but does not appear to "look forward" to visits
Marked: Subject appears neutral toward visits from family or 4
significant others. Brightens only mildly
Severe: Subject prefers no contact with or is hostile toward 5
family or significant others

Relationships with Friends and Peers

Subjects may also be relatively restricted in their relationships with
friends and peers of either sex. They may have few or no friends, make
little or no effort to develop such relationships, and choose to spend all or
most of their time alone.

Have you been spending much time with friends?
Do you enjoy spending time alone, or would you rather have more friends?

No inability to form close friendships 0

→

Questionable inability to form friendships   1
Mild, but definite inability to form friendships   2
Moderate: Subject able to interact, but sees friends/acquaintances 3
  only two to three times per month
Marked: Subject has difficulty forming and/or keeping friend-   4
  ships. Sees friends/acquaintances only one to two times per
  month
Severe: Subject has no friends and no interest in developing   5
  any social ties

Global Rating of Anhedonia–Asociality

The global rating should reflect the overall severity of the anhedonia–asociality complex, taking into account the norms appropriate for the subject's age, sex, and family status.

No evidence of anhedonia–asociality   0
Questionable evidence of anhedonia–asociality   1
Mild, but definite evidence of anhedonia–asociality   2
Moderate evidence of anhedonia–asociality   3
Marked evidence of anhedonia–asociality   4
Severe evidence of anhedonia–asociality   5

ATTENTION

Attention is often poor in schizophrenics. The subject may have trouble focusing his attention, or he may only be able to focus sporadically and erratically. He may ignore attempts to converse with him, wander away while in the middle of an activity or task, or appear to be inattentive when engaged in formal testing or interviewing. He may or may not be aware of his difficulty in focusing his attention.

Social Inattentiveness

While involved in social situations or activities, the subject appears inattentive. He looks away during conversations, does not pick up the topic during a discussion, or appears uninvolved or unengaged. He may abruptly terminate a discussion or a task without any apparent reason. He may seem "spacy" or "out of it." He may seem to have poor concentration when playing games, reading, or watching TV.

No indication of inattentiveness   0
Questionable signs   1

Mild, but definite signs of inattentiveness   2
Moderate: Subject occasionally misses what is happening in the   3
    environment
Marked: Subject often misses what is happening in the environ-   4
    ment; has trouble with reading comprehension
Severe: Subject unable to follow conversation, remember what   5
    he's read, or follow TV plot

Inattentiveness during Mental Status Testing

The subject may perform poorly on simple tests of intellectual functioning in spite of adequate education and intellectual ability. This should
be assessed by having the subject spell "world" backward and by serial 7's
(at least a tenth-grade education) or serial 3's (at least a sixth-grade education) for a series of five subtractions. A perfect score is 10.

No errors   0
Questionable: No errors but subject performs in a halting man-   1
    ner or makes/corrects an error
Mild, but definite (one error)   2
Moderate (two errors)   3
Marked (three errors)   4
Severe (more than three errors)   5

Global Rating of Attention

This rating should assess the subject's overall ability to attend or
concentrate, and include both clinical appearance and performance on
tasks.

No indications of inattentiveness   0
Questionable   1
Mild, but definite inattentiveness   2
Moderate inattentiveness   3
Marked inattentiveness   4
Severe inattentiveness   5

Scale for the Assessment of Positive Symptoms

HALLUCINATIONS

Hallucinations represent an abnormality in perception. They are false perceptions occurring in the absence of some identifiable external stimulus. They may be experienced in any of the sensory modalities, including hearing, touch, taste, smell, and vision. True hallucinations should be distinguished from illusions (which involve a misperception of an external stimulus), hypnogogic and hypnopompic experiences (which occur when the subject is falling asleep or waking up), or normal thought processes that are exceptionally vivid. If the hallucinations have a religious quality, then they should be judged within the context of what is normal for the subject's social and cultural background. Hallucinations occurring under the immediate influence of alcohol, drugs, or serious physical illness should not be rated as present. The subject should always be requested to describe the hallucination in detail.

Auditory Hallucinations

The subject has reported voices, noises, or sounds. The commonest auditory hallucinations involve hearing voices speaking to the subject or calling him names. The voices may be male or female, familiar or unfamiliar, and critical or complimentary. Typically, subjects suffering from schizophrenia experience the voices as unpleasant and negative. Hallucinations involving sounds rather than voices, such as noises or music, should be considered less characteristic and less severe.

Have you ever heard voices or other sounds when no one is around? What did they say?

None	0
Questionable	1
Mild: Subject hears noises or single words; they occur only occasionally	2
Moderate: Clear evidence of voices; they have occurred at least weekly	3
Marked: Clear evidence of voices which occur almost every day	4
Severe: Voices occur often every day	5

VOICES COMMENTING.   Voices commenting are a particular type of auditory hallucination which phenomenologists such as Kurt Schneider consider to be pathognomonic of schizophrenia, although some recent evidence contradicts this. These hallucinations involve hearing a voice that makes a running commentary on the subject's behavior or thought as it occurs. If this is the only type of auditory hallucination the subject hears, it should be scored instead of auditory hallucinations (No. 1 above). Usually, however, voices commenting will occur in addition to other types of auditory hallucinations.

Have you ever heard voices commenting on what you are thinking or doing?
What do they say?

None	0
Questionable	1
Mild: Subject hears noises or single words; they occur occasionally	2
Moderate: Clear evidence of voices; they have occurred at least weekly	3
Marked: Clear evidence of voices which occur almost every day	4
Severe: Voices occur often every day	5

VOICES CONVERSING.   Like voices commenting, voices conversing are considered a Schneiderian first-rank symptom. They involve hearing two or more voices talking with one another, usually discussing something about the subject. As in the case of voices commenting, they should be scored independently of other auditory hallucinations.

Have you heard two or more voices talking with each other?
What did they say?

None	0
Questionable	1
Mild: Subject hears noises or single words; they occur occasionally	2
Moderate: Clear evidence of voices; they have occurred at least weekly	3
Marked: Clear evidence of voices which occur almost every day	4
Severe: Voices occur often every day	5

Somatic or Tactile Hallucinations

These hallucinations involve experiencing peculiar physical sensations in the body. They include burning sensations, tingling, and perceptions that the body has changed in shape or size.

Have you ever had burning sensations or other strange feelings in your
body?

→

What were they?
Did your body ever appear to change in shape or size?

None	0
Questionable	1
Mild: Subject experiences peculiar physical sensations; they occur only occasionally	2
Moderate: Clear evidence of somatic or tactile hallucinations; they have occurred at least weekly	3
Marked: Clear evidence of somatic or tactile hallucinations which occur almost every day	4
Severe: Hallucinations occur often every day	5

Olfactory Hallucinations

The subject experiences unusual smells which are typically quite unpleasant. Sometimes the subject may believe that he himself smells. This belief should be scored here if the subject can actually smell the odor himself, but should be scored among delusions if he only believes that others can smell the odor.

Have you ever experienced any unusual smells or smells that others do not notice?
What were they?

None	0
Questionable	1
Mild: Subject experiences unusual smells; they occur only occasionally	2
Moderate: Clear evidence of olfactory hallucinations; they have occurred at least weekly	3
Marked: Clear evidence of olfactory hallucinations; they occur almost every day	4
Severe: Olfactory hallucinations occur often every day	5

Visual Hallucinations

The subject sees shapes or people that are not actually present. Sometimes these are shapes or colors, but most typically they are figures of people or human-like objects. They may also be characters of a religious nature, such as the Devil or Christ. As always, visual hallucinations involving religious themes should be judged within the context of the subject's cultural background. Hypnogogic and hypnopompic visual hallucinations (which are relatively common) should be excluded, as should visual hallucinations occurring when the subject has been taking hallucinogenic drugs.

Have you had visions or seen things that other people cannot?
What did you see?
Did this occur when you were falling asleep or waking up?

None	0
Questionable	1
Mild: Subject experiences visual hallucinations; they occur only occasionally	2
Moderate: Clear evidence of visual hallucinations; they have occurred at least weekly	3
Marked: Clear evidence of visual hallucinations which occur almost every day	4
Severe: Hallucinations occur often every day	5

Global Rating of Severity of Hallucinations

This global rating should be based on the duration and severity of hallucinations, the extent of the subject's preoccupation with the hallucinations, his degree of conviction, and their effect on his actions. Also consider the extent to which the hallucinations might be considered bizarre or unusual. Hallucinations not mentioned above, such as those involving taste, should be included in this rating.

None	0
Questionable	1
Mild: Hallucinations definitely present, but occur infrequently; at times the subject may question their existence	2
Moderate: Hallucinations are vivid and occur occasionally; they may bother him to some extent	3
Marked: Hallucinations are quite vivid, occur frequently, and pervade his life	4
Severe: Hallucinations occur almost daily and are sometime unusual or bizarre; they are very vivid and extremely troubling	5

DELUSIONS

Delusions represent an abnormality in content of thought. They are false beliefs that cannot be explained on the basis of the subject's cultural background. Although delusions are sometimes defined as "fixed false beliefs," in their mildest form they may persist for only weeks to months, and the subject may question his beliefs or doubt them. The subject's

→

behavior may or may not be influenced by his delusions. The rating of severity of individual delusions and of the global severity of delusional thinking should take into account their persistence, their complexity, the extent to which the subject acts on them, the extent to which the subject doubts them, and the extent to which the beliefs deviate from those that normal people might have. For each positive rating, specific examples should be noted in the margin.

Persecutory Delusions

People suffering from persecutory delusions believe that they are being conspired against or persecuted in some way. Common manifestations include the belief that one is being followed, that one's mail is being opened, that one's room or office is bugged, that the telephone is tapped, or that police, government officials, neighbors, or fellow workers are harassing the subject. Persecutory delusions are sometimes relatively isolated or fragmented, but sometimes the subject has a complex set of delusions involving both a wide range of forms of persecution and a belief that there is a well-designed conspiracy behind them. For example, a subject may believe that his house is bugged and that he is being followed because the government wrongly considers him a secret agent for a foreign government; this delusion may be so complex that it explains almost everything that happens to him. The ratings of severity should be based on duration and complexity.

Have people been bothering you in any way?
Have you felt that people are against you?
Has anyone been trying to harm you in any way?
Has anyone been watching or monitoring you?

None	0
Questionable	1
Mild: Delusional beliefs are simple and may be of several different types; subject may question them occasionally	2
Moderate: Clear, consistent delusion that is firmly held	3
Marked: Consistent, firmly-held delusion that the subject acts on	4
Severe: Complex well-formed delusion that the subject acts on and that preoccupies him a great deal of the time; some aspects of the delusion or his reaction may seem quite bizarre	5

Delusions of Jealousy

The subject believes that his mate is having an affair with someone. Miscellaneous bits of information are construed as "evidence." The person usually goes to great effort to prove the existence of the affair, searching for hair in the bedclothes, the odor of shaving lotion or smoke on clothing, or receipts or checks indicating a gift has been bought for the lover. Elaborate plans are often made in order to trap the two together.

Have you ever worried that your husband (wife) might be unfaithful to you? What evidence do you have?

None	0
Questionable	1
Mild: Delusion clearly present, but the subject may question it occasionally	2
Moderate: Clear consistent delusion that is firmly held	3
Marked: Consistent, firmly held delusion that the subject acts on	4
Severe: Complex, well-formed delusion that the subject acts on and that preoccupies him a great deal of the time; some aspects of the delusion or his reaction may seem quite bizarre	5

Delusions of Sin or Guilt

The subject believes that he has committed some terrible sin or done something unforgivable. Sometimes the subject is excessively or inappropriately preoccupied with things he did wrong as a child, such as masturbating. Sometimes the subject feels responsible for causing some disastrous event, such as a fire or accident, with which he in fact has no connection. Sometimes these delusions may have a religious flavor, involving the belief that the sin is unpardonable and that the subject will suffer eternal punishment from God. Sometimes the subject simply believes that he deserves punishment by society. The subject may spend a good deal of time confessing these sins to whomever will listen.

Have you ever felt that you have done some terrible thing that you deserve to be punished for?

None	0
Questionable	1
Mild: Delusional beliefs may be simple and may be of several different types; subject may question them occasionally	2
Moderate: Clear, consistent delusion that is firmly held	3
Marked: Consistent, firmly held delusion that the subject acts on	4
Severe: Complex, well-formed delusion that the subject acts on and that preoccupies him a great deal of the time; some aspects of the delusion or his reaction may seem quite bizarre	5

➤

Grandiose Delusions

The subject believes that he has special powers or abilities. He may think he is actually some famous personage, such as a rock star, Napoleon, or Christ. He may believe he is writing some definitive book, composing a great piece of music, or developing some wonderful new invention. The subject is often suspicious that someone is trying to steal his ideas, and he may become quite irritable if his ideas are doubted.

Do you have any special or unusual abilities or talents?
Do you feel you are going to achieve great things?

None	0
Questionable	1
Mild: Delusional beliefs may be simple and may be of several different types; subject may question them occasionally	2
Moderate: Clear, consistent delusion that is firmly held	3
Marked: Consistent, firmly held delusion that the subject acts on	4
Severe: Complex, well-formed delusion that the subject acts on and that preoccupies him a great deal of the time; some aspects of the delusion or his reaction may seem quite bizarre	5

Religious Delusions

The subject is preoccupied with false beliefs of a religious nature. Sometimes these exist within the context of a conventional religious system, such as beliefs about the Second Coming, the Antichrist, or possession by the Devil. At other times, they may involve an entirely new religious system or a pastiche of beliefs from a variety of religions, particularly Eastern religions, such as ideas about reincarnation or Nirvana. Religious delusions may be combined with grandiose delusions (if the subject considers himself a religious leader), delusions of guilt, or delusions of being controlled. Religious delusions must be outside the range considered normal for the subject's cultural and religious background.

Are you a religious person?
Have you had an unusual religious experiences?
What was your religious training as a child?

None	0
Questionable	1
Mild: Delusional beliefs may be simple and may be of several different types; subject may question them occasionally	2
Moderate: Clear, consistent delusion that is firmly held	3

Marked: Consistent, firmly held delusion that the subject acts on   4
Severe: Complex, well-formed delusion that the subject acts on   5
     and that preoccupies him a great deal of the time; some as-
     pects of the delusion or his reaction may seem quite bizarre

Somatic Delusions

The subject believes that somehow his body is diseased, abnormal, or changed. For example, he may believe that his stomach or brain is rotting, that his hands or penis have become enlarged, or that his facial features are unusual (dysmorphophobia). Sometimes somatic delusions are accompanied by tactile or other hallucinations, and when this occurs, both should be rated. (For example, the subject believes that ballbearings are rolling around in his head, placed there by a dentist who filled his teeth, and can actually hear them clanking against one another.)

Is there anything wrong with your body?
Have you noticed any change in your appearance?

None   0
Questionable   1
Mild: Delusional beliefs may be simple and may be of several   2
     different types; subject may question them occasionally
Moderate: Clear, consistent delusion that is firmly held   3
Marked: Consistent, firmly held delusion that the subject acts on   4
Severe: Complex, well-formed delusion that the subject acts on   5
     and that preoccupies him a great deal of the time; some as-
     pects of the delusion or his reaction may seem quite bizarre

Ideas and Delusions of Reference

The subject believes that insignificant remarks, statements, or events refer to him or have some special meaning for him. For example, the subject walks into a room, sees people laughing, and suspects that they were just talking about him and laughing at him. Sometimes items read in the paper, heard on the radio, or seen on television are considered to be special messages to the subject. In the case of ideas of reference, the subject is suspicious, but recognizes his idea is erroneous. When the subject actually believes that the statements or events refer to him, then this is considered a delusion of reference.

Have you ever walked into a room and thought people were talking about you
or laughing at you?

➤

Have you seen things in magazines or on TV that seem to refer to you or contain a special message for you?
Have people communicated with you in any unusual ways?

None	0
Questionable	1
Mild: Occasional ideas of reference	2
Moderate: Have occurred at least weekly	3
Marked: Occurs at least two to four times weekly	4
Severe: Occurs frequently	5

Delusions of Being Controlled

The subject has a subjective experience that his feelings or actions are controlled by some outside force. The central requirement for this type of delusion is an actual strong subjective experience of being controlled. It does not include simple beliefs or ideas, such as that the subject is acting as an agent of God or that friends or parents are trying to coerce him to do something. Rather, the subject must describe, for example, that his body has been occupied by some alien force that is making it move in peculiar ways, or that messages are being sent to his brain by radio waves and are causing him to experience particular feelings that he recognizes are not his own.

Have you ever felt you were being controlled by some outside force?

None	0
Questionable	1
Mild: Subject has experienced being controlled, but doubts it occasionally	2
Moderate: Clear experience of control, which has occurred on two or three occasions in a week	3
Marked: Clear experience of control, which occurs frequently; behavior may be affected	4
Severe: Clear experience of control, which occurs frequently, pervades the subject's life, and often affects his behavior	5

Delusions of Mind Reading

The subject believes that people can read his mind or know his thoughts. This is different than thought broadcasting (see below) in that it is a belief without a percept. That is, the subject subjectively experiences and recognizes that others know his thoughts, but he does not think that they can be heard out loud.

Have you ever had the feeling that people could read your mind?

None	0
Questionable	1
Mild: Subject has experienced mind reading, but doubts it occasionally	2
Moderate: Clear experience of mind reading, which has occurred on two or three occasions in a week	3
Marked: Clear experience of mind reading, which occurs frequently; behavior may be affected	4
Severe: Clear experience of mind reading, which occurs frequently, pervades the subject's life, and often affects his behavior	5

Thought Broadcasting

The subject believes that his thoughts are broadcast so that he or others can hear them. Sometimes the subject experiences his thoughts as a voice outside his head; this is an auditory hallucination as well as a delusion. Sometimes the subject feels his thoughts are being broadcast although he cannot hear them himself. Sometimes he believes that his thoughts are picked up by a microphone and broadcast on the radio or television.

Have you ever heard your own thoughts out loud, as if they were a voice outside your head?

Have you ever felt your thoughts were broadcast so other people could hear them?

None	0
Questionable	1
Mild: Subject has experienced thought broadcasting, but doubts it occasionally	2
Moderate: Clear experience of thought broadcasting, which has occurred on two or three occasions in a week	3
Marked: Clear experience of thought broadcasting, which occurs frequently; behavior may be affected	4
Severe: Clear experience of thought broadcasting, which occurs frequently, pervades the subject's life, and often affects his behavior	5

→

Thought Insertion

The subject believes that thoughts that are not his own have been inserted into his mind. For example, he may believe that a neighbor is practicing voodoo and planting alien sexual thoughts in his mind. This symptom should not be confused with experiencing unpleasant thoughts the subject recognizes as his own, such as delusions of persecution or guilt.

Have you ever felt that thoughts were being put into your head by some outside force?
Have you ever experienced thoughts that didn't seem to be your own?

None	0
Questionable	1
Mild: Subject has experienced thought insertion, but doubts it occasionally	2
Moderate: Clear experience of thought insertion, which has occurred on two or three occasions in a week	3
Marked: Clear experience of thought insertion, which occurs frequently; behavior may be affected	4
Severe: Thought insertion, which occurs frequently, pervades the subject's life, and affects behavior	5

Thought Withdrawal

The subject believes that thoughts have been taken away from his mind. He is able to describe a subjective experience of beginning a thought and then suddenly to have it removed by some outside force. This symptom does not include the mere subjective recognition of alogia.

Have you ever felt your thoughts were taken away by some outside force?

None	0
Questionable	1
Mild: Subject has experienced thought withdrawal, but doubts it occasionally	2
Moderate: Clear experience of thought withdrawal, which has occurred on two or three occasions in a week	3
Marked: Clear experience of thought withdrawal, which occurs frequently; behavior may be affected	4
Severe: Clear experience of thought withdrawal, which occurs frequently, pervades the subject's life and often affects his behavior	5

Global Rating of Severity of Delusions

The global rating should be based on duration and persistence of delusions, the extent of the subject's preoccupation with the delusions, his degree of conviction, and their effect on his actions. Also consider the extent to which the delusions might be considered bizarre or unusual. Delusions not mentioned above should be included in this rating.

None	0
Questionable	1
Mild: Delusion definitely present but, at times, the subject questions the belief	2
Moderate: The subject is convinced of the belief, but it may occur infrequently and have little effect on his behavior	3
Marked: The delusion is firmly held; it occurs frequently and affects the subject's behavior	4
Severe: Delusions are complex, well-formed, and pervasive; they are firmly held and have a major effect on the subject's behavior; they may be somewhat bizarre or unusual	5

BIZARRE BEHAVIOR

The subject's behavior is unusual, bizarre, or fantastic. For example, he may urinate in a sugar bowl, paint the two halves of his body different colors, or kill a litter of pigs by smashing their heads against a wall. The information for this item will sometimes come from the subject, sometimes from other sources, and sometimes from direct observation. Bizarre behavior due to the immediate effects of alcohol or drugs should be excluded. As always, social and cultural norms must be considered in making the ratings, and detailed examples should be elicited and noted.

Clothing and Appearance

The subject dresses in an unusual manner or does other strange things to alter his appearance. For example, he may shave off all his hair or paint parts of his body different colors. His clothing may be quite unusual; for example, he may choose to wear some outfit that appears generally inappropriate and unacceptable, such as a baseball cap backward with rubber galoshes and long underwear covered by denim overalls. He may dress in a fantastic costume representing some historical personage or a man from outer space. He may wear clothing completely inappropriate to climatic conditions, such as heavy wools in the middle of summer.

➤

Has anyone made comments about your appearance?

None	0
Questionable	1
Mild: Occasional oddities of dress or appearance	2
Moderate: Appearance or apparel are clearly unusual and would attract attention	3
Marked: Appearance or apparel are markedly odd	4
Severe: Subject's appearance or apparel are very fantastic or bizarre	5

Social and Sexual Behavior

The subject may do things that are considered inappropriate according to usual social norms. For example, he may masturbate in public, urinate or defecate in inappropriate receptacles, or exhibit his sex organs inappropriately. He may walk along the street muttering to himself, or he may begin talking to people whom he has never met about his personal life (as when riding on a subway or standing in some public place). He may drop to his knees praying and shouting in the midst of a crowd of people, or he may suddenly sit in a yoga position while in the midst of a crowd. He may make inappropriate sexual overtures or remarks to strangers.

Have you ever done anything that others might think unusual or that has called attention to yourself?

None	0
Questionable	1
Mild: Occasional instances of somewhat peculiar behavior	2
Moderate: Frequent instances of odd behavior	3
Marked: Very odd behavior	4
Severe: Extremely odd behavior, which may have a fantastic quality	5

Aggressive and Agitated Behavior

The subject may behave in an aggressive, agitated manner, often quite unpredictably. He may start arguments inappropriately with friends or members of his family, or he may accost strangers on the street and begin haranguing them angrily. He may write letters of a threatening or angry nature to government officials or others with whom he has some quarrel. Occasionally, subjects may perform violent acts such as injuring or tormenting animals, or attempting to injure or kill human beings.

Have you ever done anything to try to harm animals or people?
Have you felt angry with anyone?
How did you express your anger?

None	0
Questionable	1
Mild: Occasional instances	2
Moderate: For example, writing angry letters to strangers	3
Marked: For example, threatening people, public harangues	4
Severe: For example, mutilating animals, attacking people	5

Repetitive or Stereotyped Behavior

The subject may develop a set of repetitive actions or rituals that he must perform over and over. Frequently, he will attribute some symbolic significance to these actions and believe that they are either influencing others or preventing himself from being influenced. For example, he may eat jelly beans every night for dessert, assuming that different consequences will occur depending on the color of the jelly beans. He may have to eat foods in a particular order, wear particular clothes, or put them on in a certain order. He may have to write messages to himself or to others over and over; sometimes this will be in an unusual or occult language.

Are there any things that you feel you have to do?

None	0
Questionable	1
Mild: Occasional instances of ritualistic or stereotyped behavior	2
Moderate: For example, eating or dressing rituals lacking symbolic significance	3
Marked: For example, eating or dressing rituals with a symbolic significance	4
Severe: For example, keeping a diary in an incomprehensible language	5

Global Rating of Severity of Bizarre Behavior

In making this rating, the interviewer should consider the type of behavior, the extent to which it deviates from social norms, the subject's awareness of the degree to which the behavior is deviant, and the extent to which it is obviously bizarre.

None	0
Questionable	1

➤

Mild: Occasional instances of unusual or apparently idiosyncra-   2
  tic behavior; subject usually has some insight
Moderate: Behavior which is clearly deviant from social norms   3
  and seems somewhat bizarre; subject may have some insight
Marked: Behavior which is markedly deviant from social norms   4
  and clearly bizarre; subject may have some insight
Severe: Behavior which is extremely bizarre or fantastic; may   5
  include a single extreme act, e.g., attempting murder; subject
  usually lacks insight

POSITIVE FORMAL THOUGHT DISORDER

Positive formal thought disorder is fluent speech that tends to communicate poorly for a variety of reasons. The subject tends to skip from
topic to topic without warning, to be distracted by events in the nearby
environment, to join words together because they are semantically or
phonologically alike even though they make no sense, or to ignore the
question asked and ask another. This type of speech may be rapid, and it
frequently seems quite disjointed. It has sometimes been referred to as
"loose associations." Unlike alogia (negative formal thought disorder), a
wealth of detail is provided, and the flow of speech tends to have an
energetic, rather than an apathetic, quality to it.

In order to evaluate thought disorder, the subject should be permitted
to talk at length on some topic, particularly a topic unrelated to his psychopathology, for as long as five to ten minutes. The interviewer should
observe closely the extent to which his sequencing of ideas is well-
connected. In addition the interviewer should insist that he clarify or
elaborate further if the ideas seem vague or incomprehensible. He should
also pay close attention to how well the subject can reply to a variety of
different types of questions, ranging from simple ("Where were you
born?") to more complicated ("How do you think the present government
is doing?").

The anchor points for these ratings assume that the subject has been
interviewed for a total of approximately forty-five minutes. If the interview is shorter, the ratings should be adjusted accordingly.

Derailment (Loose Associations)

A pattern of spontaneous speech in which the ideas slip off one track
onto another that is clearly but obliquely related, or onto one that is
completely unrelated. Things may be said in juxtaposition that lack a
meaningful relationship, or the subject may shift idiosyncratically from
one frame of reference to another. At times there may be a vague connec-

tion between the ideas, and at others none will be apparent. This pattern of speech is often characterized as sounding "disjointed." Perhaps the commonest manifestation of this disorder is a slow, steady slippage, with no single derailment being particularly severe, so that the speaker gets farther and farther off the track with each derailment without showing any awareness that his reply no longer has any connection with the question that was asked. This abnormality is often characterized by lack of cohesion between clauses and sentences and unclear pronoun references. For example:

INTERVIEWER: Did you enjoy college?

SUBJECT: Um-hum. Oh, hey, well, I, oh, I really enjoyed some communities I tried it, and the, and the next day when I'd be going out, you know, um, I took control like, uh, I put, um, bleach on my hair in, in California. My roommate was from Chicago, and she was going to the junior college. And we lived in the Y.M.C.A., so she wanted to put it, um, peroxide on my hair, and she did, and I got up and looked at the mirror and tears came to my eyes. Now do you understand it, I was full aware of what was going on but why couldn't I, I … why, why the tears? I can't understand that, can you?

None	0
Questionable	1
Mild: Occasional instances of derailment, with only slight topic shifts	2
Moderate: Several instances of derailment; subject is sometimes difficult to follow	3
Marked: Frequent instances of derailment; subject is often difficult to follow	4
Severe: Derailment so frequent and/or extreme that the subject's speech is almost incomprehensible	5

Tangentiality

Replying to a question in an oblique, tangential or even irrelevant manner. The reply may be related to the question in some distant way. Or the reply may be unrelated and seem totally irrelevant. In the past tangentiality has sometimes been used as roughly equivalent to loose associations or derailment. The concept of tangentiality has been partially redefined so that it refers only to answers to questions and not to transitions in spontaneous speech. For example:

INTERVIEWER: What city are you from?

SUBJECT: That's a hard question to answer because my parents … I was born in Iowa, but I know that I'm white instead of black, so apparently I came from the North somewhere and I don't know where, you know, I

➤

really don't know whether I'm Irish or Scandinavian or I don't, I don't believe I'm Polish but I think I'm, I think I might be German or Welsh.

None	0
Questionable	1
Mild: One or two oblique replies	2
Moderate: Occasional oblique replies (three to four times)	3
Marked: Frequent oblique replies (more than four times)	4
Severe: Tangentiality so severe that interviewing the subject is extremely difficult	5

Incoherence (Word Salad, Schizophasia)

A pattern of speech that is essentially incomprehensible at times, incoherence is often accompanied by derailment. It differs from derailment in that incoherence the abnormality occurs *within* the level of the sentence or clause, which contains words or phrases that are joined incoherently. The abnormality in derailment involves unclear or confusing connections between larger units, such as sentences or clauses.

This type of language disorder is relatively rare. When it occurs, it tends to be severe or extreme, and mild forms are quite uncommon. It may sound quite similar to Wernicke's aphasia or jargon aphasia, and in these cases the disorder should only be called incoherence when history and laboratory data exclude the possibility of a past stroke, and formal testing for aphasia is negative.

Exclusions: Mildly ungrammatical constructions or idiomatic usages characteristic of a particular regional or ethnic background, lack of education, or low intelligence.

The following is an example of incoherence:

INTERVIEWER: What do you think about current political issues like the energy crisis?

SUBJECT: They're destroying too many cattle and oil just to make soap. If we need soap when you can jump into a pool of water, and then when you go to buy your gasoline, my folks always thought they should, get pop but the best thing to get, is motor oil, and, money. May, may as well go there and, trade in some, pop caps and, uh, tires, and tractors to group, car garages, so they can pull cars away from wrecks, is what I believed in.

None	0
Questionable	1
Mild: Occasional instances of incoherence	2
Moderate: Frequent bursts of incoherence	3

Marked: At least half of the subject's speech is incomprehensible   4
Severe: Almost all of the subject's speech is incomprehensible   5

Illogicality

Illogicality is expressed in a pattern of speech in which conclusions are reached that do not follow logically. This may take the form of nonsequiturs (= it does not follow), in which the subject makes a logical inference between two clauses that is unwarranted or illogical. It may take the form of faulty inductive inferences, or the form of reaching conclusions based on faulty premises without any actual delusional thinking.

Exclusions: Illogicality may either lead to or result from delusional beliefs. When illogical thinking occurs within the context of a delusional system, it should be subsumed under the concept of delusions and not considered a separate phenomenon representing a different type of thinking disorder. Illogical thinking that is clearly due to cultural or religious values or to intellectual deficit should also be excluded.

The following is an example of illogicality:

> Parents are the people that raise you. Anything that raises you can be a parent. Parents can be anything—material, vegetable, or mineral—that has taught you something. Parents would be the world of things that are alive, that are there. Rocks—a person can look at a rock and learn something from it, so that would be a parent.

None   0
Questionable   1
Mild: Occasional instances of illogicality   2
Moderate: Frequent instances of illogicality (three or four times)   3
Marked: Much of the subject's speech is illogical (more than four times)   4
Severe: Most of the subject's speech is illogical   5

Circumstantiality

Circumstantiality is a pattern of speech that is very indirect and delayed in reaching its goal idea. In the process of explaining something, the speaker brings in many tedious details and sometimes makes parenthetical remarks. Circumstantial replies or statements may last for many minutes if the speaker is not interrupted and urged to get to the point. Interviewers will often recognize circumstantiality on the basis of needing to interrupt the speaker in order to complete the process of history-taking within an allotted time. When not called circumstantial, these people are often referred to as "long-winded."

→

Exclusions: Although it may coexist with instances of poverty of content of speech or loss of goal, circumstantiality differs from poverty of content of speech in containing excessive amplifying or illustrative detail and from loss of goal in that the goal is eventually reached if the person is allowed to talk long enough. It differs from derailment in that the details presented are closely related to some particular goal or idea and that the particular goal or idea must be, by definition, eventually reached.

None	0
Questionable	1
Mild: Occasional instances of circumstantiality	2
Moderate: Frequent instances of circumstantiality	3
Marked: At least half of subject's speech is circumstantial	4
Severe: Most of the subject's speech is circumstantial	5

Pressure of Speech

The pressure of speech is an increase in the amount of spontaneous speech as compared to what is considered ordinary or socially customary. The subject talks rapidly and is difficult to interrupt. Some sentences may be left uncompleted because of eagerness to get on to a new idea. Simple questions that could be answered in only a few words or sentences are answered at great length so that the answer takes minutes rather than seconds and indeed may not stop at all if the speaker is not interrupted. Even when interrupted, the speaker often continues to talk. Speech tends to be loud and emphatic. Sometimes speakers with severe pressure will talk without any social stimulation and talk even though no one is listening. When subjects are receiving phenothiazines or lithium, their speech is often slowed down by medication, and then it can be judged only on the basis of amount, volume, and social appropriateness. If a quantitative measure is applied to the rate of speech, then a rate greater than 150 words per minute is usually considered rapid or pressured. This disorder may be accompanied by derailment, tangentiality, or incoherence, but it is distinct from them.

None	0
Questionable	1
Mild: Slight pressure of speech; some slight increase in amount, speed, or loudness of speech	2
Moderate: Usually takes several minutes to answer simple questions, may talk when no one is listening, and/or speaks loudly and rapidly	3

Marked: Frequently talks as much as three minutes to answer   4
simple questions; sometimes begins talking without social
stimulation; difficult to interrupt

Severe: Subject talks almost continually, cannot be interrupted at   5
all, and/or may shout to drown out the speech of others

Distractible Speech

During the course of a discussion or interview, the subject stops
talking in the middle of a sentence or idea and changes the subject in
response to a nearby stimulus, such as an object on a desk, the interviewer's clothing or appearance. For example, "Then I left San Francisco
and moved to ... where did you get that tie? It looks like it's left over from
the fifties. I like the warm weather in San Diego. Is that a conch shell on
you desk? Have you ever gone scuba diving?"

None   0
Questionable   1
Mild: Is distracted once during an interview   2
Moderate: Is distracted from two to four times during an inter- 3
view
Marked: Is distracted from five to ten times during an interview 4
Severe: Is distracted more than ten times during an interview   5

Clanging

Clanging is a pattern of speech in which sounds rather than meaningful relationships appear to govern word choice, so that the intelligibility of
the speech is impaired and redundant words are introduced. In addition to
rhyming relationships, this pattern of speech may also include punning
associations, so that a word similar in sound brings in a new thought. For
example, "I'm not trying to make a noise. I'm trying to make sense. If you
can made sense out of nonsense, well, have fun. I'm trying to make sense
out of sense. I'm not making sense (cents) anymore. I have to make
dollars."

None   0
Questionable   1
Mild: Occurs once during an interview   2
Moderate: Occurs from two to four times during an interview   3
Marked: Occurs five to ten times during and interview   4
Severe: Occurs more than ten times, or so frequently that the   5
interview is incomprehensible

→

Global Rating of Positive Formal Thought Disorder

In making this rating, the interviewer should consider the type of abnormality, the degree to which it affects the subject's ability to communicate, the frequency with which abnormal speech occurs, and its degree of severity.

None	0
Questionable	1
Mild: Occasional instances of disorder; subject's speech is understandable	2
Moderate: Frequent instances of disorder; subject is sometimes hard to understand	3
Marked: Subject is often difficult to understand	4
Severe: Subject is incomprehensible	5

INAPPROPRIATE AFFECT

Affect expressed is inappropriate or incongruous, not simply flat or blunted. Most typically, this manifestation of affective disturbance takes the form of smiling or assuming a silly facial expression while talking about a serious or sad subject. (Occasionally subjects may smile or laugh when talking about a serious subject which they find uncomfortable or embarrassing. Although their smiling may seem inappropriate, it is due to anxiety and therefore should not be rated as inappropriate affect.) Do not rate affective flattening or blunting as inappropriate.

Not at all: Affect is not inappropriate	0
Questionable	1
Mild: At least one instance of inappropriate smiling or other inappropriate affect	2
Moderate: Subject exhibits two to four instances of inappropriate affect	3
Marked: Subject exhibits five to ten instances of inappropriate affect	4
Severe: Subject's affect is inappropriate most of the time	5

Both scales reprinted with permission of Dr. Nancy C. Andreasen.

STRAUSS–CARPENTER LEVELS OF FUNCTIONING SCALE

Purpose and Development

Strauss and Carpenter (1975) developed the clinician-rated Levels of Functioning Scale to assess the functioning of schizophrenics, especially for the purpose of outcome evaluation. Researchers commonly use the scale for both long-term studies of schizophrenics and treatment-outcome studies (Brekke, 1992).

Strauss and Carpenter (1972) developed the 4-item scale first, and then Hawk, Strauss, and Carpenter (1975) added 5 items and modified the wording of the initial 4 items so that the time frame in the questions was flexible. We will provide the 9-item version with the modified wording, and we will identify the 4 items, now modified, that comprise the 4-item scale.

Individuals who want to read the published reports on the scale should be aware that some reports fail to make clear which version of the scale was used. Also, researchers have used varying names for the scale, including Levels of Function Scale, Outcome Scale, and Multidimensional Outcome Scale. Further, Strauss and Carpenter (1974) included similar items in a prognostic scale, so researchers occasionally cite the wrong article for the scale they used.

Administration and Scoring

The Levels of Functioning Scale requires 9 clinician ratings. Hawk et al. (1975) used mental status exams, psychiatric histories, and social data interviews to collect the relevant information. Strauss (1994) recommended the following method of calculating a total 4-item score: Calculate the average of items 2A and 2B and then the average of items 3A and 3B. Using these averages, add the first four ratings (items 1–4). As an alternative, scale users can sum the scores for items 1, 2A, 3A, and 4, which, with minor wording changes, are the 4 items set out in Strauss and Carpenter (1972). With either method, scores can range from 0 to 16, with higher scores indicating better functioning. For 9-item total scores, sum the responses to the 9 items.

Sample Scores

Hawk et al. (1975) reported a mean score of 24.8 (SD = 9.2) on the 9-item scale for 61 former inpatients assessed five years after being diagnosed schizophrenics. Strauss and Carpenter (1972) reported means for 85

TABLE A
Mean Scores of Schizophrenics on the Levels of Functioning
Scale

| | Friis et al. (1993) (N = 40) | | Strauss & Carpenter (1972) (N = 85) |
	Mean	SD	Mean
Nonhospitalization	3.2	1.5	3.0
Employment	1.1	1.6	2.7
Symptom Absence	2.0	1.5	2.3
Social Contact	1.8	1.7	2.8

schizophrenics on the original 4-item version of the scale. Friis Melle, Opjordsmoen, and Retterstol (1993) reported means and standard deviations for 40 schizophrenics on a 4-item version of the scale. Table 1 shows mean scores for the two groups.

Reliability

For the 9 items, interitem correlations ranged from .21 to .90, with most over .50 (Strauss & Carpenter, 1977). For all 9 items, interrater reliability has ranged from .82 to 1.0 (Kay & Murrill, 1990).

Validity

Strauss and Carpenter (1977) found that the sum of all 9 items correlated significantly with prognostic information collected five years before. Knesevich, Zalcman, and Clayton (1983) and Gaebel and Pietzcker (1987) found correlations between 4-item scale scores and prognostic data from one to six years before.

Researchers have found that scores on the items in the 4-item scale correlate significantly with Global Assessment Scale scores (Brekke, 1992; Friis et al., 1993), Health–Sickness Ratings Scale scores (Friis et al., 1993), Role Functioning Scale scores (Brekke, 1992), and Clinical Global Impressions ratings (Gaebel & Pietzcker, 1987). Gaebel and Pietzcker (1987) and Taylor, Tandon, Shipley, Eiser, and Goodson (1991) found that low 4-item scale scores were correlated with rapid-onset REM, a sleep characteristic previously found to be associated with severe mental illness.

STRAUSS–CARPENTER LEVELS OF FUNCTIONING SCALE

Instructions: Rate the most usual function in rating period (1 or 2 months in most instances).

1. DURATION OF NONHOSPITALIZATION FOR PSYCHIATRIC DISORDER

Describe:
Rate:

Not in hospital at all	4
Hospitalized less than 1/4 of the time	3
Hospitalized 1/4 to 1/2 of the time	2
Hospitalized over 1/2 up to 3/4 of the time	1
Hospitalized more than 3/4 of the time	0

2A. FREQUENCY OF SOCIAL CONTACTS

Describe:
Rate:
Number of Social Relations (meets with friends or does things with social groups, bowling, meetings, etc. EXCLUDE dates with opposite sex or social activities only with spouse.)

(Do not include meetings with friends at work or "over the back fence.")

Meets with friends on average of at least once a week	4
Meets with friends about once every two weeks	3
Meets with friends about once a month	2
INCLUDE ALL ACQUAINTANCES	
Does not meet with friends except "over the back fence" or at work or school	1
Does not meet with friends at all under any conditions	0

2B. QUALITY OF SOCIAL RELATIONS (In relations described in 2A, what has subject had most usually?)

One or more close relationships	4
One or more rather close relationships	3
One or more moderately close relationships	2
Only rather superficial relationships	1
Only very superficial relationships (e.g., only relationship is saying hello to neighbors)	0

→

3A. QUANTITY OF USEFUL WORK (Include as job: paid work,
    student, housewife. Exclude time in hospital. Any hospitaliz-
    ation in this period would *not* contribute to lower score.
    Working as a student for a full academic period would be
    rated "4.")

"Employed" full-time continuously	4
"Employed" for about 3/4 of the usual working hours in the period	3
"Employed" for about 1/2 of the period's working hours (e.g., employed half-time continuously or full-time for half the period)	2
"Employed" for about 1/4 of the period's working hours (e.g., half-time work for half the period)	1
No useful work	0

3B. QUALITY OF USEFUL WORK (Consider in regard to per-
    son's age, education, training, and opportunities available—
    but *not* compensating for his psychopathology, how he is
    functioning in the area of work in regard to expectable level
    of complexity and competence of which he should be ca-
    pable.)

Very competent	4
Competent	3
Moderately competent	2
Marginally competent	1
Incompetent	0

4.   ABSENCE OF SYMPTOMS

Describe:
Rate:

No signs or symptoms	4
Slight signs or symptoms most of the time or moderate signs and symptoms on rare occasions	3
Moderate signs and symptoms some of the time	2
Severe signs and symptoms some of the time or moderate signs and symptoms continuously	1
Continuous and severe signs and symptoms	0

5.   ABILITY TO MEET OWN BASIC NEEDS (feed self, keep
    clean)

Needs no help with these things	4
Needs a little help with these things	3
Needs some help with these things	2
Needs considerable help with these things	1
Needs total help with these things	0

6. FULLNESS OF LIFE

Very full life	4
Full life	3
Moderately full life	2
Relatively empty life	1
Vegetative existence	0

7. OVERALL LEVEL OF FUNCTION

Rate:
(Consider as baseline a hypothetical "normal" person with full employment, meaningful social relationships, no symptoms, etc.)

No impairment	4
Slight impairment most of the time or moderate impairment on rare occasions	3
Moderate impairment some of the time	2
Severe impairment some of the time or moderate impairment continuously	1
Continuous and severe impairment	0

Reprinted with permission of Dr. John S. Strauss and Dr. William T. Carpenter.

MAGICAL IDEATION SCALE AND PERCEPTUAL ABERRATION
SCALE

Purpose and Development

Eckblad and Chapman (1983) developed the Magical Ideation Scale, a 30-item self-report measure, to assess odd beliefs that Meehl (1964) described as common in schizophrenia-prone individuals. These beliefs, which we view as related to schizotypal personality disorder, involve forms of causality beyond the cultural norm, such as belief in mind-reading and the replacement of people by doubles.

Chapman, Chapman, and Raulin (1978) developed the Perceptual Aberration Scale, a 35-item self-report measure, to assess odd perceptions that Krepelin and Bleuler described schizophrenics as often having. These perceptions deal primarily with the respondent's own body, e.g. feeling as if "my body was melting into the surroundings," but some items involve other bizarre perceptions such as that "everything around me is tilting."

In developing the scales, the Chapmans and colleagues created items to manifest the constructs, tested the items for interitem consistency and association with measures of acquiescence and social desirability responding, and eliminated items that were did not correlate with the others or were highly influenced by response biases.

Researchers often use both scales in studies, sometimes combining all 65 items into one scale. Combining the scales into one is defensible because (a) the constructs measured are both related to schizotypal personality disorder; (b) scores on the two scales have been found to intercorrelate .68 to .84 (Bailey, West, Widiger, & Freiman, 1993; Chapman, Chapman, & Miller, 1982; Kelley & Coursey, 1992; Muntaner, Garcia-Sevilla, Fernandez, & Torrubia, 1988); and (c) the two scales show similar patterns of correlations with other measures (Bailey et al., 1992).

A version of the Magical Ideation Scale exists in Catalan (Muntaner et al., 1988); a version of the Perceptual Aberration Scale exists in German (Scherbarth & Hautzinger, 1991).

Administration and Scoring

Respondents answer true or false to each question. For a total score on the Magical Ideation Scale, count the number of "false" responses on items 4, 7, 15, 19, 22, 24, and 30, and "true" responses on the other items. Scores can range from 0 to 30, with higher scores indicating more magical ideation.

For the Perceptual Aberration Scale, count the number of "false" responses on items 6, 13, 24, and 25, and the number of "true" responses on the other items. Scale scores can range from 0 to 35, with higher scores indicating more aberration.

Cutoff and Sample Scores

Researchers have typically followed the practice of Eckblad and Chapman (1983) in considering high scorers to be individuals who score two standard deviations or more above the mean for a sample. That often has set a cutoff score in college students of about 20 on Magical Ideation and 15 on Perceptual Aberration. Researchers often intermix the items of the two scales (e.g., Muntaner et al., 1988) and use an infrequency scale to identify and eliminate as subjects individuals who earn high Magical Ideation or Aberration scores because of random responding (Chapman et al., 1978).

In groups of thousands of college students, Eckblad and Chapman (1983) and Balogh and Merritt (1990) found Magical Ideation mean scores for males and females of about 8 to 9, $SD = 5$ to 6.

In studies with almost 2,000 college students total, Chapman et al. (1978) and Lenzenweger and Moldin (1990) found mean scores of about 6.0 to 7.4, $SD =$ about 6, on the Perceptual Aberration Scale. Normals from the community averaged 5.1, $SD = 5.4$, in the study by Chapman et al. (1978) and 4.1, $SD = 4.95$, in a study by Katsanis, Iacono, and Beiser (1990). Sixty-six male schizophrenics scored an average of 7.7, $SD = 7.2$ (Chapman et al., 1978), and 118 psychotic patients scored an average of 6.4, $SD = 6.0$ (Katsanis et al., 1990). Bailey et al. (1993) found a mean of 7.9, $SD = 7.9$, for 50 personality disordered patients.

Reliability

For the Magical Ideation Scale, internal reliability as measured by Cronbach's alpha has ranged from .82 to .87 (Eckblad & Chapman, 1983; Chapman, Chapman, & Miller, 1982; Muntaner et al., 1988). Muntaner et al. (1988) reported 1-month test–retest reliability of .80, and Chapman et al. (1982) reported 6-week test–retest reliability of .80 to .82.

For the Perceptual Aberration Scale, Cronbach's alpha has ranged from .85 to .94 (Chapman et al., 1978; Chapman et al., 1982; Lenzenweger & Moldin, 1990; Muntaner et al., 1988). Muntaner et al. (1988) reported 4-week test–retest reliability of .71, and Chapman et al. (1982) reported 6-week test–retest reliability of .75 to .76.

When Zborowski and Garske (1990) used the items of both scales together, they found internal consistency as measured by the Kudor–Richardson formula to be .90.

Validity

First, we will review validity evidence for the Magical Ideation Scale. Eckblad and Chapman (1983) used the Schedule for Affective Disorders and Schizophrenia—Lifetime Form to interview college students, and found that high scorers of the Magical Ideation scale had higher interviewer ratings of schizotypal experiences, thought broadcasting, auditory psychotic-like experiences, aberrant beliefs, and reported telepathic reception.

Magical Ideation Scale scores have been found repeatedly to correlate with many measures of psychosis and schizotypal personality (Kelley & Coursey, 1992; Muntaner et al., 1988; Thaker, Moran, Adami, & Cassady, 1993), including scores on MMPI scales 2, 7, 8 and 0 (Chapman et al. 1982). Magical Ideation scores also have been associated with belief in paranormal phenomena (Tobacyk & Wilkinson, 1990); nonconformity (Stone & Schuldberg, 1990); poor eye-tracking (Van der Bosch, Rozendaal, & Mol, 1987); and poor concentration (Eckblad & Chapman, 1983).

Kaney and Bentall (1989) found that clients with persecutory delusions scored higher on the Magical Ideation Scale than depressed clients and normals. George and Neufeld (1987) found that Magical Ideation scores significantly discriminated schizophrenic patients from nonschizophrenic patients and from normals.

Bailey et al. (1992) found that the Magical Ideation Scale and the Perceptual Ideation Scale each correlated much more highly with a measure of schizotypal personality than with measures of other personality disorders such as schizoid and borderline.

For the Perceptual Aberration Scale, studies have shown that scores correlate with several MMPI measures of schizophrenic-like symptoms (Chapman et al., 1982); with various measures of schizotypal personality (Bailey et al., 1992; Lenzenweger, 1991; Lenzenweger & Korfine, 1992; Lenzenweger & Loranger, 1989; Mustaner et al., 1988; Raine, 1987; Thaker et al., 1993); with psychotic-like symptoms (Allen, Chapman, Chapman, & Vuchetich, 1987); and with social avoidance (Lenzenweger & Moldin, 1989).

Researchers have also reported significant correlations between Perceptual Aberration scores and nightmare frequency (Levin and Raulin, 1991); nonconformity (Stone & Schuldberg, 1990); and prior criticism from the respondents' parents (Edell & Kaslow, 1991).

Other studies have found that high scores on the Perceptual Aberration Scale correlated with poor sustained attention performance (Lenzenweger, Cornblatt, & Putnick, 1991); poor eye-tracking (Van der Bosch et al., 1987); and blink inhibition to a repeated startling stimulus (Simons & Giardina, 1992).

Chapman et al. (1978) found that Perceptual Aberration scores significantly discriminated schizophrenic from nonpsychotic outpatients and normals. Lenzenweger and Loranger (1989) found that high scorers on the Perceptual Aberration Scale were significantly more likely to have a relative who has been treated for schizophrenia.

Researchers who combined Magical Ideation and Perceptual Ideation items into one scale found correlations with psychotic-like symptoms (Chapman & Chapman, 1987); odd behavior (Zborowski & Garske, 1993); sexual arousal to a wide range of stimuli (Frost & Chapman, 1987); idiosyncratic responses to unfamiliar proverbs (Allen & Schuldberg, 1989); cognitive slippage (Allen, Chapman, & Chapman, 1987); inferior visual search strategies similar to those used by right-brain damaged patients (Jutai, 1989); and mixed handedness (Chapman & Chapman, 1987).

The main findings against the validity of the Magical Ideation and Perceptual Aberration scales involve undesirable correlations with acquiescence and social desirability responding (Chapman et al., 1978; Eckblad & Chapman, 1983; Peltier & Walsh, 1990). and with anxiety/neurosis and depression (Chapman et al., 1978; Eckblad & Chapman, 1983; Lenzinger & Loranger, 1989; Muntaner et al., 1988).

Further, the lack of major differences between clinical and student groups in typical mean scores on the Perceptual Aberration Scale also creates concern. Also, Thaker, Moran, Adami, and Casady (1993) and Kasanis, Iacono, and Besier (1990) found that relatives of schizophrenics scored significantly lower on the Perceptual Aberration Scale than other people. The researchers speculated that the relatives adopted a defensive response bias.

MAGICAL IDEATION SCALE AND PERCEPTUAL ABERRATION SCALE

Instructions for Both Scales

Please answer each item true or false. Please do not skip any items. It is important that you answer every item, even if you are not quite certain which is the best answer. An occasional item may refer to experiences which you have had only when taking drugs. Unless you had the experience at other times, mark it as it you have not had that experience.

Some items may sound like others, but all of them are slightly different. Answer each item individually, and don't worry about how you answered a somewhat similar previous item.

MAGICAL IDEATION SCALE

Circle T for true and F for false.

T F 1. I have occasionally had the silly feeling that a TV or radio broadcaster knew I was listening to him.

T F 2. I have felt that there were messages for me in the way things were arranged, like in a store window.

T F 3. Things sometimes seem to be in different places when I get home, even though no one has been there.

T F 4. I have never doubted that my dreams are the products of my own mind.

T F 5. I have noticed sounds on my records that are not there at other times.

T F 6. I have had the momentary feeling that someone's place has been taken by a look-alike.

T F 7. I have never had the feeling that certain thoughts of mine really belonged to someone else.

T F 8. I have wondered whether the spirits of the dead can influence the living.

T F 9. At times I perform certain little rituals to ward off negative influences.

T F 10. I have felt that I might cause something to happen just by thinking too much about it.

T F 11. At times, I have felt that a professor's lecture was meant especially for me.

T F 12. I have sometimes felt that strangers were reading my mind.

T F   13. If reincarnation were true, it would explain some unusual experiences I have had.

T F   14. I sometimes have a feeling of gaining or losing energy when certain people look at me or touch me.

T F   15. It is not possible to harm others merely by thinking bad thoughts about them.

T F   16. I have sometimes sensed an evil presence around me, although I could not see it.

T F   17. People often behave so strangely that one wonders if they are part of an experiment.

T F   18. The government refuses to tell us the truth about flying saucers.

T F   19. I almost never dream about things before they happen.

T F   20. I have sometimes had the passing thought that strangers are in love with me.

T F   21. The hand motions that strangers make seem to influence me at times.

T F   22. Good luck charms don't work.

T F   23. I have sometimes been fearful of stepping on sidewalk cracks.

T F   24. Numbers like 13 and 7 have no special powers.

T F   25. I have had the momentary feeling that I might not be human.

T F   26. I think I could learn to read others' minds if I wanted to.

T F   27. Horoscopes are right too often for it to be a coincidence.

T F   28. Some people can make me aware of them just by thinking about me.

T F   29. I have worried that people on other planets may be influencing what happens on Earth.

T F   30. When introduced to strangers, I rarely wonder whether I have known them before.

PERCEPTUAL ABERRATION SCALE

Please circle T for true and F for false.

T F   1. I sometimes have had the feeling that some parts of my body are not attached to the same person.

T F   2. Occasionally I have felt as though my body did not exist.

T F   3. Sometimes people whom I know well begin to look like strangers.

T F   4. My hearing is sometimes so sensitive that ordinary sounds become uncomfortable.

→

T F   5. Often I have a day when indoor lights seem so bright that they bother my eyes.

T F   6. My hands or feet have never seemed far away.

T F   7. I have sometimes felt confused as to whether my body was really my own.

T F   8. Sometimes I have felt that I could not distinguish my body from other objects around me.

T F   9. I have felt that my body and another person's body were one and the same.

T F 10. I have felt that something outside my body was a part of my body.

T F 11. I sometimes have had the feeling that my body is abnormal.

T F 12. Now and then, when I look in the mirror, my face seems quite different than usual.

T F 13. I have never had the passing feeling that my arms or legs have become longer than usual.

T F 14. I have sometimes felt that some part of my body no longer belongs to me.

T F 15. Sometimes when I look at things like tables and chairs, they seem strange.

T F 16. I have felt as though my head or limbs were somehow not my own.

T F 17. Sometimes part of my body has seemed smaller than it usually is.

T F 18. I have sometimes had the feeling that my body is decaying inside.

T F 19. Occasionally it has seemed as if my body had taken on the appearance of another person's body.

T F 20. Ordinary colors sometimes seem much too bright to me.

T F 21. Sometimes I have had a passing thought that some part of my body was rotting away.

T F 22. I have sometimes had the feeling that one of my arms or legs is disconnected from the rest of my body.

T F 23. It has seemed at times as if my body was melting into my surroundings.

T F 24. I have never felt that my arms or legs have momentarily grown in size.

T F 25. The boundaries of my body always seem clear.

T F 26. Sometimes I have had feelings that I am united with an object near me.

T F 27. Sometimes I have had the feeling that a part of my body is larger than it usually is.

T F 28. I can remember when it seemed as though one of my limbs took on an unusual shape.

T F 29. I have had the momentary feeling that my body has become misshapen.

T F 30. I have had the momentary feeling that the things I touch remain attached to my body.

T F 31. Sometimes I feel like everything around me is tilting.

T F 32. I sometimes have to touch myself to make sure I'm still there.

T F 33. Parts of my body occasionally seem dead or unreal.

T F 34. At times I have wondered if my body was really my own.

T F 35. For several days at a time I have had such a heightened awareness of sights and sounds that I cannot shut them out.

Reprinted with permission of Loren J. Chapman, Ph.D.

BORDERLINE SYNDROME INDEX

Purpose and Development

The Borderline Syndrome Index is a 52-item self-report scale designed to assess symptoms typical of borderline personality disorder (Conte, Plutchik, Karasu, & Jerrett, 1980). A group of clinicians experienced in working with borderline clients generated an initial pool of 70 items, which included criteria for the disorder listed in DSM-III. On the basis of the responses of a sample of patients and normal volunteers, the 52 items that best discriminated between these two groups were selected for the final scale.

Administration and Scoring

Respondents answer "yes," coded as 1, or "no," coded as 0, to each of the 52 items. The total scale score is the sum of all items. Scores can range from 0 to 52, with high scores indicating more disturbance.

Sample Scores and Cutoff Scores

Conte et al. (1980) reported scores and percentile equivalents for 35 borderline clients and 50 normal individuals. Table 1 shows an extract of these scores. Conte et al. (1980) suggest a cutoff score of 25 to identify individuals with borderline personality disorder. In their sample this cutoff would have led to correct identification of 50% of the borderlines and 100% of the normals. A cutoff of 15 would have led to correct identification of 92% of the borderlines and 94% of the normals.

Reliability

In a sample consisting of individuals with borderline personality disorder, schizophrenia, or depression, and individuals with no diagnosis, Conte et al. (1980) found internal reliability as assessed by the Kuder–Richardson formula was .92.

Validity

Several studies have found that scale scores are highly associated with other measures of borderline personality (D'Angelo, 1991; Lewis & Harder, 1991). Edell (1984) reported that higher scale scores were associated with elevations on all MMPI scale except for Masculinity/Femininity and Ma-

TABLE 1
Scores and Their Percentile
Equivalents on the Borderline
Syndrome Index for Borderline
Clients and Normal Individuals
(Conte et al., 1980)

| Raw score | Percentile | |
	Borderline	Normal
0	0	5
5	1	60
10	3	83
15	8	94
20	23	98
25	51	100
30	75	
35	88	
40	95	
45	98	
50	100	

nia. Higher scale scores have also been found to be associated with disturbances in separation and individuation (Dolan, Evans, & Norton, 1992),
worse coping mechanisms, and more eating disturbances (Fitzgibbon &
Kirschenbaum, 1990).

Conte et al. (1980) found that borderline clients' scores on the scale
were significantly higher than those of depressed clients, schizophrenic
clients, and normal individuals. Edell (1984) also reported that borderline
clients scored much higher on the scale than schizophrenic or normal
individuals.

Some research suggests that the scale may also measure symptoms of
the schizotypal and mixed personality disorders. Edell (1984) found no
difference between the scores of individuals with a diagnosis of borderline
personality disorder, schizotypal personality disorder, or mixed personality disorder, and Serban, Conte, and Plutchik (1987) confirmed this lack
of difference in scores of borderline, schizotypal, and mixed personality
disordered individuals.

Supporting the predictive validity of the scale, two studies found that
eating-disordered clients who had higher Borderline Syndrome Index
scores later showed less improvement both in the realm of eating and in
global adjustment (Johnson, Tobin, & Dennis, 1990; Sansone & Fine, 1992).

BORDERLINE SYNDROME INDEX

Please indicate whether each of the following statements describe the way you feel or act.

	Yes	No
1. I never feel as if I belong	——	——
2. I am afraid of going crazy	——	——
3. I want to hurt myself	——	——
4. I am afraid to form a close personal relationship	——	——
5. People who seem great at first often turn out to disappoint me	——	——
6. People disappoint me	——	——
7. I feel as if I can't cope with life	——	——
8. It seems a long time since I felt happy	——	——
9. I feel empty inside	——	——
10. I feel my life is out of control	——	——
11. I feel lonesome most of the time	——	——
12. I turned out to be a different kind of person than I wanted to be	——	——
13. I am afraid of anything new	——	——
14. I have trouble remembering things	——	——
15. It's hard for me to make decisions	——	——
16. I feel there is a wall around me	——	——
17. I get puzzled as to who I am	——	——
18. I am afraid of the future	——	——
19. Sometimes I feel I'm falling apart	——	——
20. I worry that I will faint in public	——	——
21. I never accomplish as much as I could	——	——
22. I feel as if I were watching myself play a role	——	——
23. My family would be better off without me	——	——
24. I am beginning to think that I'm losing out everywhere	——	——
25. I can't tell what I will do next	——	——
26. When I get into a relationship, I feel trapped	——	——
27. No one loves me	——	——
28. I can't tell the difference between what has really happened and what I have imagined	——	——
29. People treat me like "a thing"	——	——
30. Sometimes strange thoughts come into my head, and I can't get rid of them	——	——

31. I feel life is hopeless
32. I have no respect for myself
33. I seem to live in a fog
34. I am a failure
35. It scares me to take responsibility for anyone
36. I do not feel needed
37. I don't have any real friends
38. I feel that I can't run my own life
39. I feel uneasy in crowds, such as when I'm shopping or at a movie
40. I have trouble making friends
41. It's too late to try to be somebody
42. It's hard for me just to sit still and relax
43. I feel as if other people can read me like an open book
44. I feel as if something is about to happen
45. I am bothered by murderous ideas
46. I don't feel sure of my masculinity (femininity)
47. I have trouble keeping friends
48. I hate myself
49. I often have sex with persons I don't care for
50. I feel afraid in open spaces or on the streets
51. I sometimes keep talking to convince myself that I exist
52. Sometimes I am not myself

Reprinted with permission from Conte, H. R., Plutchik, R., Karasu, T. B., & Jerrett, I. (1980). A self-report borderline scale: Discriminative validity and preliminary norms. *Journal of Nervous and Mental Disease, 168,* 4–25. Copyright Williams and Wilkins, 1980.

REFERENCES

Allen, J., & Schuldberg, D. (1989). Positive though disorder in a hypothetically psychosis-prone population. *Journal of Abnormal Psychology, 90*, 491–494.

Allen, J. J., Chapman, L. J., & Chapman, J. P. (1987). Cognitive slippage and depression in hypothetically psychosis-prone college students. *Journal of Nervous and Mental Disease, 175*, 347–353.

Allen, J. J., Chapman, L. J., Chapman, J. P., Vuchetich, J. P., et al. (1987). Prediction of psychoticlike symptoms in hypothetically psychosis-prone college students. *Journal of Abnormal Psychology, 96*, 83–88.

Andreasen, N. C. (1982). Negative symptoms in schizophrenia. *Archives of General Psychiatry, 39*, 784–788.

Andreasen, N. C. (1984) *Scale for the assessment of positive symptoms*. Unpublished scale.

Andreasen, N. C. (1989). The Scale of the Assessment of Negative Symptoms (SANS): Conceptual and theoretical foundations. *British Journal of Psychiatry, 155 (supplement 7)*, 49–52.

Andreasen, N. C. (1990). Methods for assessing positive and negative symptoms. In N. C. Andreasen (Ed.), *Schizophrenia: Positive and negative symptoms and syndromes. Modern Problems in Pharmacopsychiatry* (pp. 73–88). Basel, Switzerland: Karger.

Andreasen, N. C., & Olsen, S. (1982). Negative vs. positive schizophrenia: Definition and validation. *Archives of General Psychiatry, 39*, 789–794.

Andreasen, N. C., Flaum, M., Swayze, V. W., Tyrrell, G., & Arndt, S. (1990). Positive and negative symptoms in schizophrenia: A critical reappraisal. *Archives of General Psychiatry, 47*, 615–621.

Andreasen, N. C., Swayze, V. W., Flaum, V., O'Leary, D. S., & Alliger, R. (1994). The neural mechanisms of mental phenomena. In (N. C. Andreasen, (Ed.), *Schizophrenia: From Mind to Molecule* (pp. 49–91). Washington, DC: American Psychiatric Press.

Balogh, D. W., & Merritt, R. D. (1990). Accounting for schizophrenics' Magical Ideation scores: Are college-student norms relevant? *Psychological Assessment, 2*, 326–328.

Brekke, J. S. (1992). An examination of the relationships among three outcome scales in schizophrenia. *Journal of Nervous and Mental Disease, 180*, 162–167.

Carpenter, W. T. (1994). Personal communication.

Chapman, J. P., & Chapman, L. J. (1987). Handedness of hypothetically psychosis-prone subjects. *Journal of Abnormal Psychology, 96*, 89–93.

Chapman, L. J., & Chapman, J. P. (1987). The search for symptoms predictive of schizophrenia. *Schizophrenia Bulletin, 13*, 497–503.

Conte, H. R., Plutchik, R., Karasu, T. B., & Jerrett, I. (1980). A self-report borderline scale: Discriminative validity and preliminary norms. *Journal of Nervous and Mental Disease, 168*, 4–25.

D'Angelo, E. (1991). Convergent and discriminant validity of the Borderline Syndrome Index. *Psychological Reports, 69*, 631–635.

Dolan, B. M., Evans, C., & Norton, K. (1992). The Separation-Individuation Inventory: Association with borderline phenomena. *Journal of Nervous and Mental Disease, 180*, 529–533.

Edell, W. S. (1984). The Borderline Syndrome Index: Clinical validity and utility. *Journal of Nervous and Mental Disease, 172*, 254–263.

Fenton, W. S., & McGlashan, T. H. (1991). Natural history of schizophrenia subtypes: II. Positive and negative symptoms and long-term course. *Archives of General Psychiatry, 48*, 978–986.

Fenton, W. S., & McGlashan, T. H. (1992). Testing systems for assessment of negative symptoms in schizophrenia. *Archives of General Psychiatry, 49*, 179–184.

Fitzgibbon, M. L., & Kirschenbaum, D. S. (1990). Heterogeneity of clinical presentation among obese individuals seeking treatment. *Addictive Behaviors, 15,* 291–295.

Friis, S., Melle, I. Opjordsmoen, S., & Retterstol, N. (1993). Global assessment scale and health–sickness rating scale: Problems in comparing the global functioning scores across investigations. *Psychotherapy Research, 3,* 105-114.

Frost, L. A., & Chapman, L. J. (1987). Polymorphous sexuality as an indicator of psychosis proneness. *Journal of Abnormal Psychology, 96,* 299–304.

Gaebel, W., & Pietzcker, A. (1987). Prospective study of course of illness in schizophrenia: II. Prediction of outcome. *Schizophrenia Bulletin, 13,* 299–306.

George, L., & Neufeld, R. W. (1987). Magical ideation and schizophrenia. Special Issue: Eating disorders. *Journal of Consulting and Clinical Psychology, 55,* 778– 779.

Hawk, A. B., Carpenter, W. T., & Strauss, J. S. (1975). Diagnostic criteria and five-year outcome in schizophrenia. *Archives of General Psychiatry, 32,* 343–347.

Johnson, C., Tobin, D., & Dennis, A. (1990). Differences in treatment outcomes between borderline and nonborderline bulimics at one-year follow-up. *International Journal of Eating Disorders, 9,* 617–627.

Jutai, J. W. (1989). Spatial attention in hypothetically psychosis-prone college students. *Psychiatry Research, 27,* 207–215.

Kaney, S., & Bentall, R. P. (1989). Persecutory delusions and attributional style. *British Journal of Medical Psychology, 62,* 191–198.

Katsanis, J., Iacono, W. G., & Beiser, M. (1990). Anhedonia and perceptual aberration in first-episode psychotic patients and their relatives. *Journal of Abnormal Psychology, 99,* 202–206.

Kay, S. R. (1991). *Positive and negative syndromes in schizophrenia.* New York: Brunner/Mazel.

Kay, S. R., Stanley, R., & Murrill, L. M. (1990). Predicting outcome of schizophrenia: Significance of symptom profiles and outcome dimensions. *Comprehensive Psychiatry, 31,* 91–102.

Kelley, M. P., & Coursey, R. D. (1992). Factor structure of Schizotypy Scales. *Personality and Individual Differences, 13,* 723–731.

Klimidis, S., Stuart, G. W., Minas, I. H., Copolov, D. L., & Singh, B. S. Positive and negative symptoms in the psychoses: Re-analysis of published SAPS and SANS global ratings. *Schizophrenia Research, 9,* 11–18.

Knesevich, J. W., Zalcman, S. J., & Clayton, P. J. (1983). Six-year follow-up of patients with carefully diagnosed good- and poor-prognosis schizophrenia. *American Journal of Psychiatry, 140,* 1507–1510.

Lenzenweger, M .F., & Korfine, L. (1992). Identifying schizophrenia-related personality disorder features in a nonclinical population using a psychometric approach. *Journal of Personality Disorders, 6,* 256–266.

Lenzenweger, M. F. (1991). Confirming schizotypic personality configurations in hypothetically psychosis-prone university students. *Psychiatry Research, 37,* 81–96.

Lenzenweger, M. F., Cornblatt, B. S., & Putnick, M. (1991). Schizotype and sustained attention. *Journal of Abnormal Psychology, 100,* 84–89.

Lenzenweger, M. F., & Moldin, S. O. (1990). Discerning the latent structure of hypothetical psychosis proneness through admixture analysis. *Psychiatry Research, 33,* 243–257.

Lenzenweger, M. F., & Loranger, A. W. (1989). Detection of familial schizophrenia using a psychometric measure of schizotypy. *Archives of General Psychiatry, 46,* 902–907.

Lenzenweger, M. F., & Loranger, A. W. (1989). *Journal of Abnormal Psychology, 98,* 3–8.

Levin, R., & Raulin, M. L. (1991). Preliminary evidence for the proposed relationship between frequent nightmares and schizotypal symptomatology. *Journal of Personality Disorders, 5,* 8–14.

Lewis, S. J., & Harder, D. W. (1991). A comparison of four measures to diagnose DSM-III-R borderline personality disorder in outpatients. *Journal of Nervous and Mental Diseases, 179*, 329–337.

Muntaner, C., Garcia-Sevilla, L., Fernandez, A., & Torrubia, R. 1988). Personality dimensions, schizotypal and borderline personality traits, and psychosis proneness. *Personality & Individual Differences, 9*, 257–268.

Peltier, B. D., & Walsh, J. A. (1990). *Educational and Psychological Measurement, 50*, 803–815.

Peralta, V., de Leon, J., & Cuesta, M. J. (1992). Are there more than two syndromes in schizophrenia? A critique of the positive-negative dichotomy. *British Journal of Psychiatry, 161*, 335–343.

Raine, A. (1987). Validation of schizoid personality scales using indices of schizotypal and borderline personality disorder in a criminal population. *British Journal of Clinical Psychology, 26*, 305–309.

Rosse, R. B., & Kleinberg, A. W. (1993). Positive and negative symptoms of schizophrenia as predictors of length of military service: A retrospective study. *Military Medicine, 158*, 529–533.

Sansone, R. A., & Fine, M A. (1992). Borderline personality as a predictor of outcome in women with eating disorders. *Journal of Personality Disorders, 6*, 176–186.

Scherbarth-Roschmann, P., & Hautzinger, M. (1991). Psychopathologie bei Personen mit schiotypiscen und zykolthymen Merkmalen: Plus- und Minussymptomatik. *Zeitschrift fur Klinische Psychologie. Forschung und Praxis, 20*, 371–378.

Serban, G., Conte, H. R., & Plutchik, R. (1987). Borderline and schitzotypal personality disorders: Mutually exclusive or overlapping. *Journal of Personality Assessment, 51*, 15–22.

Silk, K. R., & Tandon, R. (1991). Negative symptom rating scales. In J. F. Greden & R. Tandon (Eds.), *Negative schizophrenic symptoms: Pathophysiology and clinical implications* (pp. 63–77). Washington, DC: American Psychiatric Press.

Stone, B. L., & Schuldberg, D. (1990). Perceptual aberration, magical ideation, and the Jackson Personality Research Form. *Journal of Nervous and Mental Disease, 178*, 396.

Strauss, J. S., & Carpenter, W. T. (1972). The prediction of outcome in schizophrenia. *Archives of General Psychiatry, 27*, 739–746.

Strauss, J. S., & Carpenter, W. T. (1974). The prediction of outcome in schizophrenia: II. Relationship between predictor and outcome variables. *Archives of General Psychiatry, 31*, 37–42.

Strauss, J. S., & Carpenter, W. T. (1977). The prediction of outcome in schizophrenia: III. 5-year outcome and its predictors. *Archives of General Psychiatry, 34*, 159–163.

Strauss, J. S., Carpenter, W. T., & Bartko, J. (1974). The diagnosis and understanding of schizophrenia, III: Speculations on the processed that underlie schizophrenic symptoms and signs. *Schizophrenia Bulletin, 1*, 61–69.

Taylor, S. F., Tandon, R., Shipley, J. E., Eiser, A. S., & Goodson, J. (1991). Sleep onset REM periods in schizophrenic patients. *Biological Psychiatry, 30*, 205–209.

Thaker, G., Moran, M., Adami, H., & Cassady, S. (1993). Psychosis Proneness Scales in schizophrenia spectrum personality disorders: Familial vs. nonfamilial samples. *Psychiatry Research, 46*, 47–57.

Tobacyk, J. J., & Wilkinson, L. V. (1990). Magical thinking and paranormal beliefs. *Journal of Social Behavior and Personality, 5*, 255–264.

Van den Bosch, R. J., Rozendaal, N., & Mol, J. M. (1987). Symptom correlates of eye-tracking dysfunction. *Biological Psychiatry, 22*, 919–921.

Zborowski, M. J., & Garske, J. P. (1993). Interpersonal deviance and consequent social impact in hypothetically schizophrenia-prone men. *Journal of Abnormal Psychology, 102*, 482–489.

CHAPTER 5

Mood Disorders

CENTER FOR EPIDEMIOLOGICAL STUDIES—DEPRESSION SCALE (CES-D)

Purpose and Development

The CES-D, as it is almost always called, is a 20-item measure of depression developed by Radloff (1977) for use in survey research. It can be used as an interview schedule or a questionnaire. Radloff generated the items on the basis of items used in previously validated depression scales such as the Beck Depression Inventory and the Zung Depression Scale. She chose the items to represent six major components of depression identified in clinical writings and factor analyses: "depressed mood, feelings of guilt and worthlessness, feelings of helplessness and hopelessness, psychomotor retardation, loss of appetite, and sleep disturbance" (Radloff, 1977, p. 386). The scale has recently been used for quick screening of medical patients as well as epidemiological research.

There are now French (Fuhrer & Ruoillon, 1989), German (Weyerer, Geiger-Kabisch, Denzinger, & Pfeifer-Kurda, 1992), Korean (Noh, Avison, & Kaspar, 1992), and Spanish (Roberts and Vernon, 1983) versions of the scale.

Administration and Scoring

The response to each item is scored on a 0 to 3 scale. Items 4, 8, 12, and 16 are reverse scored. Scale scores can range from 0 to 60, with higher scores indicating more depression.

The instructions for use as an interview schedule vary slightly from those given below as part of the questionnaire presentation. For interview-

117

ing, give the respondent a printed form of the response options and the items. Radloff (1977) indicated that, instead of asking the respondent to circle a response, say, "Below is a list of the ways you might have felt or behaved. Please tell me how often you have felt this way during the past week."

Cutoff and Sample Scores

Radloff (1977) found that a cutoff score of 16 or greater correctly identified every person in a group of 35 severely depressed outpatients. Weissman, Sholomskas, Pottenger, Prusoff, & Locke (1977) found that this cutoff correctly classified over 99% of 147 acutely depressed outpatients.

As part of a community survey, Myers and Weissman (1980) tested the CES-D cutoff score of 16 against diagnoses based on interviews following the lengthy Schedule for Affective Disorders and Schizophrenia. Of the individuals classified by the SADS criteria as having major depression, 94% met the CES-D criteria. Of the individuals classified by the SADS criteria as not depressed, 64% did not meet the CES-D criteria.

In another community sample, Roberts and Vernon (1983) tested the CES-D against the SADS, with the SADS administered one to two weeks after the CES-D. The study found that 84% of the individuals classified by the SADS as having major depression met the CES-D criteria, and 60% of the individuals classified by the SADS as not having major depression did not meet the CES-D criteria.

Schulberg, Saul, McClelland, Ganguli, Christry, & Frank (1985) tested the cutoff score of 16 against DSM-III diagnoses based on the Diagnostic Interview Schedule in a sample of mental health center clients and found that 84% of clients diagnosed as having major depression met the CES-D criterion of 16 and that 44% who were not diagnosed as depressed did not meet the CES-D criterion. The study also found that in a sample of primary care medical patients, 96% of the patients diagnosed as depressed met the CES-D criterion and 38% not diagnosed as depressed scored under the CES-D cutoff. Using the same interview schedule with relatives of psychiatric patients, Zimmerman & Coryell (1994) found 88% identification of depressives and 92% identification of nondepressives.

Breslau (1985) tested the accuracy of a cutoff of 16 against Diagnostic Interview Schedule diagnoses of major depression in a group of 310 mothers of children with chronic disabilities and found that the CES-D correctly identified 88% of the depressives and 73% of the nondepressives. The study also found that the CES-D did almost as well in identifying mothers with generalized anxiety disorder, suggesting that the scale is not specific to depression.

Schulberg et al. (1985) tested the accuracy of other cutoff points and concluded that it was most accurate to classify scores at 27 or over as indicating major depression. Costello and Devins (1989) applied a cutoff score of 13 to a sample of primary care female patients because it led to identification of all 68 women who received a DSM-III diagnosis of major depression based on an interview schedule. In another sample of women patients the researchers found that a cutoff of 27 produced the most accurate classifications. Zich, Attkisson, and Greenfield (1990) likewise found in a sample of 34 medical outpatients who were assessed for depression with the Diagnostic Interview Schedule that a cutoff of 27 led to more accurate classifications that 16.

The cutoff studies together do not point to any one specific cutoff score as the best for all types of respondents. Users of the scale will have to make cutoff decisions on the basis of on their own weighing of the relative risks of false-positive versus false-negative errors in their group of respondents.

Radloff (1977) reported mean scores of about 8 to 9, SD = about 8, for groups of hundreds of individuals in community samples and 39 (no SD given) for 35 persons admitted to outpatient treatment for depression. Husaini, Neff, Harrington, Hughes, and Stone (1980) reported mean scores of 6.9, SD = 7.9, for 707 individuals in a rural community sample and 30.8, SD = 11.6 for a sample of 33 mental health center outpatients who were diagnosed as depressed. Weissman et al. (1977) reported a mean score of 38.1, SD = 9.0, for 148 outpatients who were diagnosed as depressed.

Reliability

Radloff (1977) reported internal consistency as measured by Cronbach's alpha ranged from .84 to .90 for general population and patient samples. Interview–reinterview reliability for periods from three to 12 months ranged from .32 for three months to .54 for six months. In a sample of high school students, Roberts, Andrews, Lewinsohn, and Hops (1990) found one-month test–retest reliability of .49 to .60 for a self-administered CES-D.

Validity

Studies have repeatedly found that scale scores correlate highly with clinician-rating measures of depression, such as the Hamilton Depression Rating Scale and global ratings (Radloff, 1977), and with other self-report measures, such as the Beck Depression Inventory and the Zung Self-Rating Depression Scale (Berndt, 1990), as well as the SCL-90 depression subscale (Weissman et al., 1977). Radloff (1977) also found that scale scores correlated with admitting a need for help with an emotional problem and with having several major recent life events such as becoming separated from a spouse.

Radloff (1977) reported that CES-D scores discriminated significantly between psychiatric inpatients and general population groups. Weissman et al. (1977) found much lower scale scores in drug addicts, alcoholics, and schizophrenics than in depressed patients.

Radloff (1977) found that CES-D scores decreased significantly and substantially after four weeks of outpatient treatment for severe depression. Finally, Radloff reported that scale scores correlated only $-.18$, albeit significantly, with a measure of social desirability responding.

CENTER FOR EPIDEMIOLOGICAL STUDIES—DEPRESSION SCALE

Circle the number of each statement which best describes how often you felt or behaved this way—DURING THE PAST WEEK.

	Rarely or none of the time (Less than 1 day)	Some or a little of the time (1–2 days)	Occasionally or a moderate amount of the time (3–4 days)	Most or all of the time (5–7 days)
DURING THE PAST WEEK:				
1. I was bothered by things that usually don't bother me	0	1	2	3
2. I did not feel like eating; my appetite was poor	0	1	2	3
3. I felt that I could not shake off the blues even with help from my family or friends	0	1	2	3
4. I felt that I was just as good as other people	0	1	2	3
5. I had trouble keeping my mind on what I was doing	0	1	2	3
6. I felt depressed	0	1	2	3
7. I felt that everything I did was an effort	0	1	2	3
8. I felt hopeful about the future	0	1	2	3
9. I thought my life had been a failure	0	1	2	3
10. I felt fearful	0	1	2	3
11. My sleep was restless	0	1	2	3
12. I was happy	0	1	2	3
13. I talked less than usual	0	1	2	3
14. I felt lonely	0	1	2	3
15. People were unfriendly	0	1	2	3
16. I enjoyed life	0	1	2	3

→

17. I had crying spells	0	1	2	3
18. I felt sad	0	1	2	3
19. I felt that people disliked me	0	1	2	3
20. I could not get "going"	0	1	2	3

Scale in public domain.

Zung Self-Rating Depression Scale

Purpose and Uses

The Zung Self-Rating Depression Scale (Zung, 1965) is a 20-item self-report measure of depression developed to assess aspects of depression identified in prior factor analytic studies. Its content overlaps almost entirely with the Hamilton Depression Rating Scale and DSM-III criteria for depression (Zung, 1986). Berndt (1990) described the scale as one of the most used depression scales. Non-English versions of the scale have been used in many countries, including Czechlosvakia, Germany, India, Japan, Korea, the Netherlands, and Sweden (Zung, 1986). Most recently, a Spanish-language version has been used in several studies in Mexico (e.g., Ramos-Brieva, Lafuetne-Lopez, Montejo-Iglesias, & Moreno-Sarmiento, 1991), and an Italian version has also been used (d'Amato, 1988).

Administration and Scoring

Respondents use a 4-point rating scale to complete each of the 20 items. Ten items are scored as indicators of depression (1, 3, 4, 7, 8, 9, 10, 13, 15, 19); the other ten are positively worded and hence are reverse-scored (2, 5, 6, 11, 12, 14, 16, 17, 18, 20). Total scores can range from 20 to 80, with higher scores indicating more depression.

Cutoff and Sample Scores

Zung (1986) recommended using 50 or above as a cutoff for depression. In a group of chronic pain patients, Turner and Romano (1984) compared this cutoff to clinician DSM-III diagnoses based on interviews. The scale correctly identified 83% of the patients who were diagnosed as depressed and correctly identified 81% of the patients not diagnosed as depressed.

In a review of sample scores, Zung (1986) concluded that ordinary people between ages 20 and 64 score on average 39 on the scale (no standard deviation was provided), while older and younger people tend to score higher; that U.S. patients with depressive disorders score an average of 64, $SD = 12$; and that mean scores for samples of depressives in Austria, Czechlosvakia, England, Germany, India, Japan, Korea, the Netherlands, and Sweden varied from 56 to 70 (SD from 6 to 24).

Reliability

Zung (1986) reported finding internal consistency of .92 as measured by Cronbach's alpha. Knight, Waal-Manning, and Spears (1983) reported an alpha of .79.

Validity

Scale scores have been found to correlate from .59 to .64 with the MMPI-Depression Scale (Zung, 1967; Zung, Richards, & Short, 1965); .73 to .77 with the Beck Depression Inventory (Davies, Burrows, & Poynton, 1975; Griffin & Kogut, 1988); and from .62 to .80 with the Hamilton Depression Rating Scale (Davies et al., 1975; Brown & Zung, 1972; Biggs, Wylie, & Zeigler, 1978); and highly also with less well known observer and self-report measures of depression (Bramley, Easton, Morley, & Snaith, 1988; Marone & Lubin, 1968) and interviewer-based DSM-III diagnoses of depression (Griffin & Kogut, 1988).

Validation studies have shown that scale scores (a) differentiated among groups of depressed inpatients, inpatients diagnosed with other disorders, and nonpatients (Zung, 1965); (b) differentiated a group of outpatients diagnosed as depressed from three groups with different diagnoses (anxiety, personality disorder, and situational adjustment reaction) (Zung, 1967); and (c) differentiated between clients diagnosed with depression and clients with anxiety disorders (Bramley et al., 1988). However, in one study the scale did not discriminate between inpatient and outpatient groups of depressives (Carroll, Fielding, & Blashki, 1973).

Finally, Zung (1965) found that scale scores significantly decreased for depressed inpatients during the course of their treatment for depression.

ZUNG SELF-RATING DEPRESSION SCALE

Please put a mark in the appropriate column for each item to indicate how true it is for you now.

	A little of the time	Some of the time	Good part of the time	Most of the time
1. I feel downhearted, blue, and sad				
2. Morning is when I feel the best				
3. I have crying spells or feel like it				
4. I have trouble sleeping through the night				
5. I eat as much as I used to				
6. I enjoy looking at, talking to, and being with attractive women/men				
7. I notice that I am losing weight				
8. I have trouble with constipation				
9. My heart beats faster than usual				
10. I get tired for no reason				
11. My mind is as clear as it used to be				
12. I find it easy to do the things I used to				
13. I am restless and can't sleep				
14. I feel hopeful about the future				

15. I am more irritable than usual				
16. I find it easy to make decisions				
17. I feel that I am useful and needed				
18. My life is pretty full				
19. I feel that others would be better off if I were dead				
20. I still enjoy the things I used to do				

HAMILTON DEPRESSION RATING SCALE

Purpose and Development

Hamilton (1960, 1967) developed a rating scale to be used to measure the severity of depression in individuals already diagnosed as suffering from depressive disorder. Berndt (1990) recently described it as the most widely used rating scale for depression.

The National Institute of Mental Health (NIMH) converted the scale into a checklist with less scoring information (Guy, 1976), but Hamilton always preferred his version (Hamilton & Shapiro, 1990), and NIMH later reverted to the more detailed version (Hamilton, 1986).

The scale has been translated into almost all the European languages and Korean (Hamilton, 1986).

Administration and Scoring

Hamilton (1986) recommended that the scale be used by experienced clinicians on the basis of an "easygoing" interview, and, when available, information from family, close friends, nurses, and records. The relevant time period for the ratings is the prior 7 or 10 days (Hamilton, 1986). Hamilton (1986) noted that information used for rating one item should not be used for rating another item. There are no specific interview questions to ask.

Only the first 17 items are scored for a depression severity score. Four additional items (18–21) are included in the scale to provide information relevant not to severity but to ancillary symptoms that might require specific treatment: diurnal variation (melancholia), depersonalization, paranoia, and obsessions (Hamilton, 1967).

Hamilton (1960) recommended that the severity score be calculated by doubling the score of one rater or by adding the score of two independent raters. We agree with Thompson (1989) that there is in general no good reason to either double the score or use two raters. It is simplest to add a rater's scores for the 17 items and consider that the scale score. For purposes of comparison or publication, users of the scale should be aware that studies using the scale sometimes do not make clear whether the reported scores are doubled. Without the doubling, scores can range from 0 to 50, with higher scores indicating more depression.

Over the years Hamilton modified slightly the wording of the 2-point and 4-point rating scales used with the items. We provide below the scale wording of Hamilton (1967).

Hamilton (1967) provided supplemental information for rating females on five scale items, 1, 7, 11, 13, and 14. Some of that information is now outdated (e.g., "Most women are housewives."), and some has little practical value (e.g., "[T]hree symptoms appear to be more common in women than in men."). However, the supplemental information for item 7 is valuable for rating males as well as females because it makes clear that the item covers loss of interest in housework and "hobbies" as well as in "work and activities." Scale users may want to disregard the less valuable supplemental information regarding the other items.

Sample Scores

Altshuler, Post and Fedio (1991) recommended considering non-doubled scores of 0–6 as normal, 7–17 as mild depression, 18–24 as moderate depression, and over 24 as severe depression. Altshuler et al. (1991) noted that a minimum score of 18 is often required for a person to be included in a depression study. Rehm (1987) reviewed several studies and concluded that normals often score around 6, depressed outpatients 24 to 27, and depressed inpatients from 32 to 42.

Reliability

Item-total correlations ranged from .21 to .78 in two studies described by McNamara (1992) and from virtually 0 to .91 in two other studies reported by Bech and Rafaelsen (1980). Interrater reliability ranged from .87 to .98 in several studies (Thompson, 1989).

Validity

The Hamilton Depression Rating Scale has become the standard against which other purported measures of depression are measured (Rabkin & Klein, 1987). Scores on the scale have been repeatedly found to correlate .58 to .84 with psychiatrists' global ratings of depression and with scores on many other rater and self-report measures of depression (Thompson, 1989). The scale has also been found repeatedly to distinguish between medical and depressed patients and to distinguish among general medical practice depressed patients, day-care depressed patients, and depressed inpatients (Thompson, 1989).

Other studies have found that scale scores decrease after treatment for depression (McNamara, 1992) and change after treatment proportionately to changes in cognitive performance (Fudge, Perry, Garvey, & Kelly, 1990).

McNamara (1992) noted that because the scale focuses on somatic problems, it may not be as sensitive to change in mildly depressed individuals as in the more depressed.

HAMILTON DEPRESSION RATING SCALE

Scale for items scored 0–2:
0 = absent
1 = doubtful or trivial
2 = clearly present

Scale for items scored 0–4:
0 = absent
1 = doubtful or trivial
2 = mild
3 = moderate
4 = severe

THE RATING OF MALE PATIENTS

(1) Depression (0–4)

Depressed mood is not easy to assess. One looks for a gloomy attitude, pessimism about the future, feelings of hopelessness, and a tendency to weep. As a guide, occasional weeping could count as 2, frequent weeping as 3, and severe symptoms allotted 4 points. When patients are severely depressed they may 'go beyond weeping'. It is important to remember that patients interpret the word 'depression' in all sorts of strange ways. A useful common phrase is 'lowering of spirits'.

(2) Guilt (0–4)

This is fairly easy to assess but judgment is needed, for the rating is concerned with pathological guilt. From the patient's point of view, some action of his which precipitated a crisis may appear as a 'rational' basis for self-blame, which persists even after recovery from his illness. For example, he may have accepted a promotion, but the increased responsibility precipitated his breakdown. When he 'blames himself' for this, he is ascribing a cause and not necessarily expressing pathological guilt. As a guide to rating, feelings of self-reproach count 1, ideas of guilt 2, belief that the illness might be a punishment 3, and delusions of guilt, with or without hallucinations, 4 points.

(3) Suicide (0–4)

The scoring ranges from feeling that life is not worth living 1, wishing he were dead 2, suicidal ideas and half-hearted attempts 3, serious at-

→

tempts 4. Judgement must be used when the patient is considered to be concealing this symptom, or conversely, when he is using suicidal threats as a weapon, to intimidate others, obtain help and so on.

(4), (5), (6) Insomnia (initial, middle, and delayed) (0–2)

Mild, trivial, and infrequent symptoms are given 1 point, obvious and severe symptoms are rated 2 points; both severity and frequency should be taken into account. Middle insomnia (disturbed sleep during the night) is the most difficult to assess, possibly because it is an artifact of the system rating. When insomnia is severe, it generally affects all phases. Delayed insomnia (early morning wakening) tends not to be relieved by hypnotic drugs and is not often present without other forms of insomnia.

(7) Work and interests (0–4)

It could be argued that the patient's loss of interest in his work and activities should be rated separately from his decreased performance, but it has been found too difficult to do so in practice. Care should be taken not to include fatiguability and lack of energy here; the rating is concerned with loss of efficiency and the extra effort required to do anything. When the patient has to be admitted to hospital because his symptoms render him unable to carry on, this should be rated 4 points, but not if he has been admitted for investigation or observation. When the patient improves he will eventually return to work, but when he does so may depend on the nature of his work; judgement must be used here.

(8) Retardation (0–4)

Severe forms of this symptom are rare, and mild forms are difficult to perceive. A slight flattening of affect and fixity of expression rate as 1, a monotonous voice, a delay in answering questions, a tendency to sit motionless count as 2. When retardation makes the interview extremely prolonged and almost impossible, it is rated 3, and 4 is given when an interview is impossible (and symptoms cannot be rated). Although some patients may say that their thinking is slowed or their emotional responsiveness has been diminished, questions about these manifestations usually produce misleading answers.

(9) Agitation (0–4)

Severe agitation is extremely rare. Fidgetiness at interview rates as 1, obvious restlessness with picking at hands and clothes should count as 2. If the patient has to get up during the interview he is given 3, and 4 points are given when the interview has to be conducted 'on the run', with the patient pacing up and down, picking at his face and hair and tearing at his clothes. Although agitation and retardation may appear to be opposed forms of behaviour, in mild form they can co-exist.

(10) Anxiety (psychic symptoms) (0–4)

Many symptoms are included here, such as tension and difficulty in relaxing, irritability, worrying over trivial matters, apprehension and feelings of panic, fears, difficulty in concentration and forgetfulness, 'feeling jumpy'. The rating should be based on pathological changes that have occurred during the illness and an effort should be made to discount the features of a previous anxious disposition.

(11) Anxiety (somatic symptoms (0–4)

These consist of the well-recognized effects of autonomic overactivity in the respiratory, cardiovascular, gastrointestinal and urinary systems. Patients may also complain of attacks of giddiness, blurring of vision, and tinnitus.

(12) Gastrointestinal symptoms (0–2)

The characteristic symptom in depression is loss of appetite and this occurs very frequently. Constipation also occurs but is relatively uncommon. On rare occasions patients will complain of 'heavy feelings' in the abdomen. Symptoms of indigestion, wind and pain, etc. are rated under Anxiety.

(13) General somatic symptoms (0–2)

These fall into two groups: the first is fatiguability, which may reach the point where the patients feel tired all the time. In addition, patients complain of 'loss of energy', which appears to be related to difficulty in starting up an activity. The other type of symptom consists of diffuse muscular achings, ill-defined and often difficult to locate, but frequently in the back and sometimes in the limbs; these may also feel 'heavy'.

(14) Loss of libido (0–2)

This is a common and characteristic symptom of depression, but it is difficult to assess in older men and especially those, e.g., unmarried, whose sexual activity is usually at a low level. The assessment is based on a pathological change, i.e., a deterioration obviously related to the patient's illness. Inadequate or no information should be rated as zero.

→

pathological change, i.e., a deterioration obviously related to the patient's illness. Inadequate or no information should be rated as zero.

(15) Hypochondriasis (0–4)

The severe states of this symptom, concerning delusions and hallucinations of rotting and blockages, etc., which are extremely uncommon in men, are rated as 4. Strong convictions of the presence of some organic disease which accounts for the patient's condition are rated 3. Much preoccupation with physical symptoms and with thoughts of organic disease are rated 2. Excessive preoccupation with bodily functions is the essence of a hypochondriacal attitude and trivial or doubtful symptoms count as 1 point.

(16) Loss of insight (0–2)

This is not necessarily present when the patient denies that he is suffering from mental disorder. It may be that he is denying that he is insane and may willingly recognize that he has a 'nervous' illness. In case of doubt, enquiries should be directed to the patient's attitude to his symptoms of Guilt and Hypochondriasis.

(17) Loss of weight (0–2)

The simplest way to rate this would be to record the amount of loss, but many patients do not know their normal weight. For this reason, an obvious or severe loss is rated as 2 and a slight or doubtful loss as 1 point.

(18) Diurnal variation (0–2)

This symptom has been excluded from the rating scale as it indicates the type of illness, rather than presenting an addition to the patient's disabilities. The commonest form consists of an increase of symptoms in the morning, but this is only slightly greater than worsening in the evening. A small number of patients insist that they feel worse in the afternoon. The clear presence of diurnal variation is rated as 2 and the doubtful presence is 1 point.

The following three symptoms were excluded from the rating of symptoms because they occur with insufficient frequency, but they are of interest in research.

(19) Derealization and Depersonalization (0–4)

The patient who has this symptom quickly recognizes the questions asked of him; when he has difficulty in understanding the questions it usually signifies that the symptom is absent. When the patient asserts that he has this symptom it is necessary to question him closely; feelings of 'distance' usually mean nothing more than that the patient lacks concentration or interest in his surroundings. It would appear that the severe forms of this symptom are extremely rare in patients diagnosed as depressive.

(20) Paranoid symptoms (0–4)

These are uncommon, and affirmative answers should always be checked carefully. It is of no significance if the patient says that others talk about him, since this is usually true. What is important in the mild symptom is the patient's attitude of suspicion, and the malevolence imputed to others. Doubtful or trivial suspicion rates as 1, thoughts that others wish him harm rates as 2, delusions that others wish him harm or are trying to do so rates as 3, and hallucinations are given 4 points. Care should be taken not to confuse this symptom with that of guilt, e.g., 'people are saying that I am wicked'.

(21) Obsessional symptoms (0–2)

These should be differentiated from preoccupations with depressive thoughts, ideas of guilt, hypochondriacal preoccupations and paranoid thinking. Patients usually have to be encouraged to admit to these symptom, but their statements should be checked carefully. True obsessional thoughts are recognized by the patient as coming from his own mind, as being alien to his normal outlook and feelings, and as causing great anxiety; he always struggles against them.

THE RATING OF FEMALE PATIENTS

The same general principles apply to the rating of women as of men, but there are special problems which need to be considered in detail.

(1) Depression (0–4)

It is generally believed that women weep more readily than men, but there is little evidence that this is true in the case of depressive illness. There is no reason to believe, at the moment, that an assessment of the frequency of weeping could be misleading when rating the intensity of depression in women.

(7) Work and interests (0–4)

Most women are housewives and therefore their work can be varied, both in quantity and intensity, to suit themselves. Women do not often

→

complain of work being an effort, but they say they have to take things easily, or neglect some of their work. Other members of the family may have to increase the help they give. It is rare for a housewife to stop looking after her home completely. If she has an additional job outside the home she may have to change it to part-time, or reduce her hours of work or even give it up completely. Women engage in hobbies less frequently than men. Loss of interest, therefore, may not be as obvious. Patients may complain of inability to feel affection for their families. This could be rated here, but it could be rated under other symptoms, depending upon its meaning and setting. Care should be taken not to rate it in two places. It is a very valuable and important symptom if the patient mentions it spontaneously but could be very misleading as a reply to a question.

(11) Anxiety (somatic) (0–4)

These last three symptoms appear to be more common in women than in men.

(13) Somatic symptoms (general) (0–2)

It is not uncommon for women to complain of backache and to ascribe it to a pelvic disorder. This symptom requires careful questioning.

(14) Loss of libido (0–2)

In women whose sexual experience is satisfactory, this symptom will appear as increasing frigidity, progressing to active dislike of sexual intercourse. Women who are partially or completely frigid find that their customary toleration of sex also changes to active dislike. It is difficult to rate this symptom in women who have had no sexual experience or, indeed, in widows since loss of libido in women tends to appear not so much as a loss of drive but as a loss of responsiveness. In the absence of adequate information of a pathological change a zero rating should be given.

Disturbed menstruation and amenorrhoea have been described in women suffering from severe depression, but they are very rare. Despite the difficulties in rating, it has been found that the mean score for women is negligibly less than men.

Reprinted with permission of the British Psychological Society from Hamilton, M. (1960). A rating scale for depression. *Journal of Neurology, Neurosurgery and Psychiatry, 23*, 56–62.

The Bech–Rafaelsen Melancholia Scale

Purpose and Development

The Bech–Rafaelsen Melancholia Scale is an 11-item interviewer rating scale that represents an extensive modification of the Hamilton Depression Rating Scale. Bech and Rafaelsen (1980) set out to create a new depression scale that would have higher internal consistency than the Hamilton.

Marcos and Salamero (1990) found through factor analysis that the scale items constituted a single factor. Other studies have found that the items are homogeneous with various samples (Bech & Rafaelsen, 1986; Chambon, Cialdella, Kiss, Poncet, & Milani-Bachman,1990).

There are versions of the scale in several languages (Bech & Rafaelsen, 1986; Chambon et al., 1990).

Administration and Scoring

Interviewers are free to ask whatever questions they deem appropriate in order to make the 11 ratings required for the scale. Bech (1993) described some closed-ended questions an interviewer might use for each item.

Clinicians use a 0–4 continuum to make each rating. Scale scores, which are the sum of the 11 ratings, can range from 0 to 44, with higher scores indicating more depression.

Bech (1993) recommended the following cutoff scores: 0–5: no depression; 6–9: mild depression; 10–15: less than major depression; 16–29: major depression; 30 or more: more than major depression.

Bech and Rafaelsen (1980) reported a mean scale score of 20.5, SD = 5.7, for 31 unselected depressed inpatients. For samples of 130 and 48 acutely depressed inpatients, Maier, Phillip, Heuser, Schlegel, Buller, & Wetzel (1988) reported mean scores of 15.9 (SD = 7.5) and 19.6 (SD = 9.0).

Reliability

Bech and Rafaelsen (1980) reported coefficients ranging from .52 to .88 for correlations between scale items and the sum of the other items, but other studies have found lower correlations clustering around .50 (Bech & Rafaelsen, 1986). Chambon et al. (1990) found a Cronbach's alpha of .70 for the French version of the scale. Reported interrater correlations for scale scores have ranged from .71 to .93 (Bech, Gjerris, Andersen, Bojholm, Kramp, Bolwig, Kastrup, Clemmesen, & Rafaelsen, 1985; Bech & Rafaelsen, 1986; Danish University Antidepressant Group, 1990; Maier, Phillip, Heuser, Schlegel, Buller, & Wetzel, 1988).

Validity

Scale scores have been found to correlate highly with the Raskin Depression Scale and the Global Assessment Scale, and correlate significantly more highly with another measure of depression than with a measure of anxiety (Maier et al., 1988). Further, Schlegel, Maier, Philipp, Aldenhoff, Heuser, Kretzschmar, and Benkert (1989) found that the size of ventricles (brain cavities) correlated with Bech–Rafaelsen scores but not with Hamilton Depression Rating Scale scores. Schegel, Nieber, Herrmann, and Bakauski (1991) found that the latency of an auditory event-related potential in the brain (slow brain activity) correlated with the Bech–Rafaelsen scale but not the Hamilton.

Other studies have found that scale scores discriminate significantly between major depressive episode with melancholia and without melancholia (Bech et al., 1986; Maier, Heuser, Philipp, Frommberger, & Demuth, 1988). Other research has found that scores decrease with appropriate treatment (e.g., Danish University Antidepressant Group, 1990).

The Bech–Rafaelsen Melancholia Scale

General Remarks. The interview should assess the presence and intensity of the 11 items covering a minimum period of the preceding three days. In many cases the last week is considered. Hence, the time frame should be specified. During the interview it is not mandatory to follow the order of items as indicated in the scoring sheet. However, this order is suggested because experience has shown that the items follow each other in a logical way. On the other hand, the questions and the rank order depend of course on the condition of the patient. When the interviewer is in doubt of an item, information should be solicited from relatives, or if hospitalized from ward personnel.

Item 1. Work and interests

0: No difficulties
1: Mild insufficiencies in the day-to-day activities, e.g., the patient expresses some difficulties in carrying out his or her usual activities (work and/or homework)
2: Clear but still moderate insufficiencies
3: Difficulties in starting simple routine activities which are carried out with great efforts
4: Unable to perform anything without help

Item 2. Lowered mood

0: Not present
1: Very mild tendencies to lowered spirits
2: The patient is more clearly concerned by unpleasant experiences although he or she still lacks feelings of hopelessness
3: Moderately to markedly depressed. Some hopelessness and/or clear nonverbal signs of depression
4: Severe degree of lowered mood. Pronounced hopelessness

Item 3. Sleep disturbances

This item covers the patient's subjective experience of the duration of sleep (hours of sleep per 24-hr. periods). The rating should be based on the three preceding nights, irrespective of administration of hypnotics or sedatives. The score is the average of the past three nights.

0: Usual sleep duration
1: Duration of sleep slightly reduced
2: Duration of sleep clearly reduced but still moderate, i.e., still less than a 50% reduction ➔

3: Duration of sleep markedly reduced
4: Duration of sleep extremely reduced, e.g., as if not been sleeping at all

Item 4. Anxiety

0: Not present
1: Very mild tendencies of tenseness, worry, fear, or apprehension
2: The patient is more clearly in a state of anxiety, apprehension, or insecurity, which, however, he or she is still able to control
3: The anxiety or apprehension is at times more difficult to control. At the edge of panic
4: Extreme degree of anxiety, interfering greatly with patient's daily life

Item 5. Emotional introversion

0: Not present
1: Very mild tendencies of emotional indifferences in relation to social surroundings (colleagues)
2: The patient is more clearly emotionally introverted in relation to colleagues or other people but still glad to be with friends or family
3: Moderately to markedly introverted, i.e., less need or ability to feel warmth to friends or family
4: The patient feels isolated or emotionally indifferent even to near friends or family

Item 6. Concentration difficulties

0: Not present
1: Very mild tendencies of concentration disturbances or problems in decision making
2: Even with a major effort difficult to concentrate occasionally
3: Difficulties in concentration even in things that usually need no effort (reading a newspaper, watching television program)
4: When it is clear that the patient also during interview is showing difficulties in concentration

Item 7. Tiredness or pains

0: Not present
1: Very mild feelings of tiredness or pains
2: The patient is more clearly in a state of tiredness, weakness, pains, or somatic discomfort, but these symptoms are still without influence on the patient's daily life
3: Marked feelings of tiredness or pains which interfere occasionally with the patient's daily life

4: Extreme feelings of tiredness or pains interfering more constantly with the patient's daily life

Item 8. Guilt feelings

0: No loss of self-esteem, self-depreciation, or guilt feelings
1: Concerned with the fact of being a burden to the family, friends, or colleagues due to reduced interests, introversion, low capacity, or loss of self-esteem/self-confidence
2: Self-depreciation or guilt feelings are clearly present because the patient is concerned with incidents (minor omissions or failures) in the past prior to the current episode of depression
3: Feels that current depression is a punishment but can still intellectually see that this view is unfounded
4: Guilt feelings have become paranoid ideas

Item 9. Decreased verbal activity

0: Not present
1: Very mild tendencies to reduced verbal formulation activity
2: More pronounced inertia in conversation, e.g., a trend to longer intermissions
3: Interview is clearly colored by brief responses or long pauses
4: Interview is clearly prolonged due to decreased verbal formulation activity

Item 10. Suicidal thoughts

0: Not present
1: The patient feels that life is not worthwhile, but expresses no wish to die
2: The patient wishes to die but has no plans of taking his/her own life
3: Has probably plans actively to hurt himself/herself
4: Has definitely plans to kill himself/herself

Item 11. Decreased motor activity

0: Not present
1: Very mild tendencies to decreased motor activity, e.g., facial expression slightly retarded
2: Moderately reduced motor activity, e.g., reduced gestures
3: Markedly reduced motor activity, e.g., all movements slow
4: Severely reduced motor activity, approaching stupor

Reprinted with permission of Dr. Per Bech.

MANIC-STATE RATING SCALE

Purpose and Development

Developed by researchers at the National Institute of Health, the Manic-State Rating Scale (Beigel, Murphy, & Bunney, 1971) measures manic behavior in the prior 8-hour period. Raters indicate the frequency and intensity of 26 manic behaviors such as jumping from one subject to another and acting delusional.

The scale developers created the items on the basis of relevant literature, their own observations of manic patients, and nurses' examples of manic behavior in their patients. The scale developers used the nurses' own words as much as possible in writing the final items.

Two factor analyses of scale items found several factors but only a few that appear noteworthy. In the Beigel and Murphy (1974) unrotated factor analytic study, the first factor appeared to be a general one, while the second appeared dichotomous, with poles of elated-grandiose and paranoid-destructive. The rotated factor analytic study of Double (1990) produced a similar first factor and separate second and third factors of elated-grandiose and paranoid-destructive. However, too few subjects were used in the two studies to put much stock in the factor patterns. Although Beigel and Murphy (1974) suggested the use of subscales on the basis of their factor analysis, we believe that at this point there is inadequate psychometric support for their use.

Administration and Scoring

Scale users rate patients on 26 behaviors. The raters use a 0–5 continuum to indicate how frequent the behavior was in the past 8 hours and a 1–5 scale to indicate how intense it was. Raters then multiply frequency ratings and intensity ratings for each behavior. The cross products can range from 0 to 25 for each item. For a total scale score, raters sum the cross products for all 26 items. Total scores can range from 0 to 650, with higher scores indicating more manic behavior.

The developers of this scale originally used nurses and nurses' assistants to make the ratings, after providing them with special training in how to use the scale. However, Double (1990) noted that nurses who were used to rating patients for other reasons had no difficulty making the ratings without receiving any special training. Cohen, Khan, and Cox (1989) apparently used psychiatrists to make the ratings primarily on information from a clinical interview and information from family and friends. Nagel, Adler, Bell, Nagamoto, and Freedman (1991) used a clinical interview and information from the clinical staff about recent patient activity. In a study by Liebewitz, Rudy, Gershon, and Gillis (1976), a psychiatrist made the ratings on the basis of a clinical interview and nurses' reports.

Sample Scores

Cohen et al. (1989) reported a mean scale score of 141, $SD = 32$, for 38 newly admitted inpatients who met DSM-III criteria for bipolar disorder and later recovered with treatment. Beigel and Murphy (1971) and Murphy and Beigel (1974) reported scores for groups of 30 and 12 inpatients with an "unequivocal bipolar manic-depressive illness." For the group of 12, the scores ranged from 58 to 257 with a median (by our calculation) of 200. For the group of 30, the scores ranged from 58 to 257 with a median (by our calculation) of 196.

Reliability

Beigel et al. (1971) reported intraclass correlations of .86 to 1.0 for the individual scale items, except that the item "dresses inappropriately" had no variance, so no meaningful correlation could be calculated for it.

Validity

In studies of manic inpatients, three studies found high correlations between scale scores and psychiatrists' global mania ratings (Beigel et al., 1971; Beigel and Murphy, 1974; and Bech, Bolwig, Dein, Jacobsen, & Gram, 1975). Beigel et al. (1971) also found high correlations with scores on a symptom checklist completed by the same nurse who completed the Manic-State Rating Scale. Bech, Bolwig, Dein, Jacobsen, and Gram (1975) found significant correlations between 18 of 26 individual scale items rated by nurses and psychiatrists' global mania ratings.

Nagel et al. (1991) used lithium to treat 12 recently detoxified alcoholics who were experiencing manic-like symptoms and found that Manic-State Rating Scale scores significantly decreased. Liebowitz et al. (1976) found that scale scores demonstrated the effectiveness of lithium versus placebo in a single psychotic patient repeatedly assessed.

MANIC-STATE RATING SCALE

Frequency Scale   *Intensity Scale*
0 = None   1 = Very minimal
1 = Infrequent   2 = Minimal
2 = Some   3 = Moderate
3 = Much   4 = Marker
4 = Most   5 = Very Marked
5 = All

Frequency (How much of the time?)	THE PATIENT	Intensity (How intense is it?)	Cross product
_____	1. Looks depressed.	_____	_____
_____	2. Is talking.	_____	_____
_____	3. Moves from one place to another.	_____	_____
_____	4. Makes threats.	_____	_____
_____	5. Has poor judgment.	_____	_____
_____	6. Dresses inappropriately.	_____	_____
_____	7. Looks happy and cheerful.	_____	_____
_____	8. Seeks out others.	_____	_____
_____	9. Is distractable.	_____	_____
_____	10. Has grandiose ideas.	_____	_____
_____	11. Is irritable.	_____	_____
_____	12. Is combative or destructive.	_____	_____
_____	13. Is delusional.	_____	_____
_____	14. Verbalizes depressive feelings.	_____	_____
_____	15. Is active.	_____	_____
_____	16. Is argumentative.	_____	_____
_____	17. Talks about sex.	_____	_____
_____	18. Is angry.	_____	_____
_____	19. Is careless about dress and grooming.	_____	_____
_____	20. Has diminished impulse control.	_____	_____
_____	21. Verbalizes feelings of well-being.	_____	_____
_____	22. Is suspicious.	_____	_____

_____   23. Makes unrealistic plans.   _____   _____
_____   24. Demands contact with others.   _____   _____
_____   25. Is sexually preoccupied.   _____   _____
_____   26. Jumps from one subject to   _____   _____
              another.

                                    Total Scale Score   _____

Reprinted from Beigel, A., & Murphy, D. L. (1971). Assessing clinical characteristics of the manic state. *American Journal of Psychiatry, 128,* 688–694. Copyright 1971, American Medical Association.

References

Altshuler, L., Post, R., & Fedio, P. (1991). Assessment of affective variables in clinical trials. I. E. Mohr & P. Brouwers (Eds.), *Handbook of Clinical trials: The neurobehavioral approach.* Berwyn, PA: Swets & Zeitlinger.

Bech, P. (1993). *Rating scales for psychopathology, health status, and quality of life. A compendium on documentation in accordance with DSM-III-R and WHO systems.* Berlin: Springer.

Bech, P., Bolwig, T. G., Dein, E., Jacobsen, O., & Gram, L. F. (1975). Quantitative rating of manic states: Correlation between clinical assessment and Biegel's objective rating scale. *Acta Psychiatrica Scandinavica, 52,* 1–6.

Bech, P., Gjerris, A., Andersen, J., Bojholm, S., Kramp, P., Bolwig, T. G., Kastrup, M., Clemmesen, L., & Rafaelsen, O. J. (1985). The Melancholia Scale and the Newcastle Scales: Item-combinations and inter-observer reliability. *British Journal of Psychiatry, 143,* 58–63.

Bech, P., & Rafaelsen, O. J. (1980). The use of rating scales exemplified by a comparison of the Hamilton and Bech–Rafaelsen Melancholia Scale. *Acta Psychiatrica Scandanavica, 62 (Suppl. 285),* 128–131.

Bech, P., & Rafaelsen, O. (1986). The Melancholia Scale: Development, consistency, validity, and utility. In N. Sartorius & T. Ban (Eds.), *Assessment of depression* (pp. 259–269). New York: Springer-Verlag.

Beigel, A., & Murphy, D. L. (1971). Assessing clinical characteristics of the manic state. *American Journal of Psychiatry, 128,* 688–694.

Beigel, A., Murphy, D. L., & Bunney, W. E. (1971). The Manic-State Rating Scale: Scale construction, reliability, and validity. *Archives of General Psychiatry, 25,* 256–262.

Berndt, D. (1990). Inventories and scales. In B. Wolman & G. Stricker (Eds.), *Depressive disorders: Facts, theories, and treatment methods* (pp. 255–274). New York: Wiley.

Biggs, J. T., Wylie, L. T., & Ziegler, V. E. (1978). Validity of the Zung self-rating depression scale. *British Journal of Psychiatry, 132,* 381–385.

Bramley, P., Easton, A., Morley, S., & Snaith, R. (1988). The differentiation of anxiety and depression by rating scales. *Acta-Psychiatrica-Scandinavica, 77,* 133–138.

Breslau, N. (1985). Depressive symptoms: Major depression, and generalized anxiety: A comparison of self-report and the CES-D and results from diagnostic interviews. *Psychiatry Research, 15,* 219–229.

Brown, G. L., & Zung, W. W. K. (972). Depression scales: Self-physician-rating? A validation of certain clinically observable phenomena. *Comprehensive Psychiatry, 13,* 361–367.

Carroll, B. J., Fielding, J. M., & Blashki, T. G. (1973). Depression ratings scales: A critical review. *Archives of General Psychiatry, 28,* 361–366.

Chambon, O., Cialdella, P., Kiss, L., Poncet, F., & Milani-Bachman, D. (1990). Study of the unidimensionality of the Bech–Rafaelsen Melancholia Scale using Rasch analysis in a French sample of major depressive disorders. *Pharmacopsychiatry, 23,* 243–245.

Chambon, O., Cialdella, P., Kiss, L., Poncet, F., & Milani-Bachman, D. (1990). Study of the unidimensionality of the Bech–Rafaelsen Melancholia Scale using Rasch analysis in a French sample of major depressive disorders. *Pharmacopsychiatry, 23,* 243–245.

Cohen, S., Khan, A., & Cox, G. (1989). Demographic and clinical features predictive of recovery in acute mania. *Journal of Nervous and Mental Disease, 177,* 638–642.

Costello, C., & Devins, G. (1989). Screening for depression among women attending their family physicians. *Canadian Journal of Behavioural Science, 21,* 434–451.

d'Amato, F. (1988). Studio clinico condotto con alprazolam presso servizi dipartimentali di igiene mentale del territorio. *Psichiartria-e-Psicoterapia-Analclitica, 7,* 373–388.

Danish University Antidepressant Group (DUAG). (1990). Paroxetine: A selective serotonin reuptake inhibitor showing better tolerance, but weaker antidepressant effect than clomipramine in a controlled multicenter study. *Journal of Affective Disorders, 18,* 289–299.

Davies, B., Burrows, G., & Poynton, C. (1975). A comparative study of four depression rating scales. *Australian and New Zealand Journal of Psychiatry, 9*, 21–24.

Double, D. T. (1990). The factor structure of manic rating scales. *Journal of Affective Disorders, 18*, 113–119.

Fudge, J. L., Perry, P. J., Garvey, M. J., & Kelly, M. W. (1990). A comparison of the effect of fluoxetine and trazodone on the cognitive functioning of depressed outpatients. *Journal of Affective Disorders, 18*, 275–280.

Fuhrer, R., & Rouillon, F. (1989). La version francaise l'eschelle CES-D. *European Psychiatry, 4*, 163–166.

Hamilton, M. (1960). A rating scale for depression. *Journal of Neurology, Neurosurgery and Psychiatry, 23*, 56–62.

Hamilton, M. (1967). Development of a rating scale for primary depressive illness. *British Journal of Social & Clinical Psychology, 6*, 278–296.

Hamilton, M. (1980). Rating depressive patients. *Journal of Clinical Psychiatry, 41*, 21–24.

Hamilton, M. (1986). The Hamilton Rating Scale for Depression. In N. Sartorius & T. A. Ban (Eds.), *Assessment of depression* (pp. 143–152). New York: Springer-Verlag.

Hamilton, M., & Shapiro, C. M. (1990). Depression. In D. F. Peck & C. M. Shapiro (Eds.), *Measuring human problems: A practical guide* (pp. 25–65). New York: Wiley.

Griffin, P., & Kogut, D. (1988). Validity of orally administered Beck and Zung depression scales in a state hospital setting. *Journal of Clinical Psychology, 44*, 756–759.

Guy, W. (1976). *ECDEU assessment manual for psychopharmacology.* Rockville, MD: National Institute of Mental Health.

Husaini, B., Neff, J., Harrington, Hughes, M., & Stone, R. (1980). Depression in rural communities: Validating the CES-D Scale. *Journal of Community Psychology, 8*, 20–27.

Liebowitz, J, H., Rudy, V., Gershon, E. S., & Gillis, A. (1976). A pharmacogenetic case report: Lithium-responsive postpsychotic antisocial behavior. *Comprehensive Psychiatry, 17*, 655–660.

Maier, W., Philipp, M. Heuser, I., Schlegel, S., Buller, R., & Wetzel, H. (1988). Improving depression severity assessment: Reliability, internal validity and sensitivity to change of three observer depression scales. *Journal of Psychiatric Research, 22*, 3–12.

Maier, W., Heuser, I., Philipp, M., Frommberger, U., & Demuth, W. (1988). Improving depression severity assessment: II. Content concurrent and external validity of three observer depression scales. *Journal of Psychiatric Research, 22*, 13–19.

Marcos, T., & Salamero, M. (1990). Factor study of the Hamilton Rating Scale for Depression and Bech Melancholia Scale. *Acta Psychiatrica Scandinavica, 82*, 178–181.

Marone, J., & Lubin, B. (1968). Relationship between set 2 of the depression adjective checklists (DACL) and Zung Self-Rating Depression Scale (SDS). *Psychological Reports, 22*, 333–334.

McNamara, K. (1992). Depression assessment and intervention: Current status and future directions. In S. Brown & R. Lent, *Handbook of counseling psychology* (pp. 691–718). New York: Wiley.

Murphy, D. L., & Beigel, A. (1974). Depression, elation, and lithium carbonate responses in manic patient subgroups. *Archives of General Psychiatry, 31*, 643–648.

Myers, J., & Weissman, M. (1980). Use of a self-report symptom scale to detect depression in a community sample. *American Journal of Psychiatry, 137*, 1081–1084.

Nagel, K., Adler, L. E., Bell, J., Nagamoto, H. T., & Freedman, R. (1991). Lithium carbonate and mood disorder in recently detoxified alcoholics: A double-blind, placebo-controlled pilot study. *Alcoholism Clinical and Experimental Research, 15*, 978–981.

Noh, S., Avison, W., & Kaspar, V. (1992). Depressive symptoms among Korean immigrants: Assessment of a translation of the Center for Epidemiological Studies Depression Scale. *Psychological Assessment, 4*, 84–91.

Rabkin, J., & Klein, D. (1987). The clinical measurement of depressive disorders. In A.

Marsella, R. Hirschfeld, & M. Katz (Eds.), *The measurement of depression*. New York: Guilford.

Radloff, L. S. (1977). The CES-D Scale: A self-report depression scale for research in the general population. *Applied Psychological Measurement, 1*, 385–401.

Rehm, L. D. (1987). The measurement of behavioral aspects of depression. In A. J. Marsella, R. M. Hirschfeld, & M. M. Katz (Eds.), *The measurement of depression* (pp. 199–239). New York: Guilford.

Ramos-Brieva, J., Lafuente-Lopez, R., Montejo-Iglesias, M., Moreno-Sarmiento, A. (1991). Validez predictiva de la escala de Zung en deprimidos ancianos. *Actas-Luso-Espanolas-de-Neurologia, -Psiquiatria-y-Ciencias-Afines, 19*, 122–126.

Roberts, R., Andrews, J., Lewinsohn, P., & Hops, H. (1990). Assessment of depression in adolescents using the Center for Epidemiological Studies Depression Scale. *Psychological Assessment, 2*, 122–128.

Roberts, R., & Vernon, S. (1983). The Center for Epidemiological Studies Depression Scale: Its use in a community sample. *American Journal of Psychiatry, 140*, 41–46.

Schlegel, S., Maier, W., Phillip, M., Aldenhoff, J., Heuser, I., Kretzschmar, K., & Benkert, O. (1989). Computed tomography in depression: Association between ventricular size and psychopathology. *Psychiatry Research, 29*, 221–230.

Schlegel, S., Nieber, D., Herrmann, D., & Bakauski, E. (1991). Latencies of the P300 component of the auditory event-related potential in depression are related to the Bech–Rafaelsen Melancholia Scale but not to the Hamilton Rating Scale for Depression. *Acta Psychiatrica Scandinavica, 83*, 438–440.

Schulberg, H., Saul, M., McClelland, M., Ganguli, Christy, W., & Frank, R. (1985). Assessing depression in primary medical and psychiatric practices. *Archives of General Psychiatry, 42*, 1164–1170.

Thompson, C. (1989). Affective disorders. In C. Thompson (Ed.), *The instruments of psychiatric research* (pp. 87–126). New York: Wiley.

Turner, J. A., & Romano, J. M. (1984). Self-report screening measures for depression in chronic pain patients. *Journal of Clinical Psychology, 40*, 909–913.

Weissman, M., Sholomskas, D., Pottenger, M., Prusoff, B., & Locke, B. (1977). Assessing depressive symptoms in five psychiatric populations: A validation study. *American Journal of Epidemiology, 106*, 203–214.

Weyerer, S., Geiger-Kabisch, C., Denzinger, R., & Pfeifer-Kurda, M. (1992). Die deutsche Version der CES-D Skala. Ein geeignetes Instrument zur Erfassung von Depressionen bei alteren Menschen? *Diagnostica, 38*, 354–365.

Zich, J., Attkisson, C., & Greenfield, T. (1990). Screening for depression in primary care clinics: The CES-D and the BDI. *International Journal of Psychiatry in Medicine, 20*, 259–277.

Zimmerman, M., & Coryell, W. (1994). Screening for major depressive disorder in the community: A comparison of measures. *Psychological Assessment, 6*, 71–74.

Zung, W. W. K. (1965). A self-rating depression scale. *Archives of General Psychiatry, 12*, 63–70.

Zung, W. W. K. (1967). Factors influencing the self-rating depression scale. *Archives of General Psychiatry, 16*, 543–547.

Zung, W. (1986). Zung Self-Rating Depression Scale and Depression Status Inventory. In N. Sartorius & T. Ban (Eds.), *Assessment of depression*. New York: Springer-Verlag.

Zung, W. W. K., Richards, C, & Short, M. (1965). Self-rating depression scale in an out-patient clinic. *Archives of General Psychiatry, 13*, 508–515.

Anxiety Disorders

ANXIETY SYMPTOM QUESTIONNAIRE

Purpose and Development

The Anxiety Symptom Questionnaire assesses cognitive, somatic, and behavioral dimensions of anxiety. The scale is a 36-item self-report measure developed by Lehrer and Woolfolk (1982), who first constructed a large number of items, each of which tapped either cognitive, behavioral, or somatic anxiety and gave this pool of items to two separate large groups of subjects. The results of a factor analysis confirmed three main dimensions of somatic, cognitive, and behavioral anxiety and were used to identify 36 items, each of which loaded on one of the three factors. Scholing and Emmelkamp (1992) replicated these three original factors with several samples.

Administration and Scoring

Respondents answer each of the items using a 9-point scale of frequency. Items may be summed for a total anxiety score or the three dimensions of anxiety may be examined separately. Scores on the total anxiety scale may range from 0 to 288, and higher scores indicate more anxiety. Items 1, 2, 4, 7, 10, 13, 14, 18, 20, 23, 29, 30, 31, 33, 34, and 35 measure the somatic dimension. Items 3, 6, 9, 12, 17, 22, 25, 26, and 28 measure the behavioral dimension. Finally, items 5, 8, 11, 15, 16, 19, 21, 24, 27, 32, and 36 measure the cognitive dimension. Scores on these three dimensions can range from 0 to 128, 72, and 88 respectively, and higher scores on each of the three dimensions indicate more anxiety.

Sample Scores

Koksal, Power, and Sharp (1991) gave the scale to 29 clients with phobic disorders (social phobia, simple phobia, or agoraphobia) and 25 clients with other anxiety disorders (generalized anxiety disorder, obsessional-compulsive disorder, or panic disorder). Scholing and Emmelkamp (1992) obtained scale scores from 48 men and 60 women who sought treatment for a social phobia, 48 men and 55 women who returned the scale after they were randomly selected from the telephone directory of a city, and 279 male and 369 female adolescents selected from secondary schools. Table 1 shows mean scores for each group.

Reliability

Scholing and Emmelkamp (1992) examined the internal consistency of the subscales. In a sample of individuals with social phobias, they found a Cronbach's alpha of .92 for the somatic subscale, .88 for the behavioral subscale, and .83 for the cognitive subscale. In a sample of normal adults, they found a Cronbach's alpha of .92 for the somatic subscale, .87 for the behavioral subscale, and .83 for the cognitive subscale. In a sample of adolescents, they found a Cronbach's alpha of .88 for the somatic subscale, .81 for the behavioral subscale, and .83 for the cognitive subscale.

Validity

Lehrer and Woolfolk (1982) reported that in a group of students attending evening classes scores on all three subscales were significantly associated with scores on another anxiety inventory, a measure of neuroti-

TABLE 1
Mean Scores on the Anxiety Symptom Questionnaire

Group	Total score		Somatic subscale		Behavioral subscale		Cognitive subscale	
	M	SD	M	SD	M	SD	M	SD
Phobic anxiety*			44.0	18.6	54.1	26.2	52.3	18.1
Other anxiety*			36.7	17.4	37.8	19.5	54.2	17.6
Social phobia**	91.2	24.4	31.7	12.8	28.2	8.3	31.3	8.2
Normal adults**	62.0	15.9	23.5	7.1	16.1	6.0	22.4	6.7
Adolescents**	71.1	18.7	27.7	9.2	17.3	5.5	26.2	7.9

*Koksal et al. (1991), **Scholing and Emmelkamp (1992).

cism, and a measure of introversion. Scores on the subscales were not associated with a measure of psychopathy. In a sample of 57 clients suffering from anxiety they found that the SCL-90R somatization scale was closely related to the somatic subscale and that the SCL-90R psychoticism scale was highly correlated with the behavior and cognition subscales.

Scholing and Emmelkamp (1992) found that in a group of social phobics and a group of adolescents the somatic subscale was more highly correlated with the SCL-90-R somatic subscale than were the behavioral or the cognitive subscales. They also found a strong correlation between the behavioral subscale and the Marks and Mathews Fear Questionnaire social phobia measure, high correlations between the cognition subscale and the SCL-90-R depression and interpersonal subscales, and a moderate correlation between the cognitive subscale and a social cognition inventory.

Lehrer and Woolfolk (1982) reported that the scale seems to elicit some social desirability responding. In a sample of students who completed the scale as well as a measure of social desirability response tendency, they found that some of the variance on the subscales is related to social desirability.

Lehrer and Woolfolk (1982) reported that the scale was given to anxious college freshmen who were randomly assigned to either a behaviorally based group treatment for improving coping skills or a cognitively based treatment for improving coping skills. The students in the behavioral treatment showed a significant change only on the behavior subscale while the students in the cognitive treatment group showed a significant change only on the cognitive subscale. Scholing and Emmelkamp (1992) found a large, significant difference between the total scale scores of a group of socially phobic clients and a group of normal adults. Of the three subscales the behavioral subscale distinguished most between the two groups and the somatic subscale distinguished between them the least. Scholing and Emmelkamp (1992) tracked the group of individuals with social phobias as they went through treatment and found a decrease in anxiety as measured by all three subscales.

ANXIETY SYMPTOM QUESTIONNAIRE

Please circle the number that indicates how you feel for each item. *For example,* if you feel happy often, but not all the time, circle 6 below.

I feel happy.

0	1	2	3	4	5	6	7	8
Never							Extremely Often	

(1) My throat gets dry.

0	1	2	3	4	5	6	7	8
Never							Extremely Often	

(2) I have difficulty in swallowing.

0	1	2	3	4	5	6	7	8
Never							Extremely Often	

(3) I try to avoid starting conversations.

0	1	2	3	4	5	6	7	8
Never							Extremely Often	

(4) My heart pounds.

0	1	2	3	4	5	6	7	8
Never							Extremely Often	

(5) I picture some future misfortune.

0	1	2	3	4	5	6	7	8
Never							Extremely Often	

(6) I avoid talking to people in authority (my boss, policemen).

0	1	2	3	4	5	6	7	8
Never							Extremely Often	

(7) My limbs tremble.

0	1	2	3	4	5	6	7	8
Never							Extremely Often	

(8) I can't get some thought out of my mind.

0	1	2	3	4	5	6	7	8
Never							Extremely Often	

(9) I avoid going into a room by myself where people are already gathered and talking.

0	1	2	3	4	5	6	7	8
Never							Extremely Often	

(10) My stomach hurts.

0	1	2	3	4	5	6	7	8
Never							Extremely Often	

(11) I dwell on mistakes that I have made.

0	1	2	3	4	5	6	7	8
Never							Extremely Often	

(12) I avoid new or unfamiliar situations.

0	1	2	3	4	5	6	7	8
Never							Extremely Often	

(13) My neck feels tight.

0	1	2	3	4	5	6	7	8
Never							Extremely Often	

(14) I feel dizzy.

0	1	2	3	4	5	6	7	8
Never							Extremely Often	

(15) I think about possible misfortune to my loved ones.

0	1	2	3	4	5	6	7	8
Never							Extremely Often	

(16) I cannot concentrate at a task or job without irrelevant thoughts intruding.

0	1	2	3	4	5	6	7	8
Never							Extremely Often	

(17) I pass by school friends, or people I know but have not seen for a long time, unless they speak to me first.

0	1	2	3	4	5	6	7	8
Never							Extremely Often	

(18) I breathe rapidly.

0	1	2	3	4	5	6	7	8
Never							Extremely Often	

→

(19) I keep busy to avoid uncomfortable thoughts.

0	1	2	3	4	5	6	7	8
Never							Extremely Often	

(20) I can't catch my breath.

0	1	2	3	4	5	6	7	8
Never							Extremely Often	

(21) I can't get some pictures or images out of my mind.

0	1	2	3	4	5	6	7	8
Never							Extremely Often	

(22) I try to avoid social gatherings.

0	1	2	3	4	5	6	7	8
Never							Extremely Often	

(23) My arms or legs feel stiff.

0	1	2	3	4	5	6	7	8
Never							Extremely Often	

(24) I imagine myself appearing foolish with a person whose opinion of me is important.

0	1	2	3	4	5	6	7	8
Never							Extremely Often	

(25) I find myself staying home rather than involving myself in activities outside.

0	1	2	3	4	5	6	7	8
Never							Extremely Often	

(26) I prefer to avoid making specific plans for self-improvement.

0	1	2	3	4	5	6	7	8
Never							Extremely Often	

(27) I am concerned that others might not think well of me.

0	1	2	3	4	5	6	7	8
Never							Extremely Often	

(28) I try to avoid challenging jobs.

0	1	2	3	4	5	6	7	8
Never							Extremely Often	

(29) My muscles twitch or jump.

0	1	2	3	4	5	6	7	8
Never							Extremely Often	

(30) I experience a tingling sensation somewhere in my body.

0	1	2	3	4	5	6	7	8
Never							Extremely Often	

(31) My arms or legs feel weak.

0	1	2	3	4	5	6	7	8
Never							Extremely Often	

(32) I have to be careful not to let my real feelings show.

0	1	2	3	4	5	6	7	8
Never							Extremely Often	

(33) I experience muscular aches and pains.

0	1	2	3	4	5	6	7	8
Never							Extremely Often	

(34) I feel numbness in my face, limbs or tongue.

0	1	2	3	4	5	6	7	8
Never							Extremely Often	

(35) I experience chest pains.

0	1	2	3	4	5	6	7	8
Never							Extremely Often	

(36) I have an uneasy feeling.

0	1	2	3	4	5	6	7	8
Never							Extremely Often	

Reprinted with permission of Dr. Paul Lehrer.

HAMILTON ANXIETY SCALE

Purpose and Development

The Hamilton Anxiety Scale assesses the severity of symptoms in anxious individuals. The scale is a 14-item semistructured interview measure developed by Hamilton (1959), who generated a series of symptoms associated with anxiety and then grouped these symptoms into 14 clusters. A factor analysis of the items showed that they tapped a general anxiety factor and bipolar factors of cognitions and somatic symptoms related to anxiety (Hamilton, 1959). The scale has been widely used, especially in assessing treatment outcomes.

Administration and Scoring

An interviewer rates the individual on a 5-point scale of severity for each of the items. The interviewer is guided by symptom descriptors for each item. The ratings are summed for a total score, which can range from 0 to 56, with higher scores indicating greater anxiety. Subscale scores may also be derived for Psychic Anxiety (the sum of items 7 through 13) and Somatic Anxiety (the sum of items 1 through 6 and item 14).

Sample Scores

Maier, Buller, Phillip, and Heuser (1988) gave the scale to 97 individuals with panic disorders and 101 depressed individuals, 28 of whom also had a diagnosed anxiety disorder. Kobak, Reynolds, and Greist (1993) gave the scale to 128 depressed individuals, 78 individuals with no psychiatric diagnosis, and 86 individuals with diagnosed anxiety disorders. Of those with anxiety disorders 47 had panic disorders, 20 had generalized anxiety disorders, and 18 had obsessive-compulsive disorders. Table 1 shows the mean scores of these individuals.

Reliability

In a sample of individuals with anxiety disorders, individuals with depression, and individuals with no diagnosis, Kobak et al. (1993) found that the internal consistency of the total scale was .92 as assessed by Cronbach's alpha. One-week test–retest reliability for a subsample of this group was .96.

Hamilton (1959) found that the interrater reliability for pairs of raters was .89 for the total scale and Maier et al. (1988) found interrater reliabilities of .74 for the total scale, .73 for the psychic scale, and .70 for the somatic scale.

TABLE 1
Hamilton Anxiety Scale Scores

| Group | Total | | Psychic | Somatic |
	M	SD	M	M
Individuals with Anxiety Disorders**	18.95	8.43		
Obsessive-Compulsive Disorder	9.78	6.09		
Panic Disorder	21.24	7.88		
Generalized Anxiety Disorder	21.65	5.75		
Individuals with Panic Disorder*	25.40		14.0	11.3
Individuals with Depression*	22.00		13.9	7.9
Individuals with Depression**	20.31	6.03		
Individuals with No diagnosis**	2.40	2.47		

*Maier et al. (1988), **Kobak et al. (1993).

Validity

Other measures of anxiety have been found to correlate with the total scale (Lehrer & Woolfolk, 1982; Maier et al. 1988) and the subscales (Maier et al., 1988; Beck & Steer, 1991).

Maier et al. (1988) found that even though the depressed individuals in their study were quite anxious, total scale scores and subscale scores differentiated those who were anxious and those who were depressed. Kobak et al. (1993) found that a group of individuals with diagnosed anxiety disorders scored much higher on the scale than a group of individuals with no diagnosed psychopathology. They also found that depressed individuals scored much higher than individuals with no diagnosis and even slightly higher than individuals with anxiety disorders. Thus in the Kobak et al. (1993) study the scale did not discriminate between individuals with anxiety disorders and individuals with depression. Kobak et al. (1993) suggest that this may be because anxiety is often a symptom of depression.

Kobak et al. (1993) compared the scale scores of individuals with obsessive-compulsive disorders, panic attacks, and generalized anxiety disorders. The individuals with panic attacks and generalized anxiety had similarly high scale scores, while those with obsessive-compulsive disorders had relatively low scale scores. Kobak et al. (1993) suggested that this may be because compulsive behaviors serve to reduce anxiety.

Numerous studies have found that scale scores decreased as clients go through treatment (e.g., Enkelman, 1990; Katz, Landau, Lott, & Bystritsky, 1993; Maier et al., 1983; Malcolm, Anton, Randall, & Johnston 1992).

HAMILTON ANXIETY SCALE

Anxious mood

Worries
Anticipation of the worst
Apprehension (fearful anticipation)
Irritability

Tension

Feelings of tension
Fatiguability
Inability to relax
Startle response
Moved to tears easily
Trembling
Feelings of restlessness

Fears

Of dark, strangers
Being left alone
Large animals, etc.
Traffic
Crowds

Insomnia

Difficulty in falling asleep
Broken sleep
Unsatisfying sleep and fatigue on waking
Dreams
Nightmares
Night terrors

Intellectual (cognitive)

Difficulty in concentration
Poor memory

Depressed mood

Loss of interest
Lack of pleasure in hobbies
Depression
Early waking
Diurnal swing

General somatic (muscular)

Muscular pains and aches
Muscular stiffness
Muscular twitchings
Clonic jerks
Grinding of teeth
Unsteady voice

General somatic (sensory)

Tinnitus
Blurring of vision
Hot and cold flushes
Feelings of weakness
Pricking sensations

Cardiovascular symptoms

Tachycardia
Palpitations
Pain in chest
Throbbing of vessels
Fainting feelings
Missing beat

Respiratory symptoms

Pressure or constriction in chest
Choking feelings
Sighing
Dyspnoea

Gastro-intestinal symptoms

Difficulty in swallowing
Wind
Dyspepsia:
    pain before and after meals
    burning sensation
    fullness
    waterbrash
    nausea
    vomiting
    sinking feelings
    'working' in abdomen

Gastro-intestinal symptoms (continued)
Borborygmi
Looseness of bowels
Loss of weight
Constipation

Genito-urinary symptoms
Frequency of micturition
Urgency of micturition
Amenorrhea
Menorrhagia
Development of frigidity
Ejaculation praecox
Loss of erection
Impotence

Autonomic symptoms
Dry mouth
Flushing
Pallor
Tendency to sweat
Giddiness
Tension headache
Raising of hair

Behavior at interview (general)
Tense, not relaxed
Fidgeting: hands picking fingers,
  clenching, tics, handkerchief
Restlessness: pacing
Tremor of hands
Furrowed brow
Strained face
Increased muscular tone
Sighing respirations
Facial pallor

Behavior (physiological)
Swallowing
Belching
High resting pulse rate
Respiration rate over 20/min.
Brisk tendon jerks
Tremor
Dilated pupils
Exophthalmos
Sweating
Eye-lid twitching

Scoring
___ Anxious mood
___ Tension
___ Fears
___ Insomnia
___ Intellect
___ Depressed mood
___ Somatic general (muscular and
    sensory)
___ Cardiovascular system
___ Respiratory system
___ Gastrointestinal system
___ Genitourinary system
___ Autonomic system
___ Behavior at interview
___ Behavior (physiological)

Grades
0 is none
1 is mild
2 is moderate
3 is severe
4 is very severe,
  grossly disabling

Reprinted from Hamilton, M. (1959). The assessment of anxiety states by rating. *British Journal of Medical Psychology, 32*, 50–55, with permission of the British Psychological Society.

AGORAPHOBIC COGNITIONS QUESTIONNAIRE AND BODY
SENSATIONS QUESTIONNAIRE

Purpose and Development

The Agoraphobic Cognitions Questionnaire is a 14-item self-report
measure of thoughts related to agoraphobia and the Body Sensations
Questionnaire is a 17-item self-report measure of physical sensations associated with agoraphobia (Chambless, Caputo, Bright, & Gallagher, 1984).
Items for both measures were derived from reports of agoraphobic clients.
The Agoraphobic Cognitions Questionnaire includes subscales for fear of
loss of control and concern about physical symptoms. A factor analysis of
the responses of a sample of agoraphobic clients on the Agoraphobic
Cognitions Questionnaire confirmed that the items on this scale cluster
into these two dimensions (Chambless et al., 1984). A factor analytic study
by Arrindell (1993) also found support for the two dimensions of the
Cognitions Questionnaire and further found that the items on the Body
Sensations Questionnaire form another distinct factor.

Administration and Scoring

Respondents rate the Agoraphobic Cognitions Questionnaire items
on a 5-point scale of frequency and the Body Sensations Questionnaire
items on a 5-point scale of intensity. The 14 items on the Agoraphobic
Cognitions Questionnaire may be averaged for a total scale score or broken
into two subscales, Loss of Control and Physical Concerns. Items 6, 8, 9, 11,
12, 13, and 14 comprise the Loss of Control subscale and items 1, 2, 3, 4, 5, 7,
and 10 comprise the Physical Concerns subscale. Responses on the total
Agoraphobic Cognitions Questionnaire, the Loss of Control subscale, the
Physical Concerns subscale, and the Body Sensations Questionnaire are all
averaged; thus the possible range of scores for each scale is from one to
five, with higher scores indicating more distress.

Sample Scores

Chambless et al. (1984) gave the Agoraphobic Cognitions Questionnaire to 78 individuals requesting treatment for agoraphobia and 23 individuals with no problems and the Body Sensations Questionnaire to 53
individuals requesting treatment and 23 individuals with no problems.
Craske, Rachman, and Tallman (1986) gave the Agoraphobic Cognitions
Questionnaire to 30 agoraphobic clients, 34 clients with social phobias, 173
students, 73 relatives of students, and 58 senior citizens. Bibb (1988) ob-

tained scores on the Agoraphobic Cognitions Questionnaire from a community sample of 139 individuals and scores on the Body Sensations Questionnaire from a community sample of 89 individuals. Table 1 gives the means and standard deviations of the scale scores for these groups.

For the community sample, Bibb (1988) provided separate mean scores for the Loss of Control subscale ($M = 1.89$, $SD = .70$) and the Physical Concerns subscale ($M = 1.31$, $SD = .59$) of the Agoraphobic Cognitions Questionnaire.

Reliability

In their sample of agoraphobic clients, Chambless et al. (1984) found internal consistency as measured by Cronbach's alpha was .80 for the 14-item Agoraphobic Cognitions Questionnaire and .87 for the Body Sensations Questionnaire. In a sample consisting of agoraphobic clients, clients with social phobias, senior citizens, students, and students' relatives, Craske et al. (1986) found a split-half reliability of .85 for the Agoraphobic Cognitions Questionnaire.

In their sample of agoraphobic clients, Chambless et al. (1984) found that one month test–retest reliability was .86 for the Agoraphobic Cognitions Questionnaire and .67 for the Body Sensations Questionnaire.

Validity

Scores on the Agoraphobic Cognitions Questionnaire and the Body Sensations Questionnaire have been found to be significantly associated

TABLE 1
Scores on the Agoraphobic Cognitions Questionnaire
and the Body Sensations Questionnaire

Group	Agoraphobic cognitions		Body sensations	
	M	SD	M	SD
Agoraphobic clients*	2.32	.07	3.05	.86
Agoraphobic clients**	2.51	.80		
Social Phobia clients**	2.15	.78		
Community sample***	1.60	.46	1.80	.59
Students**	1.55	.42		
Students' relatives**	1.46	.38		
Senior citizens**	1.40	.65		
Individuals with no problems*	1.38	.34	1.52	.58

*Chambless et al. (1984), **Craske et al. (1986), ***Bibb (1988).

with other measures of agoraphobia (Ost, 1990; Arrindell, 1993) and with avoidance, panic, anxiety, depression, anger, and different types of fears (Arrindell, 1993; Chambless et al., 1984).

Chambless et al. (1984) found that scores on both scales were significantly higher for agoraphobic clients than for individuals with no reported psychological problems, and Craske et al. (1986) found that a group of agoraphobic clients scored significantly higher on the Agoraphobic Cognitions Questionnaire than groups of senior citizens, students, and students' relatives, but found no significant difference between agoraphobic clients and clients with social phobias. Chambless et al. (1984) and Waddell and Demi (1993) gave the two scales to clients who were going through treatment for agoraphobia and found significant decreases in scores on both the Agoraphobic Cognitions Questionnaire and the Body Sensations Questionnaire.

AGORAPHOBIC COGNITIONS QUESTIONNAIRE
AND BODY SENSATIONS QUESTIONNAIRE

AGORAPHOBIC COGNITIONS QUESTIONNAIRE

Below are some thoughts or ideas that may pass through your mind when you are nervous or frightened. Please indicate how often each thought occurs when you are nervous. Rate from 1–5 using the scale below.

1. Thought never occurs.
2. Thought rarely occurs.
3. Thought occurs during half of the times I am nervous.
4. Thought usually occurs.
5. Thought always occurs when I am nervous.

_____ 1. I am going to throw up.
_____ 2. I am going to pass out.
_____ 3. I must have a brain tumor.
_____ 4. I will have a heart attack.
_____ 5. I will choke to death.
_____ 6. I am going to act foolish.
_____ 7. I am going blind.
_____ 8. I will not be able to control myself.
_____ 9. I will hurt someone.
_____ 10. I am going to have a stroke.
_____ 11. I am going to go crazy.
_____ 12. I am going to scream.
_____ 13. I am going to babble or talk funny.
_____ 14. I will be paralyzed by fear.
_____ 15. Other ideas not listed (Please describe and rate them).

BODY SENSATIONS QUESTIONNAIRE

Below is a list of specific body sensations that may occur when you are nervous or in a feared situation. Please mark down how afraid you are of these feelings. Use a five point scale from not worried to extremely frightened. Please rate all items.

1. Not frightened or worried by this sensation.
2. Somewhat frightened by this sensation.

➤

3. Moderately frightened by this sensation.
4. Very frightened by this sensation.
5. Extremely frightened by this sensation.

_____ 16. Heart palpitations
_____ 17. Pressure or a heavy feeling in chest
_____ 18. Numbness in arms or legs
_____ 19. Tingling in the fingertips
_____ 20. Numbness in another part of your body
_____ 21. Feeling short of breath
_____ 22. Dizziness
_____ 23. Blurred or distorted vision
_____ 24. Nausea
_____ 25. Having "butterflies" in your stomach
_____ 26. Feeling a knot in your stomach
_____ 27. Having a lump in your throat
_____ 28. Wobbly or rubber legs
_____ 29. Sweating
_____ 30. A dry throat
_____ 31. Feeling disoriented and confused
_____ 32. Feeling disconnected from your body: Only partly present
_____ 33. Other (Please describe). _____

Reprinted with permission of Dr. Diane Chambless.

MOBILITY INVENTORY FOR AGORAPHOBIA

Purpose and Development

The Mobility Inventory for Agoraphobia is a 27-item self-report measure developed by Chambless, Caputo, Jasin, Gracely, and Williams (1985) to measure avoidance behavior and panic attacks related to agoraphobia. Items for the scale were generated on the basis of information obtained from agoraphobic clients. A factor analysis of the items showed that items group into two main factors which can be described as avoidance of public situations and avoidance of enclosed places (Kwon, Evans, and Oei, 1990).

Administration and Scoring

Respondents use a 5-point scale to rate each of 26 situations on how much they avoid the situation when they are alone and when they are with a trusted companion. Respondents also report how many panic attacks they had in the last seven days. Ratings for the 26 situations are averaged to obtain a measure of avoidance when alone and avoidance when with a companion. This results in two scores, each with a possible range of 1 to 5, with higher scores indicating more avoidance. The report of number of panic attacks is used as a separate index.

Sample Scores

Chambless et al. (1985) obtained scale scores from two groups of 94 and 83 individuals seeking treatment for agoraphobia and a group of 23 individuals reporting no anxiety related problems. Craske, Rachman, and Tallman (1986) gave the scale to 30 agoraphobic clients, 34 clients with social phobias, 173 students, 73 relatives of students, and 58 senior citizens. Table 1 shows mean scale scores for these samples.

Reliability

In two groups of agoraphobic clients, the internal consistency of the Avoidance When Alone measure was .96 and .94 as assessed by Cronbach's alpha and the internal consistency of the Avoidance When with a Companion measure was .97 and .91 (Chambless et al., 1985). In a sample consisting of agoraphobic clients, clients with social phobias, senior citizens, students, and students' relatives, Craske et al. (1986) found a split-half reliability of .94 for the overall scale.

In one sample of agoraphobic clients, Chambless et al. (1985) found a

TABLE 1
Mobility Inventory for Agoraphobia Scores

Group	Avoidance alone		Avoidance accompanied		Panic	
	M	SD	M	SD	M	SD
Agoraphobic clients*	3.35	1.06	2.64	.90	2.72	2.77
Agoraphobic clients*	3.30	.99	2.41	.70	3.21	3.98
Agoraphobic clients**	2.43	.87	3.54	.82		
Social phobia clients**	1.57	.58	2.17	.77		
Students**	1.28	.36	1.79	.53		
Students' relatives**	1.30	.33	1.65	.53		
Senior citizens**	1.60	.72	1.86	.73		
Individuals without anxiety problems*	1.25	.24	1.07	.08	.02	

*Chambless et al. (1985), **Craske et al. (1986).

one-month test–retest reliability of .89 for the Avoidance When Alone measure, .75 for the Avoidance When with a Companion measure, and .62 for the Panic Attack measure. In another sample of agoraphobic clients, Chambless et al. (1985) found a one week test–retest reliability of .90 for the Avoidance When Alone measure, .86 for the Avoidance When with a Companion measure, and .56 for the Panic Attack measure.

Validity

Chambless et al. (1985) found that in a sample of agoraphobic clients high scores on the Avoidance When Alone, Avoidance When with a Companion, and Panic Attack measures of the Mobility Inventory were all significantly associated with high scores on another agoraphobia measure, more depression, and more trait anxiety. The researchers hypothesized that because the presence of another person serves as a buffer, the associations for Avoidance When Alone would be greater than the Associations for Avoidance When with a Companion, and their results confirmed this hypothesis.

Chambless et al. (1984) found that scores on all three measures that comprise the Mobility Inventory significantly discriminated between a group of individuals with no reported anxiety problems and a group of agoraphobic clients. To test whether the Mobility Inventory is a general test of anxiety or can discriminate between different anxiety disorders, they then compared a group of clients with agoraphobia to a group of clients with another anxiety disorder (social phobia). The agoraphobic clients had higher scores on all three measures comprising the Mobility Inventory. Craske et al. (1986) also found that a group of agoraphobic clients scored significantly higher on the Mobility Inventory than groups of clients with social phobias, senior citizens, students, and students' relatives.

Chambless et al. (1984) gave the Mobility Inventory to a group of clients who were going through treatment for agoraphobia and found significant decreases on all three measures that comprise the Mobility Inventory from before to after treatment. Waddell and Demi (1993) also found that the scores of agoraphobic clients decreased as they went through treatment.

MOBILITY INVENTORY FOR AGORAPHOBIA

Please indicate the degree to which you avoid the following places or situations because of discomfort or anxiety. Rate your amount of avoidance when you are with a trusted companion and when you are alone. Do this by using the following scale.

1. Never avoid
2. Rarely avoid
3. Avoid about half the time
4. Avoid most of the time
5. Always avoid

(You may use numbers half-way between those listed when you think it is appropriate, for example, 3½ or 4½).

Write your score in the blanks for each situation or place under both conditions: when accompanied, and, when alone. Leave blank those situations that do not apply to you.

Places	When accompanied	When alone
Theaters	_____	_____
Supermarkets	_____	_____
Classrooms	_____	_____
Department stores	_____	_____
Restaurants	_____	_____
Museums	_____	_____
Elevators	_____	_____
Auditoriums or stadiums	_____	_____
Parking garages	_____	_____
High places		
Tell how high _____	_____	_____
Enclosed spaces (e.g., tunnels)	_____	_____
Open spaces		
(a) Outside (e.g., fields, wide streets, courtyards)	_____	_____
(b) Inside (e.g., large rooms, lobbies)	_____	_____
Riding in		
Buses	_____	_____
Trains	_____	_____
Subways	_____	_____
Airplanes	_____	_____

Boats   _____   _____
Driving or riding in car
  (a) At any time   _____   _____
  (b) On expressways   _____   _____
Situations
  Standing in lines   _____   _____
  Crossing bridges   _____   _____
  Parties or social gatherings   _____   _____
  Walking on the street   _____   _____
  Staying at home alone   N/A   _____
  Being far away from home   _____   _____
Other (specify) _____   _____   _____
We define a panic attack as:

(1) a high level of anxiety accompanied by
(2) strong body reactions (heart palpitations, sweating, muscle tremors, dizziness, nausea) with
(3) the temporary loss of the ability to plan, think, or reason and
(4) the intense desire to escape or flee the situation. (Note: this is different from high anxiety or fear alone.)

Please indicate the total number of panic attacks you have had in the last 7 days. _____

FEAR QUESTIONNAIRE

Purpose and Development

This 22-item self-report measure was developed by Marks and Mathews (1979) to assess avoidance in phobic clients. Clinicians at several hospitals collaborated to arrive at items that ask about the most common aspects of phobias; items were also selected on the basis of previous factor analytic research. The result was one item asking about a main target phobia, one item asking about overall phobic symptoms, 15 questions asking about frequently encountered phobias, and five questions focusing on symptoms of depression and anxiety often associated with phobic reactions. The 15 questions asking about frequently encountered phobias target fears related to agoraphobia, blood or injury, and social situations. In confirmatory and exploratory factor analyses, Trull and Hillerbrand (1990) found mixed support for the three phobia dimensions of agoraphobia, blood–injury, and social situations.

A National Institute of Mental Health conference on anxiety disorders prompted the recommendation that the questionnaire be used as a standard measure in all studies of phobias (Shear, Klosko, & Fyer, 1989).

Administration and Scoring

Respondents write a description of their main phobia. They then rate this phobia and 15 situations that commonly elicit phobic reactions on a 9-point scale of avoidance. Next they rate five depression and anxiety symptoms on a 9-point scale of severity. Finally they rate their overall phobic symptoms on a 9-point scale of severity.

The scores on the main target phobia and the overall phobic symptoms question can be used as separate indexes. Scores on each of these indexes may range from 0 to 8. The Fear Questionnaire score is the sum of items 2 to 16 and scores may range from 0 to 120. These items may be broken into subscales. Items 5, 6, 8, 12, and 15 comprise the Agoraphobia subscale. Items 2, 4, 10, 13, and 16 comprise the Blood–Injury subscale. Items 3, 7, 9, 11, and 14 comprise the Social subscale. Scores on each of these subscales may range from 0 to 40. The Anxiety–Depression score is the sum of items 18 to 22, and scores may range from 0 to 40. For each of the scales higher scores indicate more distress.

Sample Scores

Marks and Mathews (1979) gave the questionnaire to 20 phobic patients. Mizes and Crawford (1986) gave the questionnaire to 109 male and 107 female high school students, 95 male and 89 female college students, and a community sample of 73 men and 99 women. Trull and Hillerbrand (1990) gave the phobia subscales of the questionnaire to 158 female and 93 male college students, none of whom had received treatment for a phobic condition. They also gave the phobia subscales to 63 women and 48 men randomly selected from the community. Table 1 shows the average scores for these groups.

Reliability

Arrindell, Emmelkamp, and Van der End (1984) used Cronbach's alpha to assess internal consistency of the total scale and the subscales in phobic individuals, individuals from the community, and college students and found that internal consistency ranged from .66 to .85. Trull and Hillerbrand (1990) found poorer internal consistency for the subscales in a sample of normal college students and in a sample of individuals from the community; internal consistency ranged from .44 to .73. In both studies the Blood–Injury subscale tended to have the lowest consistency while the other scales had moderate consistency.

In a sample of phobic clients Marks and Mathews (1979) found a one-week test–retest reliability of .82 for the Total Phobia scale, .89 for the Agoraphobia subscale, .96 for the Blood–Injury subscale, .82 for the Social Phobia subscale, .93 for the Main Target Phobia rating, .79 for the Global Phobia rating, and .82 for Depression–Anxiety ratings.

Validity

Studies by Ost (1990) and Arrindell (1993) found that Agoraphobia subscale scores were significantly associated with other measures of agoraphobia.

Lelliot, McNamee, and Marks (1991) found that individuals with agoraphobia scored higher on the Agoraphobia subscale than individuals with social phobias, and individuals with social phobias scored higher on the Social Phobia subscale than individuals with agoraphobia. Mavissakalian (1986) found that clients with agoraphobia scored higher on the Agoraphobia subscale than on the other subscales. Trull and Hillerbrand (1990) found that Total Phobia scores, Agoraphobia subscale scores, and

TABLE 1
Fear Questionnaire Scores of Phobic Clients, College Students,
High School Students, and Individuals Drawn from the Community

Group	Total phobia		Agoraphobia		Blood–Injury		Social		Main phobia		Global rating		Anxiety/ Depression	
	M	SD	M	SD	M	SD	M	SD	M	SD	M	SD	M	SD
Phobic clients (Marks, 1979)	47	19.3	17	10.0	15	10.7	15	8.8	7	2.1	5.5	2.7	22	9.1
College students (Mizes, 1986)														
Females	32.25	13.03	7.89	5.44	11.55	6.93	12.92	5.52	1.08	2.46	1.16	1.26	11.83	6.16
Males	26.00	13.01	4.65	4.63	10.15	6.60	11.44	6.44	1.16	2.38	1.03	.94	10.75	8.06
College students (Trull, 1990)														
Females	29.3	14.0	6.1	5.0	12.5	7.3	10.7	5.4	—		—		—	
Males	25.0	11.5	4.2	4.0	10.3	6.7	10.6	4.8						
High school students (Mizes, 1986)														
Females	27.36	15.56	6.39	5.64	9.53	6.42	11.44	6.44	2.22	3.07	1.64	1.31	10.58	8.06
Males	22.00	15.40	4.10	4.61	8.42	7.81	9.42	6.12	1.00	2.22	1.22	1.20	8.92	7.64
Community sample (Mizes, 1986)														
Females	21.21	14.51	4.99	6.00	7.34	6.01	8.81	6.09	1.78	2.69	1.20	1.17	6.86	6.17
Males	22.77	14.06	4.85	5.09	9.05	6.47	8.86	5.49	1.92	2.92	1.14	.99	8.95	6.65
Community sample (Trull, 1990)														
Females	46.1	16.2	14.8	8.5	15.0	6.9	16.3	6.2	—		—		—	
Males	33.0	13.1	7.9	7.1	10.9	6.8	14.2	4.3						

Note: The above scores do not include the write-in items.

Social Phobia subscale scores were significantly higher in a group of individuals drawn from the community through a telephone survey than in a group of college students. They point out that because individuals with agoraphobia and social phobias are less likely to enter college settings, these differences provide evidence for the validity of the scales.

Marks and Mathews (1979) gave the questionnaire to a group of phobic clients and found significant decreases during treatment in the Main Target Phobia rating, the Global Phobia rating, the Depression–Anxiety subscale, the Total Phobia scale, and the Agoraphobia and Social Phobia subscales. Mavissakalian (1986) also found decreases on the Agoraphobia, Social Phobia, and Blood–Injury subscales in clients going through treatment.

FEAR QUESTIONNAIRE

Choose a number from the scale below to show how much you would avoid each of the situations listed below because of fear or other unpleasant feelings. Then write the number you chose next to each situation.

0	1	2	3	4	5	6	7	8
Would not avoid it		Slightly avoid it		Definitely avoid it		Markedly avoid it		Always avoid it

_____ 1. Main phobia you want treated (describe in your own words)
_____

_____ 2. Injections or minor surgery
_____ 3. Eating or drinking with other people
_____ 4. Hospitals
_____ 5. Traveling alone by bus or coach
_____ 6. Walking alone in busy streets
_____ 7. Being watched or stared at
_____ 8. Going into crowded shops
_____ 9. Talking to people in authority
_____ 10. Sight of blood
_____ 11. Being criticized
_____ 12. Going alone far from home
_____ 13. Thought of injury or illness
_____ 14. Speaking or acting to an audience
_____ 15. Large open spaces
_____ 16. Going to the dentist
_____ 17. Other situations (describe) _____

Now choose a number from the scale below to show how much you are troubled by each problem listed and write the number next to the problem.

0	1	2	3	4	5	6	7	8
Hardly at all		Slightly troublesome		Definitely troublesome		Markedly troublesome		Very severely troublesome

_____ 18. Feeling miserable or depressed
_____ 19. Feeling irritable or angry
_____ 20. Feeling tense or panicky
_____ 21. Upsetting thoughts coming into your mind
_____ 22. Feeling you or your surroundings are strange or unreal
_____ 23. Other feelings (describe) _____

How would you rate the present state of your phobic symptoms on the scale below? Please circle one number between 0 and 8.

0	1	2	3	4	5	6	7	8
No phobias present		Slightly disturbing/ disabling		Definitely disturbing/ disabling		Markedly disturbing/ disabling		Very severely disturbing/ disabling

Reprinted from *Behaviour Research & Therapy*, *17*, Marks, I.M., & Mathews, A.M., Brief standard self-rating for phobic patients, 263–267, Copyright 1979, with kind permission from Elsevier Science Ltd, The Boulevard, Langford Lane, Kidlington OX5 1GB, UK.

DEATH ANXIETY SCALE

Purpose and Development

The Death Anxiety Scale is a 15-item self-report measure developed by Templer (1970) to assess anxiety related to death. Templer generated a pool of 40 items and asked seven mental health professionals to rate the face validity of the items. The 31 items receiving the highest ratings were embedded in a large group of filler items and presented to 141 college students. The student ratings were in turn used to select the 15 items that contributed most to the internal consistency of the scale.

Administration and Scoring

Respondents rate whether each item is mostly true or mostly false. Scores for items 2, 3, 5, 6, 7, and 15 are reversed and then the ratings for all items are summed. Scores can range from 0 to 15, with higher scores indicating more death anxiety.

Sample Scores

Templer (1970) gave the Death Anxiety Scale to 21 psychiatric patients who had previously shown signs of preoccupation with death or fear of death and to a group of 21 psychiatric patients who were matched to the first group for diagnosis, gender, and age. Alvarado, Templer, Bresler, and Thomas-Dobson (1993) gave the Death Anxiety Scale to 114 women and 86 men drawn from the community. These individuals were recruited from among students at two colleges, employees of a county hospital, and managers and sales representatives of a company and their spouses. Stevens, Cooper, and Thomas (1980) gave the scale to a cross-sectional community sample of 295 individuals, and broke scale scores down by age and gender. Table 1 shows the average scores for individuals in these samples. More detailed information about scores in various populations was given by Templer and Ruff (1971) who presented scores for individuals from 23 separate samples.

Reliability

When given to a sample of 31 college students, the scale had an internal consistency of .76 as measured by Kuder–Richardson Formula 20 and a three-week test–retest reliability of .83 (Templer, 1970).

TABLE 1
Scores on the Death Anxiety Scale

Group	M	SD
Death-anxious clients (Templer, 1970)	11.62	1.96
Controls for death-anxious clients (Templer, 1970)	6.77	2.72
Community sample (Alvarado et al., 1993)	6.81	3.20
Community sample (Stevens et al. 1980)	6.89	3.20
Adolescents	7.50	
Young adults	7.25	
Middle-aged	6.85	
Elderly	5.75	
Females	7.06	
Males	6.55	

Validity

In a sample of 69 college students, Templer (1970) found that the Death Anxiety Scale was highly correlated with another measure of death anxiety and moderately correlated with measures of general anxiety. White and Handal (1991) found that individuals who had higher scores tended to be more distressed and less satisfied with life. Templer, Ruff, and Franks (1971) found a high correlation between the scale scores of family members.

Alverado et al. (1993) factor analyzed the items on the Templer Death Anxiety Scale and the Templer Death Depression Scale and found that the factor structure of the combined items differentiated between items assessing death anxiety and items assessing death-related depression. In a sample of 46 students, Templer (1970) found that responses on the Death Anxiety Scale were not related to a measure of social desirability responding.

Templer (1970) found that a group of psychiatric patients who had expressed fear of death or preoccupation with death scored significantly higher on the scale than a matched group of psychiatric patients who had not expressed such fears.

Henderson (1990) found that elderly individuals who were given the opportunity to increase their control over the dying process by making living wills experienced less death anxiety as measured by the scale.

DEATH ANXIETY SCALE

Directions: If a statement is true or mostly true as applied to you, circle "T". If a statement is false or mostly false as applied to you, circle "F".

T   F   34. I am very much afraid to die.
T   F   35. The thought of death seldom enters my mind.
T   F   36. It doesn't make me nervous when people talk about death.
T   F   37. I dread to think about having to have an operation.
T   F   38. I am not at all afraid to die.
T   F   39. I am not particularly afraid of getting cancer.
T   F   40. The thought of death never bothers me.
T   F   41. I am often distressed by the way time flies so very rapidly.
T   F   42. I fear dying a painful death.
T   F   43. The subject of life after death troubles me greatly.
T   F   44. I am really scared of having a heart attack.
T   F   45. I often think about how short life really is.
T   F   46. I shudder when I hear people talking about a World War III.
T   F   47. The sight of a dead body is horrifying to me.
T   F   48. I feel that the future holds nothing for me to fear.

Scale reprinted with permission of Dr. Donald Templer.

DENTAL FEAR SURVEY

Purpose and Development

The Dental Fear Survey is a 20-item self-report measure developed by Kleinknecht to assess dental anxiety. The items were selected to obtain information about specific fear stimuli, physiological arousal, and avoidance tendencies related to dentistry (Kleinknecht, Klepac, & Alexander, 1973). Factor analyses by Kleinknecht, Thorndike, McGlynn, and Harkavy (1984), McGlynn, McNeil, Gallagher, and Vrana (1987), and Milgrom, Kleinknecht, Elliot, Hsing, and Choo-Soo (1990) confirmed that the scale items group into these three aspects of dental anxiety.

The scale has been translated into Malay and Chinese (Milgrom et al., 1990).

Administration and Scoring

Respondents use a 5-point scale of intensity to rate each item. The items are summed to obtain a total score, which can range from 20 to 100. Three subscale scores may be derived as follows: the sum of items 1, 2, 8, 9, 10, 11, 12, 13, and 20 measures dental treatment avoidance and anticipatory anxiety about treatment, the sum of items 14–18 measures fear reactions to dental stimuli, and the sum of items 3–7 measures physiological arousal experienced during treatment. Scores can range from 9 to 45 for the first subscale and 5 to 25 for the other two subscales. For each scale higher scores indicate more distress.

Sample Scores

McGlynn et al. (1987) obtained scores from 1,951 female and 1,966 male college students. Table 1 shows their average scores.

Reliability

In a sample of college students, McGlynn et al. (1987) found internal consistency as calculated by Cronbach's alpha was .90 for the total scale, .91 for the avoidance subscale, .91 for the fear subscale, and .81 for the arousal subscale. Using the same sample of college students, they found an 8- to 13-week test–retest reliability of .88 for the total scale, .87 for the Avoidance subscale, .83 for the Fear subscale, and .74 for the Arousal subscale.

TABLE 1
Mean Dental Fear Survey Scores for
College Students (McGlynn et al., 1987)

	Females		Males	
	M	SD	M	SD
Total score	43.21	15.72	37.98	12.82
Avoidance	14.22	6.51	12.42	5.00
Fear	17.34	6.45	14.76	5.54
Arousal	9.46	3.70	8.91	5.85

Validity

In a sample of students, McNeil and Berryman (1989) found higher Dental Fear Scale scores were related to greater fear of pain, being closed in, and mutilation. In a sample of university students going through simulated dental treatment, Milgrom et al. (1990) found higher Dental Fear scores were related to greater trait anxiety but found no association between scale scores and state anxiety or physiological arousal. Kleinknecht and Bernstein (1978) found that responses on scale item 20 (which had a .89 correlation with the rest of the items) were significantly related to state anxiety and pain ratings of dental patients.

Milgrom et al. (1990) found that university students who had visited a dentist during the past year had significantly lower scale scores than those who had not, but failed to find differences between military conscripts in Singapore who had visited a dentist within the past two years and those who had not.

DENTAL FEAR SURVEY

DENTAL REPORT

The items in this questionnaire refer to various situations, feelings, and reactions related to dental work. Please rate your feeling or reaction on these items by circling the number (1, 2, 3, 4, or 5) or the category which most closely corresponds to your reaction.

1. Has fear of dental work ever caused you to put off making an appointment?

1	2	3	4	5
never	once or twice	a few times	often	nearly every time

2. Has fear of dental work ever caused you to cancel or not appear for an appointment?

1	2	3	4	5
never	once or twice	a few times	often	nearly every time

When having dental work done:

3. My muscles become tense ...

1	2	3	4	5
not at all	a little	somewhat	much	very much

4. My breathing rate increases ...

1	2	3	4	5
not at all	a little	somewhat	much	very much

5. I perspire ...

1	2	3	4	5
not at all	a little	somewhat	much	very much

6. I feel nauseated and sick to my stomach ...

1	2	3	4	5
not at all	a little	somewhat	much	very much

7. My heart beats faster ...

1	2	3	4	5
not at all	a little	somewhat	much	very much

Following is a list of things and situations that many people mention as being somewhat anxiety- or fear-producing. Please rate how much fear, anxiety, or unpleasantness each of them causes you. Use the numbers 1–5 from the following scale. Make a check in the appropriate space. (If it helps, try to imagine yourself in each of these situations and describe what your common reaction is.)

1	2	3	4	5
none at all	a little	somewhat	much	very much

	1	2	3	4	5
8. Making an appointment for dentistry	___	___	___	___	___
9. Approaching the dentist's office	___	___	___	___	___
10. Sitting in the waiting room	___	___	___	___	___
11. Being seated in the dental chair	___	___	___	___	___
12. The smell of the dentist's office	___	___	___	___	___
13. Seeing the dentist walk in	___	___	___	___	___
14. Seeing the anesthetic needle	___	___	___	___	___
15. Feeling the needle injected	___	___	___	___	___
16. Seeing the drill	___	___	___	___	___
17. Hearing the drill	___	___	___	___	___
18. Feeling the vibrations of the drill	___	___	___	___	___
19. Having your teeth cleaned	___	___	___	___	___
20. All things considered, how fearful are you of having dental work done	___	___	___	___	___

Reprinted with permission of Dr. Ronald Kleinknecht.

ACHIEVEMENT ANXIETY TEST

Purpose and Development

The Achievement Anxiety Test is a 19-item self-report measure developed by Alpert and Haber (1960) to assess debilitating and facilitating anxiety related to academic achievement. The authors constructed a large number of items asking about test-related anxiety. From this pool they selected the items that were related to academic performance criteria and distinguished between debilitating and facilitating anxiety. A factor analysis by Plake, Smith, and Damsteegt (1981) provided some support for separate debilitating and facilitating dimensions, though three items from the facilitating scale did not load on the appropriate factor. Watson (1988) found that it was possible to condense the factor structure to one dimension on which the debilitating and facilitating items loaded on opposite ends.

Administration and Scoring

Respondents answer each item using a 5-point scale. Items 1, 2, 5, 6, 7, 9, 11, 14, 15, 16, and 18 are reverse scored. The Debilitating scale is the sum of items 1, 3, 4, 5, 7, 11, 13, 14, 17, and 19; scores on this scale may range from 10 to 50 with higher scores indicating more debilitating anxiety. The Facilitating scale is the sum of items 2, 6, 8, 9, 10, 12, 15, 16, and 18; scores on this scale may range from 9 to 45 with higher scores indicating more facilitating anxiety. Watson (1988) suggested that by recoding facilitating items and then summing all items a total score may be derived.

Sample Scores

Alpert and Haber (1960) found a mean score of 26.33 (SD = 5.33) for the Debilitating Anxiety scale and 27.28 (SD = 4.27) for the Facilitating Anxiety scale in a sample of 323 male college students and Plake et al. (1981) reported means of 26.15 (SD = 6.05) for the Debilitating Anxiety scale and 25.31 (SD = 4.77) for the Facilitating Anxiety scale for 264 male and female college students. Watson (1988) reported mean scores of 28.7 (SD = 6.14) for the Debilitating Anxiety scale, 25.3 (SD = 4.75) for the Facilitating Anxiety scale, and 57.4 (SD = 9.49) for the total score for 378 male and female college students.

Reliability

Watson (1988) found internal consistency as measured by Cronbach's alpha was .79 for the Debilitating scale, .67 for the Facilitating scale, and .82

for the total scale. Haber and Alpert (1960) found 10-week test–retest reliability was .87 for the Debilitating scale and .83 for the Facilitating scale.

Validity

Several studies have reported associations between both the Debilitating and Facilitating scale and other measures of test anxiety and general anxiety (Alpert & Haber, 1960; Tryon, 1980; Plake et al., 1981), performance (Alpert & Haber, 1960; Watson, 1988), and confidence in academic ability (Watson, 1988). Watson (1988) also found strong associations between the total score and various measures of performance and confidence in academic ability. Several studies have found that students going through interventions to reduce test anxiety show a decrease in debilitating anxiety scores (Allen, 1973; Meichenbaum, 1972) and an increase in facilitating anxiety scores (Meichenbaum, 1972).

ACHIEVEMENT ANXIETY TEST

Instructions: Please circle the number for each item that comes closest to describing you.

1. Nervousness while taking an exam or test hinders me from doing well.

Always   Never

1   2   3   4   5

2. I work most effectively under pressure, as when the task is very important.

Always   Never

1   2   3   4   5

3. In a course where I have been doing poorly, my fear of a bad grade cuts down my efficiency.

Never   Always

1   2   3   4   5

4. When I am poorly prepared for an exam or test, I get upset, and do less well than even my restricted knowledge should allow.

This never happens to me   This practically always happens to me

1   2   3   4   5

5. The more important the examination, the less well I seem to do.

Always   Never

1   2   3   4   5

6. While I may (or may not) be nervous before taking an exam, once I start, I seem to forget to be nervous.

I always forget   I am always nervous

1   2   3   4   5

7. During exams or tests, I block on questions to which I know the answers, even though I remember them as soon as the exam is over.

                                    I never block on questions to which I know the answers

This always happens to me

1   2   3   4   5

→

8. Nervousness while taking a test helps me to do better.

It never helps   It often helps
1   2   3   4   5

9. When I start a test, nothing is able to distract me.

This is always true of me   This is never true of me
1   2   3   4   5

10. In courses in which the total grade is based mainly on one exam, I seem to do better than other people.

Never   Always
1   2   3   4   5

11. I find that my mind goes blank at the beginning of an exam, and it takes me a few minutes before I can function.

I almost always blank out at first   I never blank out at first
1   2   3   4   5

12. I look forward to exams.

Never   Always
1   2   3   4   5

13. I am so tired from worrying about an exam, that I find I almost don't care how well I do by the time I start the test.

I never feel this way   I almost always feel this way
1   2   3   4   5

14. Time pressure on an exam causes me to do worse than the rest of the group under similar conditions

Time pressure always seems to   Time pressure never seems to
make me do worse than others   make make do worse than
on an exam   others on an exam
1   2   3   4   5

15. Although "cramming" under preexamination tension is not effective for most people, I find that if the need arises, I can learn material immediately before an exam, even under considerable pressure, and successfully retain it to use on the exam.

I am always able to use the   I am never able to used the
"crammed" material successfully   "crammed" material successfully
1   2   3   4   5

16. I enjoy taking a difficult exam more than an easy one.

Always   Never
1   2   3   4   5

17. I find myself reading exam questions without understanding them, and I must go back over them so that they will make sense.

Never   Always
1   2   3   4   5

18. The more important the exam or test, the better I seem to do.

This is true of me   This is not true of me
1   2   3   4   5

19. When I don't do well on a difficult item at the beginning of an exam, it tends to upset me so that I block on very easy questions later on.

This never happens to me   This almost always happens to me
1   2   3   4   5

Reprinted with permission of Dr. Ralph Norman Haber.

INTERACTION ANXIOUSNESS SCALE

Purpose and Development

The Interaction Anxiousness Scale is a 15-item self-report measure of social anxiety developed by Leary (1983). Three researchers first generated a pool of 87 items that were theoretically based and some of which were modified items from other scales. From this pool 56 items that clearly related to self-reported anxiety in social situations were selected and given to two group of college students. Based on these subjects' responses, the items that contributed the most to internal consistency were selected for the final scale.

Administration and Scoring

Respondents are asked to rate how well each item describes them on a 5-point scale. Items 3, 6, 10, and 15 are reverse scored. Items are summed for a total score, which can range from 15 to 75. Higher scores indicate more anxiety.

Sample Scores

Leary and Kowalski (1993) reported scale scores for five large samples of university students from different regions of the United States. All samples had very similar mean scores, so just the results of the largest sample will be given here. A group of 786 students had a mean score of 38.6, $SD = 10.5$.

Reliability

Leary (1983) found that the internal consistency of the scale was .89 as measured by Cronbach's alpha, and Leary and Kowalski (1993) reported that in five further samples internal consistency ranged from .87 to .89. Leary (1983) found that 8-week test–retest reliability was .80.

Validity

Higher scale scores have been found to be associated with higher scores on a number of other scales of social anxiety, physiological arousal, observer-rated anxiety, and self-reported anxiety (Leary, 1983; Leary, 1986; Leary & Kowalski, 1993), as well as with conceptually related constructs such as self-consciousness, sociability, social avoidance, and loneliness (Leary, Atherton, Hill, & Hur, 1986; Leary & Kowalski, 1993).

Leary (1983) found that individuals who had sought counseling because of interpersonal problems related to anxiety scored higher on the scale than comparison groups. Leary (1983) also found that individuals who scored high on the scale were more interested in participating in a social-anxiety intervention program.

INTERACTION ANXIOUSNESS SCALE

Please indicate how characteristic or true each of the following statements is for you. Write a number from the scale below next to each of the items.

> 1 = not at all characteristic or true of me
> 2 = slightly characteristic or true of me
> 3 = moderately characteristic or true of me
> 4 = very characteristic or true of me
> 5 = extremely characteristic or true of me

_____ 1. I often feel nervous even in casual get-togethers.

_____ 2. I usually feel uncomfortable when I am in a group of people I don't know.

_____ 3. I am usually at ease when speaking to a member of the opposite sex.

_____ 4. I get nervous when I must talk to a teacher or boss.

_____ 5. Parties often make me feel anxious and uncomfortable.

_____ 6. I am probably less shy in social interactions than most people.

_____ 7. I sometimes feel tense when talking to people of my own sex if I don't know them very well.

_____ 8. I would be nervous if I was being interviewed for a job.

_____ 9. I wish I had more confidence in social situations.

_____ 10. I seldom feel anxious in social situations.

_____ 11. In general, I am a shy person.

_____ 12. I often feel nervous when talking to an attractive member of the opposite sex.

_____ 13. I often feel nervous when calling someone I don't know on the telephone.

_____ 14. I get nervous when I speak to someone in a position of authority.

_____ 15. I usually fell relaxed around other people, even people who are quite different from me.

Reprinted with permission of Leary, M. R. (1983). Social anxiousness: The construct and its measurement. _Journal of Personality Assessment, 47,_ 66–74.

SOCIAL INTERACTION SELF-STATEMENT TEST

Purpose and Development

The Social Interaction Self-Statement Test is a 30-item self-report measure developed by Glass, Merluzzi, Biever, and Larsen (1982) to assess positive and negative cognitions associated with social anxiety in heterosexual interactions. Glass and her colleagues generated items for the scale by asking college students to record their thoughts as they imagined themselves in various heterosexual situations. Judges then classified these statements as positive, neutral, or negative, and those statements unanimously rated positive or negative were given to raters who evaluated each statement on an 11-point negative to positive scale. The 15 most negative statements and the 15 most positive statements were then selected for the scale, and each grouping of 15 items comprises a subscale. An initial factor analysis of the items (Glass et al., 1982) did not provide clearcut support for grouping the items into these two subscales. However, a later factor analysis by Osman, Markway, and Osman (1992) showed that the items clustered into two factors that mirrored the two subscales.

Administration and Scoring

Respondents use a 5-point scale of frequency to rate each self-statement. In the original instructions respondents are asked to think about an immediately preceding interaction with a member of the opposite sex; we slightly modified these instructions to make them more general. There are separate forms for men and women, which we combined. The Positive Self-Statements subscale is comprised of items 2, 4, 6, 9, 10, 12, 13, 14, 17, 18, 24, 25, 27, 28, and 30. The Negative Self-Statements subscale is comprised of items 1, 3, 5, 7, 8, 11, 15, 16, 19, 20, 21, 22, 23, 26, and 29. Scores on each of the subscales can range from 15 to 75, with high scores indicating more positive or negative thoughts respectively.

Sample Scores

Glass et al. (1982) obtained scores for 40 college women high in social anxiety, 40 college women low in social anxiety, and 64 women and men who were selected on the basis of either androgynous, masculine, feminine, or undifferentiated scores on a sex-role inventory. Dodge, Hope, Heimberg, and Becker (1988) gave the scale to 28 individuals who sought help for problems with social anxiety. Table 1 shows the average scores for these groups.

TABLE 1
Social Interaction Self-Statement Scores

Group	Positive Self-Statements subscale		Negative Self-Statements subscale	
	M	SD	M	SD
Socially anxious clients*	36.21	11.44	54.75	12.68
College women**				
High social anxiety	49.62	7.39	38.88	9.93
Low social anxiety	54.95	7.05	33.32	8.27
College women**				
Androgynous	55.62	8.50	38.00	12.46
Masculine	55.38	6.41	35.25	8.10
Feminine	48.38	6.32	38.50	11.71
Undifferentiated	50.88	6.60	37.50	6.87
College men**				
Androgynous	51.50	8.54	46.12	11.31
Masculine	51.00	5.60	34.38	6.80
Feminine	44.50	7.03	45.12	11.33
Undifferentiated	40.12	6.77	50.12	10.71

*Dodge et al. (1988), **Glass et al. (1982).

Reliability

In a sample of college students, Glass et al. (1982) found split-half reliability was .73 for the Positive Self-Statements subscale and .86 for the Negative Self-Statements subscale. In another sample of college students, Osman et al. (1992) found internal consistency as assessed by Cronbach's alpha was .89 for the Positive Self-Statements subscale and .91 for the Negative Self-Statements subscale.

Validity

In samples of college students, Glass et al. (1982) found that higher scores on the Positive Self-Statements subscale were significantly associated with greater self-evaluated social skills and lower anxiety. Higher scores on the Negative Self-Statements subscale were significantly associated with lower self-evaluated social skills and greater anxiety. Observer-determined ratings of social skills and tension were also significantly related to subjects' scores on the Negative Self-Statements subscale but not to scores on the Positive Self-Statements subscale. In another sample of college students, Osman et al. (1992) found that lower scores on the Positive Self-Statements subscale and higher scores on the Negative Self-

Statements subscale were associated with more general psychological distress.

Studies of individuals seeking treatment for social anxiety have found that lower scores on the Positive Self-Statements subscale and higher scores on the Negative Self-Statements subscale were associated with higher scores on several other measures of social anxiety, more depression (Dodge et al., 1988; Glass & Furlong, 1990), greater social introversion (Merluzzi, Burgio, & Glass, 1984) more irrational beliefs, and more antici- pated evaluation by others (Glass & Furlong, 1990). Merluzzi et al. (1984) also found a significant correlation between clients' scale scores and clini- cians' ratings of shyness.

Glass et al. (1982) compared the scale scores of college women cate- gorized as high or low in social anxiety and found that the high anxiety women had significantly lower Positive Self-Statements subscale scores and significantly higher Negative Self-Statements subscale scores. Similar results were found in another sample of male and female college students.

SOCIAL INTERACTION SELF-STATEMENT TEST

Directions: It is obvious that people think a variety of things when they are involved in different social situations. Below is a list of things which you may have thought to yourself at some time before, during, and after interactions with a member of the opposite sex. Read each item and decide how frequently you may have been thinking a similar thought before, during, and after the interactions. Utilize the following scale to indicate the nature of your thoughts:

1 = *hardly ever* had the thought
2 = *rarely* had the thought
3 = *sometimes* had the thought
4 = *often* had the thought
5 = *very often* had the thought

Please answer as honestly as possible.

_____ 1. When I can't think of anything to say I can feel myself getting very anxious.
_____ 2. I can usually talk to girls/guys pretty well.
_____ 3. I hope I don't make a fool of myself.
_____ 4. I'm beginning to feel more at ease.
_____ 5. I'm really afraid of what she'll/he'll think of me.
_____ 6. No worries, no fears, no anxieties.
_____ 7. I'm scared to death.
_____ 8. He/She probably won't be interested in me.
_____ 9. Maybe I can put him/her at ease by starting things going.
_____ 10. Instead of worrying I can figure out how best to get to know her/him.
_____ 11. I'm not too comfortable meeting girls/guys so things are bound to go wrong.
_____ 12. What the heck, the worst that can happen is that he/she won't go for me.
_____ 13. She/He may want to talk to me as much as I want to talk to her/him.
_____ 14. This will be a good opportunity.
_____ 15. If I blow this conversation, I'll really lose my confidence.
_____ 16. What I say will probably sound stupid.
_____ 17. What do I have to lose? It's worth a try.
_____ 18. This is an awkward situation but I can handle it.

_____ 19. Wow—I don't want to do this.

_____ 20. It would crush me if he/she didn't respond to me.

Reprinted from Glass, C., Merluzzi, T., Biever, J., & Larsen, K. (1982). Cognitive assessment of social anxiety: Development and validation of a self-statement questionnaire. *Cognitive Therapy and Research, 6,* 37–55, with permission of Plenum Publishing Corp.

MAUDSLEY OBSESSIVE-COMPULSIVE INVENTORY

Purpose and Development

The Maudsley Obsessive-Compulsive Inventory is a 30-item self-report measure developed by Hodgson and Rachman (1977) to assess obsessional-compulsive symptoms related to rituals. On the basis of the literature and interviews with clients, they generated 65 items. From this pool of items they selected 30 items that differentiated between a group of obsessional clients and a group of nonobsessional clients. They performed a factor analysis using the responses of a group of obsessional clients and found that the 30 items grouped into the following four factors: checking, cleaning, slowness, and doubting. A factor analytic study by Sternberger and Burns (1990) for the most part confirmed this factor structure. The scale is the most widely used measure for obsessive-compulsive disorders (Shear, Klosko, & Fyer, 1989).

Administration and Scoring

Respondents indicate whether each of the 30 statements is true or false for them. A response of "true" is coded as 1 and a response of "false" is coded as 0. Items 5, 11, 13, 15, 16, 17, 19, 21, 22, 23, 24, 25, 26, 27, and 29 are reverse scored, and then all items are totaled. Scores can range from 0 to 30, with a high score indicating more obsessive-compulsive tendency. The items may also be used to calculate subscale scores. Because factor loadings determined to which subscale items belong, some items are used in more than one subscale. Items 2, 6, 8, 14, 15, 20, 22, 26, and 28 comprise the Checking subscale on which scores can range from 0 to 9. Items 1, 4, 5, 9, 13, 17, 19, 21, 24, 26, and 27 comprise the Cleaning subscale on which scores can range from 0 to 11. Items 2, 4, 8, 16, 23, 25, and 29 comprise the Slowness subscale on which scores can range from 0 to 7. Items 3, 7, 10, 11, 12, 18, and 30 comprise the Doubting subscale on which scores can range from 0 to 7.

Sample Scores

Hodgson and Rachman (1977) gave the scale to 100 obsessive clients and to 50 nonobsessive clients, Dent and Salkovskis (1986) gave the scale to 65 university students, 142 medical students, and 36 nonstudents, and Sternberger and Burns (1990) gave the scale to 579 university students. Table 1 shows the mean scores for these groups.

TABLE 1
Scores on the Maudsley Obsessive-Compulsive Inventory

	Total		Checking		Cleaning		Slowness		Doubting	
Group	M	SD	M	SD	M	SD	M	SD	M	SD
Obsessive clients*	18.86	4.29	6.10	2.21	5.55	3.04	3.63	1.93	5.39	1.60
Other clients*	9.27	5.43	2.84	2.29	2.38	1.97	2.27	1.09	3.69	1.99
Students**	6.32	3.92								
Medical students**	7.26	4.41								
Students***	7.58	4.28								
Nonstudents**	5.86	3.51								

*Hodgson and Rachman (1977), **Dent and Salkovskis (1986), ***Sternberger and Burns (1990).

Reliability

In their sample of obsessive clients and other clients, Hodgson and Rachman (1977) found that internal consistency of each of the subscales ranged from .7 to .8 as assessed by Cronbach's alpha. In a sample of college students, Sternberger and Burns (1990) found an overall internal consistency of .75 as assessed by Cronbach's alpha and internal consistency of .54 and .58 for the Washing and Checking subscales respectively.

In a sample of night-school students, Hodgson and Rachman (1977) found one-month test–retest reliability was .8. In another sample of students, Sternberger and Burns (1990) found 6- to 7-month test–retest reliability was .69.

Validity

Scores on the Maudsley Obsessive-Compulsive Inventory have been found to correlate significantly with scores on other measures of aspects of obsessive-compulsive disorders in obsessive-compulsive clients (Hodgson & Rachman, 1977; Emmelkamp, 1988) and in students (Sternberger & Burns, 1990). Dent and Salkovskis (1986) found that high scores on the inventory were associated with elevated anxiety and depression. Further, Sternberger and Burns (1990) presented evidence of divergent validity through their finding that the association between the inventory scores and another measure of obsessive-compulsiveness was stronger than the relationship between inventory scores and several other measures of psychopathology.

Hodgson and Rachman (1977) asked the therapists of clients who had been treated for cleaning or checking complaints to rate the clients on these complaints, then related these ratings to the clients' Checking and Cleaning subscale scores; they found a significant association between the therapists' ratings and the subscale scores. Frost, Sher, & Geen (1986) and Sher, Martin, Raskin, and Perrigo (1991) found that individuals who scored high on the checking subscale showed more general psychopathology.

Perse, Greist, Jefferson, Rosenfield, and Dar (1987) found that obsessive-compulsive clients going through treatment showed significantly lower scores on the inventory after treatment than before treatment.

MAUDSLEY OBSESSIVE-COMPULSIVE INVENTORY

Instructions: Please answer each question by putting a circle around the "True" or the "False" next to the question. There are no right or wrong answers, and no trick questions. Work quickly and do not think too long about the exact meaning of the question.

True False   1. I avoid using public telephones because of possible contamination.

True False   2. I frequently get nasty thoughts and have difficulty in getting rid of them.

True False   3. I am more concerned than most people about honesty.

True False   4. I am often late because I can't seem to get through everything on time.

True False   5. I don't worry unduly about contamination if I touch an animal.

True False   6. I frequently have to check things (e.g., gas or water taps, doors, etc.) several times.

True False   7. I have a very strict conscience.

True False   8. I find that almost every day I am upset by unpleasant thoughts that come into my mind against my will.

True False   9. I do not worry unduly if I accidently bump into somebody.

True False 10. I usually have serious doubts about the simple everyday things I do.

True False 11. Neither of my parents was very strict during my childhood.

True False 12. I tend to get behind in my work because I repeat things over and over again.

True False 13. I use only an average amount of soap.

True False 14. Some numbers are extremely unlucky.

True False 15. I do not check letters over and over again before posting them.

True False 16. I do not take a long time to dress in a morning.

True False 17. I am not excessively concerned about cleanliness.

True False 18. One of my major problems is that I pay too much attention to detail.

True False 19. I can use well-kept toilets without any hesitation.

True False 20. My major problem is repeated checking.

True False 21. I am not unduly concerned about germs and diseases.

True False 22. I do not tend to check things more than once.

➤

True   False   23. I do not stick to a very strict routine when doing ordinary things.
True   False   24. My hands do not feel dirty after touching money.
True   False   25. I do not usually count when doing a routine task.
True   False   26. I take rather a long time to complete my washing in the morning.
True   False   27. I do not use a great deal of antiseptics.
True   False   28. I spend a lot of time every day checking things over and over again.
True   False   29. Hanging and folding my clothes at night does not take up a lot of time.
True   False   30. Even when I do something very carefully I often feel that it is not quite right.

Reprinted from *Behaviour Research & Therapy*, 15, Hodgson, R., & Rachman, S., Obsessional-compulsive complaints, 389–395, Copyright 1977, with kind permission from Elsevier Science Ltd, The Boulevard, Langford Lane, Kidlington OX5 1GB, UK.

YALE–BROWN OBSESSIVE COMPULSIVE SCALE

Purpose and Development

This scale measures severity of obsessive and compulsive symptoms independently of each other (Goodman & Price, 1992). The Yale–Brown Obsessive Compulsive Scale is a semistructured interview measure described by Goodman, Price, Rasmussen, Mazure, Fleischmann, Hill, Heninger, and Charney (1989a). Items were generated by the authors on the basis of their extensive experience treating obsessive-compulsive clients. The basic scale consists of 10 items, and additional items comprise an investigational component of the scale but are not added into the total scale score. Woody, Steketee, and Chambless (1994) found that these additional items do not contribute significantly to the 10-item scale; thus all information in this review refers to the 10-item scale. The scale may be broken into two subscales which assess obsessions and compulsions separately. A factor analysis by Fals-Stewart (1992) found that responses to the scale grouped into one factor, and thus failed to confirm that the two subscales measure separate dimensions.

Administration and Scoring

The interviewer defines obsessions and compulsions and asks the client about current symptoms. Goodman has developed a checklist that may be used to obtain detailed information about symptoms. The interviewer then asks the client about 10 aspects of obsessive-compulsive symptoms. Each of these is rated on a 0 to 4 scale of severity. Total scores may range from 0 to 40. Subscale scores may be derived for obsessive symptoms by totaling the ratings for items 1 to 5 and for compulsive symptoms by totaling the ratings for items 6 to 10. Scores on each subscale can range from 0 to 20. For each scale higher scores indicate more severe symptoms.

Sample Scores

Goodman, Price, Rasmussen, Mazure, Delgado, Heninger, and Charney (1989b) obtained scale scores from 42 obsessive-compulsive clients. Kim, Dysken, and Kuskowski (1990) obtained scores from 28 obsessive-compulsive clients. Woody et al. (1994) obtained scores from 54 obsessive-compulsive clients before treatment and from 33 obsessive-compulsive clients after treatment. Table 1 shows the mean scale scores for these groups.

TABLE 1
Yale–Brown Obsessive Compulsive Scale Scores for Obsessive
Compulsive Clients

Group	Total score		Obsessions		Compulsions	
	M	SD	M	SD	M	SD
Woody et al., 1994						
pretreatment	23.8	5.0	11.4	3.8	12.4	2.6
posttreatment	15.2	6.9	7.7	3.9	7.4	3.6
Goodman et al., 1989b	25.1	6.0				
Kim et al., 1990	28.0	4.2				

Reliability

In a sample of clients with obsessive-compulsive disorder, Goodman et al. (1989a) found internal consistency of the scale to be .89 as measured by Cronbach's alpha. In another sample of clients with obsessive-compulsive disorder, Woody et al. (1994) found lower internal consistency for the scale. Cronbach's alpha was .69 for the total scale, .77 for the Obsessions subscale, and .51 for the Compulsions subscale.

Goodman et al. (1989a) asked raters to score taped interviews of clients with obsessive-compulsive disorder and found interrater reliability was .98 for the total scale score, .97 for the Obsession subscale, and .96 for the Compulsion subscale. Woody et al. (1994) also asked raters to score taped interviews and found interrater reliability was .93 for the total scale score, .94 for the Obsessions subscale, and .89 for the Compulsions subscale.

Kim et al. (1990) assessed a group of clients with obsessive-compulsive complaints using the same rater three times at one-week intervals and found an overall test–retest reliability of .90. Woody et al. (1994) assessed clients with obsessive-compulsive complaints at an average of 48-day intervals using different raters for the first and second assessment and found a test–retest reliability of .61 for the total scale, .64 for the Obsession subscale, and .56 for the Compulsions subscale.

Validity

In three samples of clients with obsessive-compulsive complaints, Goodman et al. (1989b) found that higher scores on the Yale–Brown Obsessive Compulsive scale were significantly associated with two other measures of obsessive-compulsive disorder, but not consistently associated with a third measure of the disorder. They also found that the scale was associated with anxiety and depression. Kim et al. (1990) found that scale scores were significantly related to physicians' ratings and clients' self-ratings but were not significantly related to another measure of the obsessive-compulsive disorder. Woody et al. (1994) assessed clients with obsessive-compulsive disorders through a variety of self-report and behavioral measures of obsessive-compulsive symptoms and found that the total score of the Yale–Brown Obsessive Compulsive Scale as well as the subscales were for the most part associated with other measures as expected. They also found that the scale was related to anxiety and depression. The total scale score and Compulsive subscale was more strongly related to other measures of the obsessive-compulsive disorder than to anxiety, but the Obsessions subscale correlated similarly to other measures of the obsessive disorder and to anxiety.

Goodman et al. (1989b) found that scores on the scale significantly decreased for clients receiving pharmacological treatment for obsessive-compulsive symptoms while there was no change in the scores of clients receiving a placebo treatment. In a sample of clients receiving behavioral treatment, Woody et al. (1994) found large, significant decreases for total scale scores and scores on both subscales from before to after treatment.

YALE–BROWN OBSESSIVE COMPULSIVE SCALE

"I am now going to ask several questions about your obsessive thoughts." [Make specific reference to the patient's target obsessions.]

1. TIME OCCUPIED BY OBSESSIVE THOUGHTS
   Q: How much of your time is occupied by obsessive thoughts? [When obsessions occur as brief, intermittent intrusions, it may be difficult to assess time occupied by them in terms of total hours. In such cases, estimate time by determining how frequently they occur. Consider both the number of times the intrusions occur and how many hours of the day are affected. Ask:] How frequently do the obsessive thoughts occur? [Be sure to exclude ruminations and preoccupations which, unlike obsessions, are ego-syntonic and rational (but exaggerated).]

   0 = None.
   1 = Mild, less than 1 hr/day or occasional intrusion.
   2 = Moderate, 1 to 3 hrs/day or frequent intrusion.
   3 = Severe, greater than 3 and up to 8 hrs/day or very frequent intrusion.
   4 = Extreme, greater than 8 hrs/day or near constant intrusion.

2. INTERFERENCE DUE TO OBSESSIVE THOUGHTS
   Q: How much do your obsessive thoughts interfere with your social or work (or role) functioning? Is there anything that you don't do because of them? [If currently not working determine how much performance would be affected if patient were employed.]

   0 = None.
   1 = Mild, slight interference with social or occupational activities, but overall performance not impaired.
   2 = Moderate, definite interference with social or occupational performance, but still manageable.
   3 = Severe, causes substantial impairment in social or occupational performance.
   4 = Extreme, incapacitating.

3. DISTRESS ASSOCIATED WITH OBSESSIVE THOUGHTS
   Q: How much distress do your obsessive thoughts cause you? [In most cases, distress is equated with anxiety; however, patients may report

that their obsessions are "disturbing" but deny "anxiety." Only rate anxiety that seems triggered by obsessions, not generalized anxiety or anxiety associated with other conditions.]

0 = None.
1 = Mild, not too disturbing.
2 = Moderate, disturbing, but still manageable.
3 = Severe, very disturbing.
4 = Extreme, near constant and disabling distress.

4. RESISTANCE AGAINST OBSESSIONS

Q: How much of an effort do you make to resist the obsessive thoughts? How often do you try to disregard or turn your attention away from these thoughts as they enter your mind? [Only rate effort made to resist, not success or failure in actually controlling the obsessions. How much the patient resists the obsessions may or may not correlate with his/her ability to control them. Note that this item does not directly measure the severity of the intrusive thoughts; rather, it rates a manifestation of health, i.e., the effort the patient makes to counteract the obsessions by means other than avoidance or the performance of compulsions. Thus, the more the patient tries to resist, the less impaired is this aspect of his/her functioning. There are "active" and "passive" forms of resistance. Patients in behavioral therapy may be encouraged to counteract their obsessive symptoms by not struggling against them (e.g., "just let the thoughts come"; passive opposition) or by intentionally bringing on the disturbing thoughts. For the purposes of this item, consider use of these behavioral techniques as forms of resistance. If the obsessions are minimal, the patient may not feel the need to resist them. In such cases, a rating of "0" should be given.]

0 = Makes an effort to always resist, or symptoms so minimal doesn't need to actively resist.
1 = Tries to resist most of the time.
2 = Makes some effort to resist.
3 = Yields to all obsessions without attempting to control them, but does so with some reluctance.
4 = Completely and willingly yields to all obsessions.

5. DEGREE OF CONTROL OVER OBSESSIVE THOUGHTS

Q: How much control do you have over your obsessive thoughts? How successful are you in stopping or diverting your obsessive thinking?

→

Can you dismiss them? [In contrast to the preceding item on resistance, the ability of the patient to control his obsessions is more closely related to the severity of the intrusive thoughts.]

0 = Complete control.
1 = Much control, usually able to stop or divert obsessions with some effort and concentration.
2 = Moderate control, sometimes able to stop or divert obsessions.
3 = Little control, rarely successful in stopping or dismissing obsessions, can only divert attention with difficulty.
4 = No control, experienced as completely involuntary, rarely able to even momentarily alter obsessive thinking.

"The next several questions are about your compulsive behaviors." [Make specific reference to the patient's target compulsions.]

6. TIME SPENT PERFORMING COMPULSIVE BEHAVIORS
   Q: How much time do you spend performing compulsive behaviors? [When rituals involving activities of daily living are chiefly present, ask:] How much longer than most people does it take to complete routine activities because of your rituals? [When compulsions occur as brief, intermittent behaviors, it may difficult to assess time spent performing them in terms of total hours. In such cases, estimate time by determining how frequently they are performed. Consider both the number of times compulsions are performed and how many hours of the day are affected. Count separate occurrences of compulsive behaviors, not number of repetitions; e.g., a patient who goes into the bathroom 20 different times a day to wash his hands 5 times very quickly performs compulsions 20 times a day, not 5 or 5 × 20 = 100. Ask:] How frequently do you perform compulsions? [In most cases compulsions are observable behaviors (e.g., hand washing), but some compulsions are covert (e.g., silent checking).]

   0 = None.
   1 = Mild (spends less than 1 hr/day performing compulsions), or occasional performance of compulsive behaviors.
   2 = Moderate (spends from 1 to 3 hrs/day performing compulsions), or frequent performance of compulsive behaviors.
   3 = Severe (spends more than 3 and up to 8 hrs/day performing compulsions), or very frequent performance of compulsive behaviors.
   4 = Extreme (spends more than 8 hrs/day performing compul-

sions), or near constant performance of compulsive behaviors (too numerous to count).

7. INTERFERENCE DUE TO COMPULSIVE BEHAVIORS
   Q: How much do your compulsive behaviors interfere with your social or work (or role) functioning? Is there anything that you don't do because of the compulsions? [If currently not working determine how much performance would be affected if patient were employed.]

   0 = None.
   1 = Mild, slight interference with social or occupational activities, but overall performance not impaired.
   2 = Moderate, definite interference with social or occupational performance, but still manageable.
   3 = Severe, causes substantial impairment in social or occupational performance.
   4 = Extreme, incapacitating.

8. DISTRESS ASSOCIATED WITH COMPULSIVE BEHAVIOR
   Q: How would you feel if prevented from performing your compulsion(s)? [Pause] How anxious would you become? [Rate degree of distress patient would experience if performance of the compulsion were suddenly interrupted without reassurance offered. In most, but not all cases, performing compulsions reduces anxiety. If, in the judgment of the interviewer, anxiety is actually reduced by preventing compulsions in the manner described above, then ask:] How anxious do you get while performing compulsions until you are satisfied they are completed?

   0 = None.
   1 = Mild only slightly anxious if compulsions prevented, or only slight anxiety during performance of compulsions.
   2 = Moderate, reports that anxiety would mount but remain manageable if compulsions prevented, or that anxiety increases but remains manageable during performance of compulsions.
   3 = Severe, prominent, and very disturbing increase in anxiety if compulsions interrupted, or prominent and very disturbing increase in anxiety during performance of compulsions.
   4 = Extreme, incapacitating anxiety from any intervention aimed at modifying activity, or incapacitating anxiety develops during performance of compulsions.

➤

9. RESISTANCE AGAINST COMPULSIONS

 Q: How much of an effort do you make to resist the compulsions?
 [Only rate effort made to resist, not success or failure in actually
 controlling the compulsions. How much the patient resists the compulsions may or may not correlate with his ability to control them.
 Note that this item does not directly measure the severity of the
 compulsions; rather, it rates a manifestation of health, i.e., the effort
 the patient makes to counteract the compulsions. Thus, the more the
 patient tries to resist, the less impaired is this aspect of his functioning. If the compulsions are minimal, the patient may not feel the
 need to resist them. In such cases, a rating of "0" should be given.]

 0 = Makes an effort to always resist, or symptoms so minimal
     doesn't need to actively resist.
 1 = Tries to resist most of the time.
 2 = Makes some effort to resist.
 3 = Yields to almost all compulsions without attempting to con-
     trol them, but does so with some reluctance.
 4 = Completely and willingly yields to all compulsions.

10. DEGREE OF CONTROL OVER COMPULSIVE BEHAVIOR

 Q: How strong is the drive to perform the compulsive behavior?
 [Pause] How much control do you have over the compulsions? [In
 contrast to the preceding item on resistance, the ability of the
 patient to control his compulsions is more closely related to the
 severity of the compulsions.]

 0 = Complete control.
 1 = Much control, experiences pressure to perform the behavior
     but usually able to exercise voluntary control over it.
 2 = Moderate control, strong pressure to perform behavior, can
     control it only with difficulty.
 3 = Little control, very strong drive to perform behavior, must be
     carried to completion, can only delay with difficulty.
 4 = No control, drive to perform behavior experienced as com-
     pletely involuntary and overpowering, rarely able to even
     momentarily delay activity.

Reprinted with permission of Dr. Wayne K. Goodman.

Leyton Obsessional Inventory

Purpose and Development

This scale assesses obsessional traits and symptoms, the degree to which individuals try to resist these symptoms, and how much interference the symptoms create in the individual's life. The Leyton Obsessional Inventory is a 69-item self-report measure developed by Cooper (1970), who created a pool of items asking about obsessional symptoms and a pool of items asking about obsessive traits and then selected the items that distinguished best between those who scored high and those who scored low on the pool of items.

The original measure was a card-sort procedure with different versions for women and men (Cooper, 1970). Scores on a less cumbersome pencil-and-paper self-report version using the same items for men and women were highly correlated with scores on the original version (Snowdon, 1980; Stanley, Prather, Beck, Brown, Wagner, & Davis, 1993). The scale presented in the present review is the newer pencil and paper version using the same items for men and women.

Administration and Scoring

Respondents first indicate whether each of the items apply to them. The first 46 items on the inventory comprise the Obsessive Symptoms subscale and the last 23 items comprise the Obsessive Personality Traits subscale. Scores for the Obsessive Symptoms subscale can range from 0 to 46 and scores on the Obsessive Personality Traits subscale can range from 0 to 23. The respondent also rates the items he or she endorsed within a subset of 39 items on a 0–3 scale of how much he or she resists the symptom or trait and a 0–3 scale of how much interference with other activities the symptom or trait creates. The Resistance subscale score assesses the amount of resistance to obsessional symptoms; scores can range from 0 to 117. The Interference subscale score indicates the amount of interference with other activities the obsessive symptoms create; scores can range from 0 to 117. Higher scores on each of the four scales indicate more disturbance.

Sample and Cutoff Scores

Cooper (1970) reported scores on the inventory given in its card-sort format for 17 clients with a diagnosis relating to obsessive symptoms, 25 female homemakers who had been identified by case workers as having obsessive or perfectionistic tendencies, 19 husbands of the homemakers, and community samples of 60 women and 41 men. Stanley et al. (1993) gave the pencil-and-paper version to 18 clients with obsessive-compulsive disorders and 59 clients with other anxiety disorders. Table 1 shows the average scores for these groups.

Because Stanley et al. (1993) found that the Interference subscale scores were the strongest predictors of whether an individual had been diagnosed with obsessive-compulsive disorder, they developed cutoff scores for this scale. A score of 10 or greater on the Interference scale correctly identified 100% of the obsessive clients but only correctly identified 68% of the nonobsessive clients. A score of 20 or greater correctly identified 76.5% of the obsessive clients and 96.5% of the nonobsessive clients.

Reliability

In a sample of clients Stanley et al. (1993) found that internal consistency as measured by Cronbach's alpha was .88 for the Symptom scale, .75 for the Trait scale, .88 for the Resistance scale, and .90 for the Interference scale. Cooper (1970) found test–retest reliability over an unspecified length of time was .87 for the Symptom subscale and .91 for the Trait subscale.

Validity

In a sample of clients Stanley et al. (1993) found that scores on all subscales but the Trait subscale were associated with another measure of

TABLE 1
Leyton Obsessional Inventory Scores

Group	Symptom scale		Trait scale		Resistance scale		Interference scale	
	M	SD	M	SD	M	SD	M	SD
Obsessional clients*	33.3	7.7	11.0	3.2	36.0	11.2	36.7	18.4
Obsessive clients**	22.6	7.1	10.1	5.2	24.3	12.9	26.8	11.3
Obsessive homemakers*	19.7	8.7	7.6	3.5	16.1	11.8	10.7	12.4
Clients with anxiety**	15.2	7.5	8.6	3.9	11.2	9.3	7.9	6.7
Homemakers' husbands*	12.5	6.3	6.9	3.6	5.9	3.0	4.1	3.1
Community sample*								
Females	11.4	6.7	5.1	3.5	7.3	6.1	3.8	4.3
Males	8.7	5.6	5.1	3.8	4.4	3.9	3.6	3.8

*Cooper (1970), **Stanley et al. (1993).

obsessive-compulsiveness and all subscales were associated with neuroticism.

Cooper (1970) compared the four subscale scores of obsessive clients, obsessive homemakers, and a community sample of men and women. He found that the obsessive clients scored significantly higher than the obsessive homemakers on all four subscales and that the obsessive homemakers scored significantly higher than the individuals in the community sample on all four subscales. Stanley et al. (1993) found that the Symptom, Interference, and Resistance subscales differentiated between obsessive-compulsive clients, but that the Trait subscale did not differentiate between them.

Foa and Goldstein (1978) and Emmelkamp, van der Helm, van Zanten, and Plochg (1980) found that scores on the subscales decreased in clients going through treatment for obsessive-compulsive disorder.

LEYTON OBSESSIONAL INVENTORY

First mark "yes" or "no" for each of the items. For some of the items you mark "yes" you will also be asked to circle one phrase that describes your feelings about the behavior and circle one phrase that describes how the behavior influences your life.

1. Are you often inwardly compelled to do certain things even though your reason tells you it is not necessary?

Yes   No

2. Do unpleasant or frightening thoughts or words ever keep going over and over in your mind?

Yes   No

3. Do you ever have persistent imaginings that someone close to you (e.g., children or parents) might be having an accident or that something might have happened to them?

Yes   No

If you answered "yes," do you (please circle one phrase)

believe this is sensible	believe this is habit	try to stop this	try very hard to stop this

If you answered "yes," does this (please circle one phrase)

not interfere with other activities	interfere a little	interfere moderately	interfere a great deal

4. Have you ever been troubled by certain thoughts or ideas of harming yourself or persons in your family—thoughts which come and go without any particular reason?

Yes   No

If you answered "yes," do you (please circle one phrase)

believe this is sensible	believe this is habit	try to stop this	try very hard to stop this

If you answered "yes," does this (please circle one phrase)

not interfere with other activities	interfere a little	interfere moderately	interfere a great deal

5. Do you often have to check things several times?

Yes   No

6. Do you ever have to check gas or water taps or light switches after you have already turned them off?

Yes   No

If you answered "yes," do you (please circle one phrase)

| believe this is sensible | believe this is habit | try to stop this | try very hard to stop this |

If you answered "yes," does this (please circle one phrase)

| not interfere with other activities | interfere a little | interfere moderately | interfere a great deal |

7. Do you ever have to go back and check doors, cupboards or windows to make sure that they are really shut?

Yes   No

If you answered "yes," do you (please circle one phrase)

| believe this is sensible | believe this is habit | try to stop this | try very hard to stop this |

If you answered "yes," does this (please circle one phrase)

| not interfere with other activities | interfere a little | interfere moderately | interfere a great deal |

8. Do you hate dirt and dirty things?

Yes   No

9. Do you ever feel that if something has been used, touched, or knocked by someone else it is in some way spoiled for you?

Yes   No

If you answered "yes" do you (please circle one phrase)

| believe this is sensible | believe this is habit | try to stop this | try very hard to stop this |

If you answered "yes," does this (please circle one phrase)

| not interfere with other activities | interfere a little | interfere moderately | interfere a great deal |

➤

10. Do you dislike brushing against people or being touched in any way?

Yes   No

If you answered "yes," do you (please circle one phrase)

believe this is sensible	believe this is habit	try to stop this	try very hard to stop this

If you answered "yes," does this (please circle one phrase)

not interfere with other activities	interfere a little	interfere moderately	interfere a great deal

11. Do you feel that even a slight contact with bodily secretions (such as sweat, saliva, urine, etc.) is unpleasant or dangerous, or liable to contaminate your clothes or belongings?

Yes   No

If you answered "yes," do you (please circle one phrase)

believe this is sensible	believe this is habit	try to stop this	try very hard to stop this

If you answered "yes," does this (please circle one phrase)

not interfere with other activities	interfere a little	interfere moderately	interfere a great deal

12. Do you worry if you go through a day without having your bowels open?

Yes   No

13. Are you ever worried by the thoughts of pins, needles, or bits of hair that might have been left lying about?

Yes   No

If you answered "yes," do you (please circle one phrase)

believe this is sensible	believe this is habit	try to stop this	try very hard to stop this

If you answered "yes," does this (please circle one phrase)

not interfere with other activities	interfere a little	interfere moderately	interfere a great deal

14. Do you worry about household things that might chip or splinter if they were to be knocked or broken?

Yes   No

If you answered "yes," do you (please circle one phrase)

believe this is sensible	believe this is habit	try to stop this	try very hard to stop this

If you answered "yes," does this (please circle one phrase)

not interfere with other activities	interfere a little	interfere moderately	interfere a great deal

15. Does the sight of knives, hammers, hatchets, or other possibly dangerous things in your home ever upset you or make you feel nervous?

Yes   No

If you answered "yes," do you (please circle one phrase)

believe this is sensible	believe this is habit	try to stop this	try very hard to stop this

If you answered "yes," does this (please circle one phrase)

not interfere with other activities	interfere a little	interfere moderately	interfere a great deal

16. Do you tend to worry a bit about personal cleanliness or tidiness?

Yes   No

17. Are you fussy about keeping your hands clean?

Yes   No

If you answered "yes," do you (please circle one phrase)

believe this is sensible	believe this is habit	try to stop this	try very hard to stop this

If you answered "yes," does this (please circle one phrase)

not interfere with other activities	interfere a little	interfere moderately	interfere a great deal

18. Do you ever wash and iron clothes or ask for this to be done when they are not obviously dirty in order to keep them extra clean and fresh?

Yes   No

If you answered "yes," do you (please circle one phrase)

believe this is sensible	believe this is habit	try to stop this	try very hard to stop this

➤

If you answered "yes," does this (please circle one phrase)

| not interfere with other activities | interfere a little | interfere moderately | interfere a great deal |

19. Do you take care that the clothes you are wearing are always clean and neat, whatever you are doing?

Yes   No

If you answered "yes," do you (please circle one phrase)

| believe this is sensible | believe this is habit | try to stop this | try very hard to stop this |

If you answered "yes," does this (please circle one phrase)

| not interfere with other activities | interfere a little | interfere moderately | interfere a great deal |

20. Do you like to put your personal belongings in set places or patterns?

Yes   No

If you answered "yes," do you (please circle one phrase)

| believe this is sensible | believe this is habit | try to stop this | try very hard to stop this |

If you answered "yes," does this (please circle one phrase)

| not interfere with other activities | interfere a little | interfere moderately | interfere a great deal |

21. Do you take great care in hanging and folding your clothes at night?

Yes   No

If you answered "yes," do you (please circle one phrase)

| believe this is sensible | believe this is habit | try to stop this | try very hard to stop this |

If you answered "yes," does this (please circle one phrase)

| not interfere with other activities | interfere a little | interfere moderately | interfere a great deal |

22. Are you very strict about the house (or apartment or room) always being kept very clean?

Yes   No

If you answered "yes," do you (please circle one phrase)

| believe this is sensible | believe this is habit | try to stop this | try very hard to stop this |

If you answered "yes," does this (please circle one phrase)

| not interfere with other activities | interfere a little | interfere moderately | interfere a great deal |

23. Do you dislike having a room untidy or not quite clean for even a short time?

Yes   No

If you answered "yes," do you (please circle one phrase)

| believe this is sensible | believe this is habit | try to stop this | try very hard to stop this |

If you answered "yes," does this (please circle one phrase)

| not interfere with other activities | interfere a little | interfere moderately | interfere a great deal |

24. Do you sometimes get angry that children or other people spoil your nice clean and tidy room(s)?

Yes   No

25. Do you like furniture or ornaments to be in exactly the same place always?

Yes   No

If you answered "yes," do you (please circle one phrase)

| believe this is sensible | believe this is habit | try to stop this | try very hard to stop this |

If you answered "yes," does this (please circle one phrase)

| not interfere with other activities | interfere a little | interfere moderately | interfere a great deal |

26. Do your easy chairs have cushions which you like to keep exactly in position?

Yes   No

27. If you notice any bits or specks on the floor or furniture do you have to remove them at once before the next regular cleaning?

Yes   No

→

If you answered "yes," do you (please circle one phrase)

| believe this is sensible | believe this is habit | try to stop this | try very hard to stop this |

If you answered "yes," does this (please circle one phrase)

| not interfere with other activities | interfere a little | interfere moderately | interfere a great deal |

28. Do you ever clean or dust rooms that haven't had time to get dirty, just to make sure that they are really clean?

Yes   No

If you answered "yes," do you (please circle one phrase)

| believe this is sensible | believe this is habit | try to stop this | try very hard to stop this |

If you answered "yes," does this (please circle one phrase)

| not interfere with other activities | interfere a little | interfere moderately | interfere a great deal |

29. Do you ever have to clean, dust, sweep, or wash things over again several times just to make sure they are really clean?

Yes   No

If you answered "yes," do you (please circle one phrase)

| believe this is sensible | believe this is habit | try to stop this | try very hard to stop this |

If you answered "yes," does this (please circle one phrase)

| not interfere with other activities | interfere a little | interfere moderately | interfere a great deal |

30. Do you have to keep to strict timetables or routines for doing ordinary things?

Yes   No

If you answered "yes," do you (please circle one phrase)

| believe this is sensible | believe this is habit | try to stop this | try very hard to stop this |

If you answered "yes," does this (please circle one phrase)

not interfere with activities	interfere a little	interfere moderately	interfere a great deal

31. Do you have to keep a certain order for undressing and dressing, or washing and bathing?

Yes   No

If you answered "yes," do you (please circle one phrase)

believe this is sensible	believe this is habit	try to stop this	try very hard to stop this

If you answered "yes," does this (please circle one phrase)

not interfere with other activities	interfere a little	interfere moderately	interfere a great deal

32. Do you get a bit upset if you cannot do your work and/or household jobs at set times or in a certain order?

Yes   No

If you answered "yes," do you (please circle one phrase)

believe this is sensible	believe this is habit	try to stop this	try very hard to stop this

If you answered "yes," does this (please circle one phrase)

not interfere with other activities	interfere a little	interfere moderately	interfere a great deal

33. Do you ever have to do things over again a certain number of times before they seem quite right?

Yes   No

If you answered "yes," do you (please circle one phrase)

believe this is sensible	believe this is habit	try to stop this	try very hard to stop this

If you answered "yes," does this (please circle one phrase)

not interfere with other activities	interfere a little	interfere moderately	interfere a great deal

→

34. Do you ever have to count things several times or go through numbers in your mind?

Yes   No

If you answered "yes," do you (please circle one phrase)

believe this	believe this	try to	try very hard
is sensible	is habit	stop this	to stop this

If you answered "yes," does this (please circle one phrase)

not interfere with	interfere	interfere	interfere a
other activities	a little	moderately	great deal

35. Do you ever get behind with work and/or household jobs because you have to do something over again several times?

Yes   No

If you answered "yes," do you (please circle one phrase)

believe this	believe this	try to	try very hard
is sensible	is habit	stop this	to stop this

If you answered "yes," does this (please circle one phrase)

not interfere with	interfere	interfere	interfere a
other activities	a little	moderately	great deal

36. Are you a person who often has a guilty conscience over quite ordinary things?

Yes   No

37. Are you the sort of person who has to pay a great deal of attention to details?

Yes   No

If you answered "yes," do you (please circle one phrase)

believe this	believe this	try to	try very hard
is sensible	is habit	stop this	to stop this

If you answered "yes," does this (please circle one phrase)

not interfere with	interfere	interfere	interfere a
other activities	a little	moderately	great deal

38. Are you ever over-conscientious or very strict with yourself?

Yes   No

39. Do you ever waste time by doing a thing more thoroughly than is really necessary just to see it is really finished?

Yes   No

If you answered "yes," do you (please circle one phrase)

| believe this is sensible | believe this is habit | try to stop this | try very hard to stop this |

If you answered "yes," does this (please circle one phrase)

| not interfere with other activities | interfere a little | interfere moderately | interfere a great deal |

40. Even when you have done something carefully, do you often feel that it is somehow not quite right or complete?

Yes   No

If you answered "yes," do you (please circle one phrase)

| believe this is sensible | believe this is habit | try to stop this | try very hard to stop this |

If you answered "yes," does this (please circle one phrase)

| not interfere with other activities | interfere a little | interfere moderately | interfere a great deal |

41. Do you feel unsettled or guilty if you haven't been able to do something exactly as you would like?

Yes   No

If you answered "yes," do you (please circle one phrase)

| believe this is sensible | believe this is habit | try to stop this | try very hard to stop this |

If you answered "yes," does this (please circle one phrase)

| not interfere with other activities | interfere a little | interfere moderately | interfere a great deal |

42. Do you always fail to explain things properly, in spite of having planned beforehand exactly what to say?

Yes   No

43. Do you have difficulty in making up your mind?

Yes   No

→

If you answered "yes," do you (please circle one phrase)

| believe this is sensible | believe this is habit | try to stop this | try very hard to stop this |

If you answered "yes," does this (please circle one phrase)

| not interfere with other activities | interfere a little | interfere moderately | interfere a great deal |

44. Do you have to turn things over and over in your mind for a long time before being able to decide about what to do?

Yes   No

If you answered "yes," do you (please circle one phrase)

| believe this is sensible | believe this is habit | try to stop this | try very hard to stop this |

If you answered "yes," does this (please circle one phrase)

| not interfere with other activities | interfere a little | interfere moderately | interfere a great deal |

45. Do you ask yourself questions or have doubts about a lot of things you do?

Yes   No

If you answered "yes," do you (please circle one phrase)

| believe this is sensible | believe this is habit | try to stop this | try very hard to stop this |

If you answered "yes," does this (please circle one phrase)

| not interfere with other activities | interfere a little | interfere moderately | interfere a great deal |

46. Are there any particular things that you try to keep away from or that you avoid doing, because you know that you would be upset by them?

Yes   No

If you answered "yes," do you (please circle one phrase)

| believe this is sensible | believe this is habit | try to stop this | try very hard to stop this |

If you answered "yes," does this (please circle one phrase)

| not interfere with other activities | interfere a little | interfere moderately | interfere a great deal |

47. Do you find it difficult to throw things away?

                    Yes   No

If you answered "yes," do you (please circle one phrase)

| believe this | believe this | try to | try very hard |
| is sensible | is habit | stop this | to stop this |

If you answered "yes," does this (please circle one phrase)

| not interfere with | interfere | interfere | interfere a |
| other activities | a little | moderately | great deal |

48. Do you keep rather a lot of empty boxes, paper bags, old newspapers, or empty tins in case they come in useful one day?

                    Yes   No

If you answered "yes," do you (please circle one phrase)

| believe this | believe this | try to | try very hard |
| is sensible | is habit | stop this | to stop this |

If you answered "yes," does this (please circle one phrase)

| not interfere with | interfere | interfere | interfere a |
| other activities | a little | moderately | great deal |

49. Does your stock of soap, detergents, or cleaning materials ever get large because you find yourself buying more than you actually use?

                    Yes   No

50. Do you regard cleanliness as a virtue in itself?

                    Yes   No

51. Do you get more pleasure from saving money than from spending it?

                    Yes   No

52. Are you more careful with money than most people you know?

                    Yes   No

53. Do you keep regular accounts of the money you spend every day?

                    Yes   No

54. Do you usually look on the gloomy side of things?

                    Yes   No

→

55. Do people often get on your nerves and make you feel irritable?

Yes   No

56. When you feel critical of someone, do you usually say what you are thinking?

Yes   No

57. Do you get angry or irritated if people don't do things carefully or correctly?

Yes   No

58. Do you try to avoid changes in your house or work or in the way you do things?

Yes   No

59. Do you try to avoid changing your mind once you have made a decision about something?

Yes   No

60. Are you a person who likes to stick to principles and decisions whatever the opposition or difficulties?

Yes   No

61. Do you pride yourself on thinking things over very carefully before making decisions?

Yes   No

62. Do you think that regular daily bowel movements are important for your health?

Yes   No

63. Do you often get scared that you might be developing some sort of serious illness or cancer?

Yes   No

64. Are you very systematic and methodical in your daily life?

Yes   No

65. Do you like to get things done exactly right, down to the smallest detail?

Yes   No

66. Do you think it is important to follow rules and regulations exactly?

Yes   No

67. Do you like to have set times or orders for doing your work and/or household jobs?

Yes   No

68. Are you ever late because you just can't seem to get through everything in time?

Yes   No

If you answered "yes," do you (please circle one phrase)

| believe this is sensible | believe this is habit | try to stop this | try very hard to stop this |

If you answered "yes," does this (please circle one phrase)

| not interfere with other activities | interfere a little | interfere moderately | interfere a great deal |

69. If you have to catch a train or keep an important appointment, do you have to plan out how to do it beforehand in great detail?

Yes   No

If you answered "yes," do you (please circle one phrase)

| believe this is sensible | believe this is habit | try to stop this | try very hard to stop this |

If you answered "yes," does this (please circle one phrase)

| not interfere with other activities | interfere a little | interfere moderately | interfere a great deal |

Cooper, J. (1970). The Leyton Obsessional Inventory. *Psychological Medicine, 1,* 48–64. Reprinted with the permission of Cambridge University Press.

COMPULSIVE ACTIVITY CHECKLIST

Purpose and Development

The Compulsive Activities Checklist is a 38-item instrument developed by Freund, Steketee, and Foa (1987) to measure obsessive-compulsive symptoms by assessing specific behaviors. It can be used as an interview or as a self-report measure. Freund et al. (1987) arrived at the items by modifying several previous versions of compulsive activities checklists through rewording, deleting, and adding items. In a factor analytic study of the responses of a clinical sample, Freund et al. (1987) found that the items grouped into two main factors, one of which related to washing compulsions, the other of which related to checking compulsions. In a factor analysis of the responses of a nonclinical sample, Sternberger and Burns (1990) found overall support for the original factor structure, although some of the items from the original washing factor loaded highly on a third factor, which they labeled hygiene.

Steketee and Freund (1993) developed a 28-item version of the scale. In the Administration and Scoring section we give the items for the abbreviated scale.

Cottraux, Bouvard, Defyolle, and Messy (1988) have developed a French version of the checklist.

Administration and Scoring

Because Freund et al. (1987) developed the scale to be used for either assessor-ratings or self-ratings, we slightly modified the instructions for assessors so that instructions are valid for either type of rating. Each behavioral item is rated on a 0 to 3 scale of how much impairment obsessive and compulsive symptoms present. A total score for the checklist is created by summing the ratings for the items. Scores can range from 0 to 114. The Washing subscale contains items 2–14, 16–20, and 31–36. Scores on this subscale can range from 0 to 72. The Checking subscale contains items 1, 15, 21–30, 37, and 38. Scores on this subscale can range from 0 to 42. For each scale higher scores indicate more impairment.

For the 28-item version of the scale, items 7 and 8 are combined and items 20, 24, 27, 30, 31, 32, 34, 35, and 37 are eliminated.

Sample Scores

Freund et al. (1987) gave the checklist to 39 obsessive-compulsive clients who had been identified by therapists as having primarily washing rituals and 24 obsessive-compulsive clients who had been identified as having primarily checking rituals. They also used the checklist to assess 25 clients before and after they went through treatment. Sternberger and Burns (1990) gave the checklist to 579 university students. Table 1 shows average scores for these groups.

Steketee and Freund (1993) gave the 28-item version of the scale to 173 university students and found a mean score of 4.38 (*SD* = 5.61).

Reliability

In a sample of obsessive-compulsive clients, Freund et al. (1987) found that internal consistency as measured by Cronbach's alpha was .91 for the total score, .91 for the Washing subscale, and .98 for the Checking subscale. In a sample of students, Sternberger and Burns (1990) found internal consistency as measured by Cronbach's alpha was .86 for the total score and .78 for both subscales.

Freund et al. (1987) asked two independent raters to complete the checklist for clients on the same day and found an interrater reliability of .62. When they asked a rater and the client to fill out the checklist on the same day, they found a correlation of .94.

Freund et al. (1987) asked two different raters to assess clients at an average of 37 days apart and found a test–retest reliability of .63. Because two raters were used this relatively low test–retest reliability may be an artifact of the low interrater reliability of the checklist. In a sample of students who completed the checklist themselves, Sternberger and Burns (1990) found that six- to seven-month test–retest reliability was .74.

TABLE 1
Compulsive Activity Checklist Scores

Group	Total Score		Washing		Checking	
	M	*SD*	*M*	*SD*	*M*	*SD*
Obsessive-Compulsive clients*						
Pretreatment	43.66	18.94				
Posttreatment	19.18	15.17				
Clients with different rituals*						
Washing			33.24	13.68	12.00	7.68
Checking			8.95	5.59	16.48	9.44
University students**	10.44	8.76				

*Freund et al. (1987); ** Sternberger and Burns (1990).

Validity

In a sample of obsessive compulsive clients, Freund et al. (1987) found that total scores on the checklist were significantly associated with four other measures of obsessive-compulsive symptoms, four measures of life-functioning, and a measure of phobic tendencies. In a sample of college students, Sternberger and Burns (1990) found an association between checklist scores and two other measures of obsessive-compulsiveness. Freund et al. (1987) found no significant association between checklist scores and rituals assessed by a rater and also no significant correlation between checklist scores and several measures of depression and anxiety.

Freund et al. (1987) found that as expected the Washing subscale score was significantly associated with the Cleanliness subscale of another measure and the Checking subscale was significantly associated with the checking subscale of another measure.

Freund et al. (1987) compared the subscale scores of clients who had been identified as either having predominantly washing rituals or checking rituals. They found that clients in the washing rituals group had significantly higher Washing subscale scores while clients in the checking rituals group had significantly higher Checking subscale scores.

COMPULSIVE ACTIVITY CHECKLIST

Instructions: Rate each activity on the scale below according to how much impairment is present due to obsessive and compulsive symptoms.

0—No problem with activity—takes about same time as for average person. No need to repeat it or avoid it.

1—Activity takes about twice as long as for most people, or it must be repeated twice, or there is a tendency to avoid it.

2—Activity takes about three times as long as for most people, or it must be repeated three or more times, or it is usually avoided.

3—Unable to complete or attempt activity.

0	1	2	3	1. Retracing steps
0	1	2	3	2. Having a bath or shower
0	1	2	3	3. Washing hands and face
0	1	2	3	4. Care of hair (e.g., washing, combing, brushing)
0	1	2	3	5. Brushing teeth
0	1	2	3	6. Dressing and undressing
0	1	2	3	7. Using toilet to urinate
0	1	2	3	8. Using toilet to defecate
0	1	2	3	9. Touching people or being touched
0	1	2	3	10. Handling garbage or waste basket
0	1	2	3	11. Washing clothing
0	1	2	3	12. Washing dishes
0	1	2	3	13. Handling or cooking food
0	1	2	3	14. Cleaning house
0	1	2	3	15. Keeping things neat and orderly
0	1	2	3	16. Bed making
0	1	2	3	17. Cleaning shoes
0	1	2	3	18. Touching door handles
0	1	2	3	19. Touching your genitals, petting, or sexual intercourse
0	1	2	3	20. Visiting a hospital
0	1	2	3	21. Switching lights and spigots on or off
0	1	2	3	22. Locking or closing doors or windows
0	1	2	3	23. Checking electrical appliances
0	1	2	3	24. Doing arithmetic or accounts
0	1	2	3	25. Getting ready for work
0	1	2	3	26. Doing your work
0	1	2	3	27. Writing

➤

0 1 2 3   28. Form filling
0 1 2 3   29. Mailing letters
0 1 2 3   30. Reading
0 1 2 3   31. Walking down the street
0 1 2 3   32. Traveling by bus train or car
0 1 2 3   33. Touching the floor
0 1 2 3   34. Eating in restaurants
0 1 2 3   35. Going to cinemas or theaters
0 1 2 3   36. Using public bathrooms
0 1 2 3   37. Keeping appointments
0 1 2 3   38. Throwing things away

IMPACT OF EVENT SCALE

Purpose and Development

The Impact of Event Scale assesses subjective distress related to a traumatic life event and is often used with individuals thought to be suffering from posttraumatic stress disorder or from a stress reaction. The scale is a 15-item self-report measure developed by Horowitz, Wilner, and Alvarez (1979). Items relating to intrusion and avoidance were selected through a cluster analysis of a large pool of items generated by individuals who experienced a traumatic event. A factor analysis by Zilberg, Weiss, and Horowitz (1982) confirmed that the items grouped into these two dimensions.

Administration and Scoring

A respondent selects his or her most stressful recent life event, then uses this event as a referent when rating each of the scale items on a 0–3 scale of frequency of occurrence during the past week. The ratings for all 15 items may be summed to obtain a total distress score. The items also may be used to calculate two components of distress: (a) unwanted intrusion of thoughts or images related to the event and (b) avoidance or denial of elements of the event. Items 1, 4, 5, 6, 10, 11, and 14 comprise the Intrusion subscale and items 2, 3, 7, 8, 9, 12, 13, and 15 comprise the Avoidance subscale. Scores may range from 0 to 45 on the total scale, from 0 to 21 on the Intrusion subscale, and from 0 to 24 on the Avoidance subscale. Higher scores indicate more distress.

Horowitz et al. (1979) found a moderate correlation between the two subscales and Zilberg et al. (1982) found moderate to high correlations between the subscales in several nondistressed groups, but found no significant association between the subscales in a pretreatment client group. Because of this finding and Horowitz's stress response syndrome theory, Zilberg et al. (1982) recommend not combining the subscales into a total distress score.

Sample Scores

Horowitz et al. (1979) obtained scores from 50 women and 16 men who sought treatment for distress related to a major trauma and from 35 female and 75 male medical students. Zilberg et al. (1982) gave the scale to 35 clients who sought treatment after the death of a parent and 37 individuals who did not seek treatment after the death of a parent. Hetherington (1993) gave the scale to 306 road patrol officers who dealt with traumatic traffic accidents. Davidson and Baum (1986) gave the scale to 52 individuals living near the Three Mile Island nuclear accident and 35 individuals living some distance away. Table 1 shows the mean scores for these groups.

Reliability

Horowitz et al. (1979) found a split-half reliability of .86 for the total scale in their sample of clients seeking treatment for the aftereffects of a traumatic life event. For this same sample the internal consistency of the intrusion subscale was .78 and the internal consistency of the avoidance subscale was .82. In a sample of individuals who had suffered the loss of a parent Zilberg et al. (1982) found the internal consistency of the Intrusion subscale was .86 and the internal consistency of the Avoidance subscale was .88. In a sample of physical therapy students Horowitz et al. (1979) found a one week test–retest reliability of .87 for the total scale score, .89 for the intrusion subscale, and .79 for the avoidance subscale.

Validity

Davidson and Baum (1986) found Impact of Event Scale scores were associated with a variety of measures of chronic stress including somatic

TABLE 1
Impact of Event Scale Scores

Group	Total Score M	SD	Intrusion M	SD	Avoidance M	SD
Clients*						
Males	35.3	22.6	21.2	12.5	14.2	12.0
Females	42.1	16.7	21.4	8.6	20.6	11.3
Parental death**						
Clients			21.2	7.9	20.8	10.2
Nonclients			13.5	9.1	9.4	9.6
Road patrol officers***	22.8	14.4	11.8	8.2	11.1	7.9
Nuclear accident****						
Close	18.9	17.0	10.3	9.2	8.5	8.6
Distant	11.2	12.6	5.43	8.0	5.8	6.4
Students*						
Males	6.9	6.8	2.5	3.0	4.4	5.3
Females	12.7	10.8	6.1	5.3	6.6	7.0

*Horowitz et al. (1979), **Zilberg et al. (1982), ***Hetherington (1993), ****Davidson and Baum (1986).

complaints, impaired concentration, impaired interpersonal relationships, depression, anxiety, anger, fear, alienation, and several physiological measures. Several studies used the scale with veterans suffering from posttraumatic stress and found the total scale score as well as the subscale scores were associated with other measures of posttraumatic stress (Weisenberg, Solomon, Schwarzwald, & Mukulincer, 1987; McFall, Smith, MacKay, & Tarver, 1990; McFall, Smith, Roszell, Tarver, & Malas, 1990).

Horowitz et al. (1979) compared the responses of individuals who had sought treatment for the aftereffects of a traumatic life event with those of individuals who experienced no major trauma and found that those who sought treatment scored significantly higher on the total scale and on the two subscales. Zilberg et al. (1982) found that individuals who sought treatment after the loss of a parent had significantly higher subscale scores than individuals who did not seek treatment.

Horowitz et al. (1979) and Zilberg et al. (1982) asked clients to complete the scale before and after therapy focused on helping them overcome the effects of a traumatic experience and found a significant decrease in scale scores. The scale is also sensitive to the amelioration of symptoms as time passes after a traumatic event (Zilberg et. al., 1982; Seidner, Amick, & Kilpatrick, 1988; Sloane, 1988).

IMPACT OF EVENT SCALE

Please report the recent life event that was most stressful for you.

On _____ you experienced _____
     (*date*)   (*life event*)

Below is a list of comments made by people after stressful life events. Please check each item, indicating how frequently these comments were true for you DURING THE PAST SEVEN DAYS. If they did not occur during that time, please mark the "not at all" column.

	FREQUENCY			
	Not at all	Rarely	Sometimes	Often
1. I thought about it when I didn't mean to.	____	____	____	____
2. I avoided letting myself get upset when I thought about it or was reminded of it.	____	____	____	____
3. I tried to remove it from memory.	____	____	____	____
4. I had trouble falling asleep or staying asleep, because of pictures or thoughts about it that came into my mind.	____	____	____	____
5. I had waves of strong feelings about it.	____	____	____	____
6. I had dreams about it.	____	____	____	____
7. I stayed away from reminders of it.	____	____	____	____
8. I felt as if it hadn't happened or it wasn't real.	____	____	____	____
9. I tried not to talk about it.	____	____	____	____

10. Pictures about it popped into my mind. ____ ____ ____ ____

11. Other things kept making me think about it. ____ ____ ____ ____

12. I was aware that I still had a lot of feelings about it, but I didn't deal with them. ____ ____ ____ ____

13. I tried not to think about it. ____ ____ ____ ____

14. Any reminder brought back feelings about it. ____ ____ ____ ____

15. My feelings about it were kind of numb. ____ ____ ____ ____

Reprinted with permission of Horowitz, M., Wilner, N., & Alvarez, W. (1979). Impact of Event Scale: A measure of subjective stress. *Psychosomatic Medicine, 41*(3), 209–218.

MISSISSIPPI SCALE FOR COMBAT-RELATED POSTTRAUMATIC STRESS DISORDER

Purpose and Development

The Mississippi Scale assesses posttraumatic stress disorder in combat veterans. The scale is a 35-item self-report measure developed by Terence Keane. Items are based on the symptoms of posttraumatic stress disorder given in the DSM-III and features related to these symptoms (Keane, Caddell, & Taylor, 1988). In his comprehensive review of available instruments, Watson (1990) recommended the scale as the best scale for use with combat related posttraumatic stress disorder.

Clinical psychologists experienced in working with posttraumatic stress disorder clients generated the initial pool of 200 items. The items judged as most representative of the symptoms of posttraumatic stress disorder were then selected for the scale. A factor analytic study by McFall, Smith, MacKay, and Tarver (1990a) indicated that the items group into three main factors they labeled: intrusive reexperiencing and emotional numbing, anger dyscontrol and emotional lability, and social alienation.

Administration and Scoring

Respondents rate each of the 35 items on a 5-point scale. Items 2, 6, 11, 17, 19, 22, 24, 27, 30, and 34 are scored in reverse order. The ratings for all items are summed, resulting in a total score ranging from 35–175, with higher scores indicating more posttraumatic stress symptoms.

Sample Scores and Cutoff Scores

Keane (1994; Keane et al. 1988) obtained scale scores from 30 Vietnam veterans with an established diagnosis of posttraumatic stress disorder (PTSD), scale scores from 30 Vietnam veterans with another psychiatric diagnosis, and scale scores from 32 well-adjusted Vietnam veterans. The means for these groups were 130 (SD = 18) for the PTSD veterans, 86 (SD = 26) for the veterans with another psychiatric diagnosis, and 75 (SD = 18) for the well-adjusted veterans. Keane et al. (1988) established a cutting score of 107 for diagnosing PTSD. This cutoff score correctly identified 93% of veterans with PTSD and correctly identified 89% of veterans who did not have PTSD.

McFall et al. (1990a) gave the scale to 101 Vietnam veterans with posttraumatic stress disorder, M = 129.6 (SD = 17.7) and 102 veterans with substance abuse problems but no posttraumatic stress disorder, M = 81.0

(SD = 18.1). They used a cutting score of 100, which correctly identified 93% of those with PTSD and correctly identified 88.2% of those who did not.

Reliability

In a sample of male Vietnam veterans, Keane et al. (1988) found the Cronbach alpha coefficient assessing internal consistency of the items was .94. In a sample of veterans with PTSD and veterans with substance abuse problems, McFall et al. (1990) found the internal consistency of the scale was .96 as assessed by Cronbach's alpha.

In a sample of male Vietnam veterans, Keane et al. (1988) found a one-week test–retest reliability of .97.

Validity

McFall et al. (1990a) and McFall, Smith, Roszell, Tarver, and Malas (1990b) found that scale scores were associated with several other measures of PTSD, anger, aggressive tendencies, and irritability.

Both Keane et al. (1988) and McFall et al. (1990a) found large, significant differences between the scale scores of Vietnam veterans with an established diagnosis of PTSD and Vietnam veterans with no diagnosis of PTSD. Keane et al. (1988) also found that those who had experienced more combat scored significantly higher on the scale, a finding in line with previous research indicating that more combat experience is associated with a greater likelihood of PTSD.

MISSISSIPPI SCALE FOR COMBAT-RELATED POSTTRAUMATIC STRESS DISORDER

Please circle the number that best describes how you feel about each statement.

1. Before I entered the military, I had more close friends than I have now.

1	2	3	4	5
Not at all true	Slightly true	Somewhat true	Very true	Extremely true

2. I do not feel guilt over things that I did in the military.

1	2	3	4	5
Never true	Rarely true	Sometimes true	Usually true	Always true

3. If someone pushes me too far, I am likely to become violent.

1	2	3	4	5
Very unlikely	Unlikely	Somewhat unlikely	Very likely	Extremely likely

4. If something happens that reminds me of the military, I become very distressed and upset.

1	2	3	4	5
Never	Rarely	Sometimes	Frequently	Very frequently

5. The people who know me best are afraid of me.

1	2	3	4	5
Never	Rarely	Sometimes	Frequently	Very frequently

6. I am able to get emotionally close to others.

1	2	3	4	5
Never	Rarely	Sometimes	Frequently	Very frequently

7. I have nightmares of experiences in the military that really happened.

1	2	3	4	5
Never	Rarely	Sometimes	Frequently	Very frequently

8. When I think of some of the things I did in the military, I wish I were dead.

1	2	3	4	5
Never true	Rarely true	Sometimes true	Frequently true	Very frequently true

9. It seems as if I have no feelings.

1	2	3	4	5
Not at all true	Rarely true	Sometimes true	Frequently true	Very frequently true

10. Lately, I have felt like killing myself.

1	2	3	4	5
Not at all true	Slightly true	Somewhat true	Very true	Extremely true

11. I fall asleep, stay asleep and awaken only when the alarm goes off.

1	2	3	4	5
Never	Rarely	Sometimes	Frequently	Very frequently

12. I wonder why I am still alive when others died in the military.

1	2	3	4	5
Never	Rarely	Sometimes	Frequently	Very frequently

13. Being in certain situations makes me feel as though I am back in the military.

1	2	3	4	5
Never	Rarely	Sometimes	Frequently	Very frequently

14. My dreams at night are so real that I waken in a cold sweat and force myself to stay awake.

1	2	3	4	5
Never	Rarely	Sometimes	Frequently	Very frequently

15. I feel like I cannot go on.

1	2	3	4	5
Not at all true	Rarely true	Sometimes true	Very true	Almost always true

→

16. I do not laugh or cry at the same things other people do.

1	2	3	4	5
Not at all true	Rarely true	Somewhat true	Very true	Extremely true

17. I still enjoy doing many things that I used to enjoy.

1	2	3	4	5
Never true	Rarely true	Sometimes true	Very true	Always true

18. Daydreams are very real and frightening.

1	2	3	4	5
Never true	Rarely true	Sometimes true	Frequently true	Very frequently true

19. I have found it easy to keep a job since my separation from the military.

1	2	3	4	5
Not at all true	Slightly true	Somewhat true	Very true	Extremely true

20. I have trouble concentrating on tasks.

1	2	3	4	5
Never true	Rarely true	Sometimes true	Frequently true	Very frequently true

21. I have cried for no good reason.

1	2	3	4	5
Never true	Rarely true	Sometimes true	Frequently true	Very frequently true

22. I enjoy the company of others.

1	2	3	4	5
Never true	Rarely true	Sometimes true	Frequently true	Very frequently true

23. I am frightened by my urges.

1	2	3	4	5
Never true	Rarely true	Sometimes true	Frequently true	Very frequently true

24. I fall asleep easily at night.

1	2	3	4	5
Never true	Rarely true	Sometimes true	Frequently true	Very frequently true

25. Unexpected noises make me jump.

1	2	3	4	5
Never true	Rarely true	Sometimes true	Frequently true	Very frequently true

26. No one understands how I feel, not even my family.

1	2	3	4	5
Not at all true	Rarely true	Somewhat true	Very true	Extremely true

27. I am an easy-going, even-tempered person.

1	2	3	4	5
Never	Rarely	Sometimes	Usually	Very much so

28. I feel there are certain things that I did in the military that I can never tell anyone, because no one would ever understand.

1	2	3	4	5
Not at all true	Slightly true	Somewhat true	True	Very true

29. There have been times when I used alcohol (or other drugs) to help me sleep or to make me forget about things that happened while I was in the service.

1	2	3	4	5
Never	Infrequently	Sometimes	Frequently	Very frequently

30. I feel comfortable when I am in a crowd.

1	2	3	4	5
Never	Rarely	Sometimes	Usually	Always

31. I lose my cool and explode over minor everyday things.

1	2	3	4	5
Never	Rarely	Sometimes	Frequently	Very frequently

→

32. I am afraid to go to sleep at night.

1	2	3	4	5
Never	Rarely	Sometimes	Frequently	Almost always

33. I try to stay away from anything that will remind me of things which happened while I was in the military.

1	2	3	4	5
Never	Rarely	Sometimes	Frequently	Almost always

34. My memory is as good as it ever was.

1	2	3	4	5
Not at all true	Rarely true	Somewhat true	Usually true	Almost always

35. I have a hard time expressing my feelings, even to the people I care about.

1	2	3	4	5
Not at all true	Rarely true	Somewhat true	Usually true	Almost always

---

Reprinted with permission of Dr. Terence Keane.

REFERENCES

Allen, G. J. (1973). Treatment of test anxiety by group-administered relaxation and study counseling. *Behavior Therapy, 4,* 349–360.

Alpert, R., & Haber, R. N. (1960). Anxiety in academic achievement situations. *Journal of Abnormal and Social Psychology, 61,* 207–215.

Alvarado, K., Templer, D., Bresler, C., & Thomas-Dobson, S. (1993). Are death anxiety and death depression distinct entities? *Omega, 26,* 113–118.

Arrindell, W. A. (1993). The fear of fear concept: Evidence in favour of multidimensionality. *Behaviour Research and Therapy, 31,* 507–518.

Arrindell, W. A., Emmelkamp, P. M., & Van der End, J. (1984). Phobic dimensions: Reliability and generalizability across samples, gender, and nations. *Advances in Behaviour Research and Therapy, 6,* 207–254.

Beck, A. T., & Steer, R. A. (1991). Relationship between the Beck Anxiety Inventory and the Hamilton Anxiety Rating Scale with anxious patients. *Journal of Anxiety Disorders, 5,* 213–223.

Bibb, J. L (1988). *Parental bonding, pathological development, and fear of losing control among agoraphobics and normals.* Unpublished doctoral dissertation, the American University, Washington, DC.

Chambless, D., Caputo, G. C., Bright, P., & Gallagher, R. (1984). Assessment of fear in agoraphobics: The Body Sensations Questionnaire and the Agoraphobic Cognitions Questionnaire. *Journal of Consulting and Clinical Psychology, 52,* 1090–1097.

Chambless, D., Caputo, G. C., Jasin, S., Gracely, E., & Williams, C. (1985). The Mobility Inventory for Agoraphobia. *Behaviour Research and Therapy, 23,* 35–44.

Cooper, J. (1970). The Leyton Obsessional Inventory. *Psychological Medicine, 1,* 48–64.

Cottraux, J., Bouvard, M., Defyolle, M., & Messy, P. (1988). Validity and factor structure of the Compulsive Activity Checklist. *Behavior Therapy, 19,* 45–53.

Craske, M., Rachman, S. J., & Tallman, K. (1986). Mobility, cognitions, and panic. *Journal of Psychopathology and Behavioral Assessment, 8,* 199–210.

Davidson, L. M., & Baum, A. (1986). Chronic stress and posttraumatic stress disorders. *Journal of Consulting and Clinical Psychology, 54,* 303–308.

Dent, H. R., & Salkovskis, P. M. (1986). Clinical measures of depression, anxiety, and obsessionality in non-clinical populations. *Behaviour Research and Therapy, 24,* 689–691.

Dodge, C. S., Hope, D. A., Heimberg, R. G., & Becker, R. E. (1988). Evaluation of the Social Interaction Self-Statement Test with a social phobic population. *Cognitive Therapy and Research, 12,* 211–222.

Emmelkamp, P. (1988). Maudsley Obsessional-Compulsive Inventory. In M. Hersen & A. Bellack (Eds.), *Dictionary of Behavioral Assessment Techniques* (pp. 294–296). New York: Pergamon.

Emmelkamp, P., van der Helm, M., van Zanten, B. L., & Plochg, I. (1980). Treatment of obsessive-compulsive patients: The contribution of self-instructional training to the effectiveness of exposure. *Behaviour Research and Therapy, 18,* 61–66.

Enkelman, R. (1990). Alprazolam versus buspirone in the treatment of outpatients with generalized anxiety disorder. *Psychopharmacology, 105* (3), 428–432.

Fals-Stewart, W. (1992). A dimensional analysis of the Yale–Brown Obsessive Compulsive Scale. *Psychological Reports, 70,* 239–240.

Foa, E. B., & Goldstein, A. (1978). Continuous exposure and complete response prevention in the treatment of obsessive-compulsive neurosis. *Behavior Therapy, 9,* 821–829.

Freund, B., Steketee, G., & Foa, E. (1987). Compulsive Activity Checklist (CAC): Psychometric analysis with obsessive-compulsive disorder. *Behavioral Assessment, 9,* 67–79.

Frost, R. O., Sher, K. J., & Geen, T. (1986). Psychopathology and personality characteristics of nonclinical compulsive checkers. *Behaviour Research and Therapy, 24,* 133–143.

Glass, C. R., & Furlong, M. (1990). Cognitive Assessment of social anxiety: Affective and behavioral correlates. *Cognitive Therapy and Research, 14,* 365–384.

Glass, C. R., Merluzzi, T. V., Biever, J., & Larsen, K. (1982). Cognitive assessment of social anxiety: Development and validation of a self-statement questionnaire. *Cognitive Therapy and Research, 6,* 37–55.

Goodman, W. K., & Price, L. (1992). Assessment of severity and change in obsessive compulsive disorder. *Psychiatric Clinics of North America, 15,* 861–869.

Goodman, W., Price, L., Rasmussen, S., Mazure, C., Delgado, P., Heninger, G., & Charney, D. (1989b). The Yale–Brown Obsessive Scale: II. Validity. *Archives of General Psychiatry, 46,* 1012–1016.

Goodman, W., Price, L., Rasmussen, S., Mazure, C., Fleischman, R., Hill, C., Heninger, G., & Charney, D. (1989a). The Yale–Brown Obsessive Compulsive Scale: I. Development, use, and reliability. *Archives of General Psychiatry, 46,* 1006–1011.

Hamilton, M. (1959). The assessment of anxiety states by rating. *British Journal of Medical Psychology, 32,* 50–55.

Henderson, M. (1990). Beyond the living will. *Gerontologist, 30,* 480–485.

Hetherington, A. (1993). Traumatic stress on the roads. In R. D. Allen (Ed.), *Handbook of Post Disaster Interventions* (pp. 369–376). Corte Madera, CA: Select Press.

Hodgson, R. J., & Rachman, S. (1977). Obsessional-compulsive complaints. *Behaviour Research and Therapy, 15,* 389–395.

Horowitz, M., Wilner, N., & Alvarez, W. (1979). Impact of Event Scale: A measure of subjective stress. *Psychosomatic Medicine, 41,* 209–218.

Katz, R. J., Landau, P. S., Lott, M., & Bystritsky, A. (1993). Serotonergic (5-HT-sub-2) mediation of anxiety-therapeutic effects of serazepine in generalized anxiety disorder. *Biological Psychiatry, 34,* 41–44.

Keane, T. (1994). Scoring Procedures for the Mississippi Scale for Combat Related PTSD. Department of Veterans Affairs, Boston VA Medical Center.

Keane, T., Caddell, J., & Taylor, K. (1988). Mississippi Scale for combat related posttraumatic stress disorder: Three studies in reliability and validity. *Journal of Consulting and Clinical Psychology, 56,* 85–90.

Kim, S., Dysken, M., & Kuskowski, M. (1990). The Yale–Brown Obsessive-Compulsive Scale: A reliability and validity study. *Psychiatry Research, 41,* 37–44.

Kleinknecht, R. A., & Bernstein, D. (1978). The assessment of dental fear. *Behavior Therapy, 9,* 626–634.

Kleinknecht, R. A., Klepac, R., & Alexander, L. (1973). Origins and characteristics of fear of dentistry. *Journal of the American Dental Association, 86,* 842–848.

Kleinknecht, R. A., Thorndike, R., McGlynn, F. D., & Harkavy, J. (1984). Factor analysis of the dental fear survey with cross validation. *Journal of the American Dental Association, 108,* 59–61.

Kobak, K. A., Reynolds, W. M., & Greist, J. H. (1993). Development and validation of a computer-administered version of the Hamilton Anxiety Scale. *Psychological Assessment, 5,* 487–492.

Koksal, F., Power, K. G., & Sharp, D. M. (1991). Profiles of DSM anxiety disorders on the somatic, cognitive, behavioral and feeling components of the four systems anxiety questionnaire. *Personality and Individual Differences, 12,* 643–651.

Kwon, S., Evans, L., & Oei, T. (1990). Factor structure of the Mobility Inventory for Agoraphobia: A validation study with Australian samples of agoraphobic patients. *Journal of Psychopathology and Behavioral Assessment, 12,* 365–374.

Leary, M. R. (1983). Social anxiousness: The construct and its measurement. *Journal of Personality Assessment, 47,* 66–74.

Leary, M. R. (1986). The impact of interactional impediments on social anxiety and self-presentation. *Journal of Experimental Social Psychology, 22,* 122–135.

Leary, M. R., Atherton, S. C., Hill, S., & Hur, C. (1986). Attributional mediators of social inhibition and avoidance. *Journal of Personality, 54,* 188–200.

Leary, M. R., & Kowalski, R. M. (1993). The Interaction Anxiousness Scale: Construct and criterion-related validity. *Journal of Personality Assessment, 61,* 136–146.

Lehrer, P., & Woolfolk, R. (1982). Self-report assessment of anxiety: Somatic, cognitive, and behavioral modalities. *Behavioral Assessment, 4,* 167–177.

Lelliot, P., McNamee, G., & Marks, I. (1991). Features of agoraphobia, social, and related phobias and validation of the diagnosis. *Journal of Anxiety Disorders, 5,* 313–322.

Maier, W., Buller, R., Phillip, M., & Heuser, I. (1988). The Hamilton Anxiety Scale: Reliability, validity, and sensitivity to change in anxiety and depressive disorders. *Journal of Affective Disorders, 14,* 61–68.

Malcolm, R., Anton, R. F., Randall, C. L., & Johnston, A. (1992). A placebo-controlled trial of buspirone in anxious inpatient alcoholics. *Alcoholism: Clinical and Experimental Research, 16,* 1007–1013.

Marks, I. M., & Mathews, A. M. (1979). Brief standard self-rating for phobic patients. *Behaviour Research and Therapy, 17,* 263–267.

Mavissakalian, M. (1986). The Fear Questionnaire: A validity study. *Behaviour Research and Therapy, 24,* 83–85.

McFall, M. E., Smith, D. S., MacKay, P. W., & Tarver, D. J. (1990). Reliability and validity of the Mississippi Scale for Combat-Related Posttraumatic Stress Disorder. *Psychological Assessment: A Journal of Consulting and Clinical Psychology, 2,* 114–121.

McFall, M. E., Smith, D. S., Roszell, D. K., Tarver, D. J., & Malas, K. L. (1990). Convergent validity of measures of PTSD in Vietnam combat veterans. *American Journal of Psychiatry, 147,* 645–648.

McGlynn, F. D., McNeil, D., Gallagher, S., & Vrana, S. (1987). Factor structure, stability, and internal consistency of the dental fear survey. *Behavioral Assessment, 9,* 57–66.

McNeil, D. W., & Berryman, M. L. (1989). Components of dental fear in adults. *Behaviour Research and Therapy, 27,* 233–236.

Meichenbaum, D. H. (1972). Cognitive modification of test anxious college students. *Journal of Consulting and Clinical Psychology, 39,* 370–380.

Merluzzi, T. V., Burgio, K. L., & Glass, C. R. (1984). Cognition and psychopathology: An analysis of social introversion and self-statements. *Journal of Consulting and Clinical Psychology, 52,* 1102–1103.

Milgrom, P., Kleinknecht, R. A., Elliot, J., Hsing, L. H., & Choo-Soo, T. (1990). *Behaviour Research and Therapy, 28,* 227–233.

Mizes, J. S., & Crawford, J. (1986). Normative values on the Marks and Mathews Fear Questionnaire: A comparison as a function of age and sex. *Journal of Psychopathology and Behavioral Assessment, 8,* 253–262.

Osman, A., Markway, K., & Osman, J. R. (1992). Psychometric properties of the Social Interaction Self-Statement Test in a college sample. *Psychological Reports, 71,* 1171–1177.

Ost, L. G. (1990). The Agoraphobia Scale: An evaluation of its reliability and validity. *Behaviour Research and Therapy, 28,* 323–329.

Perse, T. L., Greist, J. H., Jefferson, J. W., Rosenfield, R., & Dar, R. (1987). Fluvoxamine treatment of obsessive-compulsive disorder. *American Journal of Psychiatry, 144,* 1543–1548.

Plake, B. S., Smith, E. P., & Damsteegt, D. C. (1981). A validity investigation of the achievement anxiety test. *Educational and Psychological Measurement, 41,* 1215–1222.

Scholing, A., & Emmelkamp, P. (1992). Self-report assessment of anxiety: A cross-validation of the Lehrer Woolfolk anxiety symptom questionnaire in three populations. *Behaviour Research & Therapy, 30,* 521–531.

Seidner, A. L., Amick, A. E., & Kilpatrick, D. G. (1988). Impact of Event Scale. In M. Hersen & A. Bellack (Eds.), *Dictionary of Behavioral Assessment Techniques* (pp. 255–257). New York: Pergamon.

Shear, K. M., Klosko, J., & Fyer, M. R. (1989). Assessment of anxiety disorders. In S. Wetzler (Ed.), *Measuring mental illness: Psychometric Assessment for clinicians* (pp. 114–138). New York: American Psychiatric Press.

Sher, K.S., Martin, E. D., Raskin, G., & Perrigo, R. (1991). Prevalence of DSM-III-R disorders among nonclinical compulsive checkers and noncheckers in a college-student sample. *Behaviour Research and Therapy, 29,* 479–483.

Sloane, P. (1988). Posttraumatic stress in survivors of an airplane crash-landing: A clinical and exploratory research intervention. *Journal of Traumatic Stress, 1,* 211–229.

Snowdon, J. (1980). A comparison of the written and postbox forms of the Leyton Obsessional Inventory. *Psychological Medicine, 10,* 165–170.

Stanley, M. A., Prather, R. C., Beck, J. G., Brown, T. C., Wagner, A. L., & Davis, M. L. (1993). Psychometric analysis of the Leyton Obsessional Inventory in patients with obsessive-compulsive and other disorders. *Psychological Assessment, 5,* 187–192.

Steketee, G., & Freund, B. (1993). Compulsive Activity Checklist (CAC): Further psychometric analyses and revision. *Behavioural Psychotherapy, 21,* 13–25.

Sternberger, L. G., & Burns, G. L. (1990). Compulsive Activity Checklist and the Obsessional-Compulsive Inventory: Psychometric properties of two measures of obsessive-compulsive disorder. *Behavior Therapy, 21,* 117–127.

Stevens, S. J., Cooper, P. E., & Thomas, L. E. (1980). Age norms for Templer's Death Anxiety Scale. *Psychological Reports, 46,* 205–206.

Templer, D. (1970). The construction and validation of a death anxiety scale. *Journal of General Psychology, 82,* 165–177.

Templer, D. I., & Ruff, C. F. (1971). Death Anxiety Scale means, standard deviations, and embeddings. *Psychological Reports, 29,* 173–174.

Templer, D. I., Ruff, C. F., & Franks, C. M. (1971). Death anxiety: Age, sex, and parental resemblance in diverse populations. *Developmental Psychology, 4,* 108.

Trull, T., & Hillerbrand, E. (1990). Psychometric properties and factor structure of the Fear Questionnaire Phobia Subscale items in two normative samples. *Journal of Psychopathology and Behavioral Assessment, 12,* 285–297.

Tryon, G. S. (1980). The measurement and treatment of test anxiety. *Review of Educational Research, 50,* 343–372.

Waddell, K. L., & Demi, A. S. (1993). Effectiveness of an intensive partial hospitalization program for treatment of anxiety disorders. *Archives of Psychiatric Nursing, 7,* 2–10.

Watson, C. G. (1990). Psychometric posttraumatic stress disorder measurement techniques: A review. *Psychological Assessment, 2,* 460–469.

Watson, J. M. (1988). Achievement Anxiety Test: Dimensionality and utility. *Journal of Educational Psychology, 80,* 585–591.

Weisenberg, M., Solomon, Z., Schwarzwald, J., & Mikulincer, M. (1987). Assessing the severity of posttraumatic stress disorder: Relationship between dichotomous and continuous measures. *Journal of Consulting and Clinical Psychology, 55,* 432–434.

White, W., & Handal, P. J. (1991). The relationship between death anxiety and mental health/distress. *Omega Journal of Death and Dying, 22,* 13–24.

Woody, S., Steketee, G., & Chambless, D. (1994). Measures for obsessive-compulsive disorder: The Yale–Brown Obsessive Compulsive Scale and the Symptom Checklist-90-R. Unpublished manuscript.

Zilberg, N. J., Weiss, D. S.., & Horowitz, M. J. (1982). Impact of Event Scale: A cross-validation study and some empirical evidence supporting a conceptual model of stress response syndromes. *Journal of Consulting and Clinical Psychology, 50,* 407–414.

Chapter 7

Somatoform Disorders and Measurement of Pain and Related Phenomena

ILLNESS BEHAVIOUR QUESTIONNAIRE

Purpose and Development

This 62-item self-report measure developed by Pilowsky and Spence (1983) assesses seven aspects of abnormal illness behavior: hypochondriasis, disease conviction, psychological versus somatic concerns, affective inhibition, affective disturbance, denial, and irritability. Lloyd (1990) suggested that the scale be used to evaluate clients in whom there is a discrepancy between medical disorder and behavioral response. An earlier version of the seven subscales was derived from a factor analysis of pain patients' and psychiatric clients' responses to 52 items asking about attitudes, feelings, and perceptions relating to illness (Pilowsky & Spence, 1975). Also embedded in the questionnaire was a second measure of hypochondriasis, the Whitley Index. Because this scale seems to measure essentially the same phenomena as the general Hypochondriasis subscale of the questionnaire, no more mention will be made of the Whitley Index in this review. The 62-item questionnaire was developed by adding items to the earlier, 52-item version of the questionnaire so that all subscales consist of at least five items (Pilowsky, 1993; Pilowsky & Spence, 1983). Factor analytic studies of the questionnaire (Main & Waddell, 1987; Pilowsky, 1993; Pilowsky & Spence, 1983; Zonderman, Heft & Costa, 1985) have to varying degrees confirmed the separateness of the seven subscales.

Administration and Scoring

Respondents indicate "yes" or "no" whether each of the 62 items apply to them. Items 4, 7, 8, 16, 22, 27, 31, 35, 43, 46, 58, and 60 are reverse coded. The Hypochondriasis subscale consists of the sum of items 9, 20, 21, 24, 29, 30, 32, 37, and 38. Scores on this subscale can range from 0 to 9, with higher scores indicating phobic concerns about health. The Disease Conviction subscale consists of items 2, 3, 7, 10, 35, and 41. Scores on this subscale can range from 0 to 6, with higher scores indicating an affirmation of the existence of disease and preoccupation with symptoms. The Psychological versus Somatic Concerns subscale consists of items 11, 16, 44, 46, and 57. Scores on this subscale can range form 0 to 5, with high scores indicating that the individual feels responsible for his or her illness and feels the need for psychological treatment for the illness. The Affective Inhibition subscale consists of items 22, 36, 53, 58, and 62. Scores on this subscale can range form 0 to 5, with high scores indicating difficulty in expressing personal feelings. The Affective Disturbance subscale consists of items 12, 18, 47, 54, and 59. Scores on this subscale can range from 0 to 5, with high scores indicating feelings of anxiety or sadness. The Denial subscale consists of items 27, 31, 43, 55, and 60. Scores on this subscale can range from 0 to 5, with high scores indicating denial of life problems and a tendency to blame all problems on the effects of illness. The Irritability subscale consists of items 4, 17, 51, 56, 61, and being less than 40 years of age (a point is given if the individual is less than 40). Scores on this scale can range from 0 to 6, with high scores indicating angry feelings and interpersonal friction.

Sample Scores

Pilowsky (1992) and Pilowsky and Spence (1983) collected extensive normative data for the questionnaire from pain clinic patients, other medical patients, and psychiatric clients. Table 1 presents the scores Pilowsky (1992) collected from 826 pain clinic patients and 750 psychiatric inpatients as well as the scores Pilowsky and Spence (1983) collected from two samples of 153 and 77 general medical practice patients. For more sample scores see Pilowsky (1992) and Pilowsky and Spence (1983).

Reliability

Pilowsky and Spence (1983) assessed the test–retest reliability of the scale by asking respondents to complete the questionnaire again a week to 12 weeks after the first administration. They found test–retest reliabilities of .87 for the Hypochondriasis subscale, .76 for the Disease Conviction

TABLE 1
Scores on the Illness Behaviour Questionnaire

Group	Hypochondriasis		Disease conviction		Psychological vs. somatic		Affective inhibition		Affective disturbance		Denial		Irritability	
	M	SD	M	SD	M	SD	M	SD	M	SD	M	SD	M	SD
Pain clinic patients (Pilowsky, 1992)	1.83	1.97	3.61	1.56	.68	.92	2.56	1.65	2.67	1.79	3.73	1.47	2.67	2.02
Adelaide general practice (Pilowsky, 1983)	1.42	1.84	1.58	1.37	2.01	.80	2.46	1.57	2.33	1.64	2.91	1.73	2.81	1.60
Seattle general practice (Pilowsky, 1983)	1.14	1.23	1.54	1.25	1.93	.99	2.00	1.53	1.93	1.61	1.98	1.51	1.55	1.19
Psychiatric clients (Pilowsky, 1992)	3.13	2.41	3.39	1.68	2.10	1.30	3.10	1.56	3.64	1.57	2.75	1.68	3.05	1.92

subscale, .76 for the Psychological versus Somatic Concerns subscale, .67 for the Affective Inhibition subscale, .87 for the Affective Disturbance subscale, .86 for the Denial subscale, and .84 for the Irritability subscale.

Validity

Pilowsky and Spence (1983) asked the spouses of patients to use the questionnaire to rate the patients and asked these same patients to rate themselves. They found a significant correlation between the spouses' ratings and the patients' ratings for each of the seven subscales. Wilson-Barnett and Trimble (1985) found neuroticism and depression were related to lower scores on denial and higher scores on each of the other subscales. Pilowsky and Spence (1983) also found a high correlation between patients' scores on the Affective Disturbance subscale and their scores on two different measures of depression.

Pilowsky and Spence (1983) compared the scores of pain clinic patients to the scores of general medical practice patients and psychiatric clients. As they had predicted, the pain clinic patients scored higher than the general medical practice patients on the Hypochondriasis, Disease Conviction, and Denial subscales and lower on the Psychological versus Somatic Focus subscale. The pain clinic patients also scored higher than the psychiatric clients on the Disease Conviction and Denial subscales and lower on the Hypochondriasis, Psychological versus Somatic Focus, Affective Inhibition, and Affective Disturbance subscales. Wilson-Barnett and Trimble (1985) found that the Affective Inhibition, Affective Disturbance, Denial, and Irritability subscales distinguished between clients with hysteria, neurological disorders, and psychiatric disorders. However, there was no difference between the groups on the Hypochondriasis, Disease Conviction, or Psychological versus Somatic subscales. Another study also found that the Affective Disturbance and Affective Inhibition subscales distinguished between pain patients with or without a psychiatric diagnosis, but that the other subscales did not differentiate between them (Tyrer, Capon, Peterson, Charlton, & Thompson, 1989).

The Disease Conviction and Hypochondriasis scales seem to be most important for treatment outcome. Waddell et al. (1989) found that the Disease Conviction scores of surgical patients who improved after surgery differed from those who did not improve, but did not find differences on the remaining subscales. In a study of the effectiveness of different treatments for chronic pain, pretreatment scores on the Disease Conviction and Hypochondriasis subscale scores predicted treatment outcome.

ILLNESS BEHAVIOUR QUESTIONNAIRE

Here are some questions about you and your illness. Circle either "Yes" or "No" to indicate your answer to each question.

Yes No 1. Do you worry a lot about your health?

Yes No 2. Do you think there is something seriously wrong with your body?

Yes No 3. Does your illness interfere with your life a great deal?

Yes No 4. Are you easy to get on with when you are ill?

Yes No 5. Does your family have a history of illness?

Yes No 6. Do you think you are more liable to illness than other people?

Yes No 7. If the doctor told you that he could find nothing wrong with you would you believe him?

Yes No 8. Is it easy for you to forget about yourself and think about all sorts of other things?

Yes No 9. If you feel ill and someone tells you that you are looking better, do you become annoyed?

Yes No 10. Do you find that you are often aware of various things happening in your body?

Yes No 11. Do you ever think of your illness as a punishment for something you have done wrong in the past?

Yes No 12. Do you have trouble with your nerves?

Yes No 13. If you feel ill or worried, can you be easily cheered up by the doctor?

Yes No 14. Do you think that other people realize what it's like to be sick?

Yes No 15. Does it upset you to talk to the doctor about your illness?

Yes No 16. Are you bothered by many pains and aches?

Yes No 17. Does your illness affect the way you get on with your family or friends a great deal?

Yes No 18. Do you find that you get anxious easily?

Yes No 19. Do you know anybody who has had the same illness as you?

Yes No 20. Are you more sensitive to pain than other people?

Yes No 21. Are you afraid of illness?

Yes No 22. Can you express your personal feelings easily to other people?

Yes No 23. Do people feel sorry for you when you are ill?

→

Yes No 24. Do you think that you worry about your health more than most people?

Yes No 25. Do you find that your illness affects your sexual relations?

Yes No 26. Do you experience a lot of pain with your illness?

Yes No 27. Except for your illness, do you have any problems in your life?

Yes No 28. Do you care whether or not people realize you are sick?

Yes No 29. Do you find that you get jealous of other people's good health?

Yes No 30. Do you ever have silly thoughts about your health which you can't get out of your mind, no matter how hard you try?

Yes No 31. Do you have any financial problems?

Yes No 32. Are you upset by the way people take your illness?

Yes No 33. Is it hard for you to believe the doctor when he tells you there is nothing for you to worry about?

Yes No 34. Do you often worry about the possibility that you have got a serious illness?

Yes No 35. Are you sleeping well?

Yes No 36. When you are angry, do you tend to bottle up your feelings?

Yes No 37. Do you often think that you might suddenly fall ill?

Yes No 38. If a disease is brought to your attention (through the radio, television, newspapers, or someone you know) do you worry about getting it yourself?

Yes No 39. Do you get the feeling that people are not taking your illness seriously enough?

Yes No 40. Are you upset by the appearance of your face or body?

Yes No 41. Do you find that you are bothered by many different symptoms?

Yes No 42. Do you frequently try to explain to others how you are feeling?

Yes No 43. Do you have any family problems?

Yes No 44. Do you think there is something the matter with your mind?

Yes No 45. Are you eating well?

Yes No 46. Is your bad health the biggest difficulty of your life?

Yes No 47. Do you find that you get sad easily?

Yes No 48. Do you worry or fuss over small details that seem unimportant to others?

Yes No 49. Are you always a cooperative patient?

Yes No 50. Do you often have the symptoms of a very serious disease?

Yes No 51. Do you find that you get angry easily?
Yes No 52. Do you have any work problems?
Yes No 53. Do you prefer to keep your feelings to yourself?
Yes No 54. Do you often find that you get depressed?
Yes No 55. Would all your worries he over if you were physically healthy?
Yes No 56. Are you more irritable toward other people?
Yes No 57. Do you think that your symptoms may be caused by worry?
Yes No 58. Is it easy for you to let people know when you are cross with them?
Yes No 59. Is it hard for you to relax?
Yes No 60. Do you have personal worries which are not caused by physical illness?
Yes No 61. Do you often find that you lose patience with other people?
Yes No 62. Is it hard for you to show people your personal feelings?

Reprinted with permission of Dr. I. Pilowsky.

WEST HAVEN–YALE MULTIDIMENSIONAL PAIN INVENTORY

Purpose and Development

The West Haven–Yale Multidimensional Pain Inventory assesses psychosocial variables related to the experience of chronic pain. This 52-item, 12 subscale, self-report measure developed by Kerns, Turk, and Rudy (1985) has the following three parts: Part I, which assesses perceived interference of pain in important realms of life, support and concern from others, pain severity, control over daily living, and affective distress; Part II, which assesses others' responses to complaints about pain; and Part III, which assesses participation in common daily activities. Kerns et al. (1985) developed the items on the basis of theoretical models, interviews with those close to chronic pain patients, and previously used lists of activities and goals. Factor analytic studies confirmed the item selection for the subscales in Part I and determined the final item selection for the subscales in Parts II and III.

Administration and Scoring

Respondents rate all items on 7-point scales of severity or frequency. The scores may be used in two ways. Subscale scores give insight into an individual's pain experience. The calculation of subscale scores is explained below. Also, Turk and Rudy (1988, 1990) developed a profile of scores that divides pain sufferers into the categories of Dysfunctional, Interpersonally Distressed, and Adaptive Copers. A detailed explanation of the classification process is beyond the scope of this review, and the reader is referred to the articles by Turk and Rudy (1988, 1990) for further information.

Subscale scores are calculated by summing items and then dividing by the number of items. Item 6 in Part I is reverse scored. The "effect of pain" subscales in Part I are as follows: Interference (items 2, 3, 4, 8, 9, 13, 14, 17, and 19), Support (items 5, 10, and 15), Pain Severity (items 1, 7, and 12), Life-Control (items 11 and 16), and Affective Distress (items 6, 18, and 20).

The "other's responses" subscales in Part II are as follows: Negative Responses (items 1, 4, 7, and 10), Solicitous Responses (items 2, 5, 8, 11, 13, and 14), and Distracting Responses (items 3, 6, 9, and 12).

The "participation in activities" subscales in Part III are as follows: Household Chores (items 1, 5, 9, 13, and 17), Outdoor Work (items 2, 6, 10, 14, and 18), Activities Away from Home (items 3, 7, 11, and 15), and Social

Activities (items 4, 8, 12, and 16). A General Activities score may be obtained by summing all items in this section and dividing by 18.

Sample Scores

Kerns and Haythornthwaite (1988) reported scale scores, except for Affective Distress Scores, for chronic pain patients who had been referred to a rehabilitation program. Table 1 shows the average scores for 43 nondepressed and 46 depressed individuals from this group.

Reliability

Kerns et al. (1985) explored the internal consistency of the subscales in a sample of chronic pain patients and found the five scales in Part I had alphas ranging from .72 to .90, the three scales in Part II had alphas ranging from .74 to .84, and the four scales in Part III had alphas ranging from .70 to .86. When they asked patients to fill the scale out twice at two-week intervals, they found test–retest reliability of .69 to .86 for the scales in Part I, .62 to .89 for the scales in Part II, and .83 to .91 for the scales in Part III.

Validity

In a sample of chronic pain patients Kearns et al. (1985) found that scores on the Affective and Control scales were associated with measures

TABLE 1
Scores on the West Haven–Yale Multidimensional
Pain Inventory (Kerns & Haythornthwaite, 1990)

	Nondepressed	Depressed
Interference	3.22 ± 1.40	4.36 ± .97
Support	4.31 ± 1.47	3.86 ± 1.40
Pain severity	3.44 ± 1.14	3.94 ± .99
Life control	4.51 ± 1.07	2.33 ± 1.47
Negative responses	.75 ± .84	1.53 ± 1.14
Solicitous responses	2.71 ± 1.13	2.42 ± 1.17
Distracting responses	1.66 ± .92	1.62 ± 1.14
Household chores	2.53 ± 1.33	2.46 ± 1.42
Outdoor work	1.12 ± 1.00	.88 ± .89
Activities away from home	1.98 ± .68	1.46 ± .80
Social activities	2.27 ± .84	1.62 ± .98

Values are Mean ± SD.

of depression and anxiety. Scores on the Solicitous Responses, Distracting Responses, Support Responses, and Punishing Responses scales were associated with a measure of marital satisfaction. Scores on the Pain Severity and Interference scales were associated with another measure of pain intensity.

Two studies which examined the relationship between chronic pain patients' responses on the scales of Part II of the questionnaire and the severity of their pain found that the Negative and Solicitous scale scores were related to pain severity (Flor, Kerns, & Turk, 1987; Kerns, Haythornthwaite, Southwick, & Giller, 1990). Kerns, Southwick, Giller, Haythornthwaite, Jacob, and Rosenberg (1991) further found that scores on the Solicitous, Distracting, and Negative Responses scales were related to the type of pain behavior chronic pain patients manifest.

In a sample of chronic pain patients going through a rehabilitation program that taught coping skills, Kerns and Haythornthwaite (1988) found significant decreases on the Pain Severity, Distracting Responses, and Interference scales but not on the other scales.

Kerns and Jacob (1992) reviewed a number of studies that tested an empirically derived taxonomy of chronic pain patients. Three reliable categories—dysfunctional, interpersonally distressed, and adaptive copers—were identified and validated in patient groups with various types of pain.

WEST HAVEN–YALE MULTIDIMENSIONAL PAIN INVENTORY

SECTION 1

In the following 20 questions, you will be asked to describe your pain and how it affects your life. Under each question is a scale to record your answer. Read each question carefully and then *circle* a number on the scale under that question to indicate how that specific question applies to you.

1. Rate the level of your pain at the present moment.

   0   1   2   3   4   5   6
   No pain   Very intense pain

2. In general, how much does your pain problem interfere with your day-to-day activities?

   0   1   2   3   4   5   6
   No interference   Extreme interference

3. Since the time you developed a pain problem, how much has your pain changed your ability to work?

   0   1   2   3   4   5   6
   No change   Extreme change

   _____ Check here, if you have retired for reasons other than your pain problem.

4. How much has your pain changed the amount of satisfaction or enjoyment you get from participating in social and recreational activities?

   0   1   2   3   4   5   6
   No change   Extreme change

5. How supportive or helpful is your spouse (significant other) to you in relation to your pain?

   0   1   2   3   4   5   6
   Not at all supportive   Extremely supportive

6. Rate your overall mood during the *past week*.

   0   1   2   3   4   5   6
   Extremely low mood   Extremely high mood

→

7. On the average, how severe has your pain been during the *last week*?

0	1	2	3	4	5	6
Not at all severe					Extremely severe	

8. How much has your pain changed your ability to participate in recreational and other social activities?

0	1	2	3	4	5	6
No change					Extreme change	

9. How much has your pain changed the amount of satisfaction you get from family-related activities?

0	1	2	3	4	5	6
No change					Extreme change	

10. How worried is your spouse (significant other) about you in relation to your pain problem?

0	1	2	3	4	5	6
Not at all worried					Extremely worried	

11. During the *past week*, how much control do you feel that you have over your life?

0	1	2	3	4	5	6
Not at all in control					Extremely in control	

12. How much *suffering* do you experience because of your pain?

0	1	2	3	4	5	6
No suffering					Extreme suffering	

13. How much has your pain changed your marriage and other family relationships?

0	1	2	3	4	5	6
No change					Extreme change	

14. How much has your pain changed the amount of satisfaction or enjoyment you get from work?

0	1	2	3	4	5	6
No change					Extreme change	

_____ Check here, if you are not presently working.

15. How attentive is your spouse (significant other) to your pain problem?

0	1	2	3	4	5	6
Not at all attentive					Extremely attentive	

16. During the *past week*, how much do you feel that you've been able to deal with your problems?

0	1	2	3	4	5	6
Not at all					Extremely well	

17. How much has your pain changed your ability to do household chores?

0	1	2	3	4	5	6
No change					Extreme change	

18. During the past week, how irritable have you been?

0	1	2	3	4	5	6
Not at all irritable					Extremely irritable	

19. How much has your pain changed your friendships with people other than your family?

0	1	2	3	4	5	6
No change					Extreme change	

20. During the *past week*, how tense or anxious you been?

0	1	2	3	4	5	6
Not at all tense or anxious					Extremely tense or anxious	

SECTION 2

In this section, we are interested in knowing how your spouse (significant other) responds to you when he or she knows that you are in pain. On the scale listed below each question, *circle* a number to indicate *how often* your spouse (or significant other) generally responds to you in that particular way *when you are in pain*. Please answer *all* of the 14 questions.

Please identify the relationship between you and the person you are thinking of. _____

→

1. Ignores me.

0	1	2	3	4	5	6
Never						Very often

2. Asks me what he/she can do to help.

0	1	2	3	4	5	6
Never						Very often

3. Reads to me.

0	1	2	3	4	5	6
Never						Very often

4. Expresses irritation at me.

0	1	2	3	4	5	6
Never						Very often

5. Takes over my jobs or duties.

0	1	2	3	4	5	6
Never						Very often

6. Talks to me about something else to take my mind off the pain.

0	1	2	3	4	5	6
Never						Very often

7. Expresses frustration at me.

0	1	2	3	4	5	6
Never						Very often

8. Tries to get me to rest.

0	1	2	3	4	5	6
Never						Very often

9. Tries to involve me in some activity.

0	1	2	3	4	5	6
Never						Very often

10. Expresses anger at me.

0	1	2	3	4	5	6
Never						Very often

11. Gets me some pain medications.

0	1	2	3	4	5	6
Never						Very often

12. Encourages me to work on a hobby.

0	1	2	3	4	5	6
Never						Very often

13. Gets me something to eat or drink.

0	1	2	3	4	5	6
Never						Very often

14. Turns on the TV to take my mind off my pain.

0	1	2	3	4	5	6
Never						Very often

SECTION 3

Listed below are 18 common daily activities. Please indicate *how often* you do each of these activities by *circling* a number on the scale listed below each activity. Please complete *all* 18 questions.

1. Wash dishes.

0	1	2	3	4	5	6
Never						Very often

2. Mow the lawn.

0	1	2	3	4	5	6
Never						Very often

3. Go out to eat.

0	1	2	3	4	5	6
Never						Very often

→

4. Play cards or other games.

0	1	2	3	4	5	6
Never						Very often

5. Go grocery shopping.

0	1	2	3	4	5	6
Never						Very often

6. Work in the garden.

0	1	2	3	4	5	6
Never						Very often

7. Go to a movie.

0	1	2	3	4	5	6
Never						Very often

8. Visit friends.

0	1	2	3	4	5	6
Never						Very often

9. Help with the house cleaning.

0	1	2	3	4	5	6
Never						Very often

10. Work on the car.

0	1	2	3	4	5	6
Never						Very often

11. Take a ride in a car.

0	1	2	3	4	5	6
Never						Very often

12. Visit relatives.

0	1	2	3	4	5	6
Never						Very often

13. Prepare a meal.

0	1	2	3	4	5	6
Never						Very often

14. Wash the car.

0	1	2	3	4	5	6
Never						Very often

15. Take a trip.

0	1	2	3	4	5	6
Never						Very often

16. Go to a park or beach.

0	1	2	3	4	5	6
Never						Very often

17. Do a load of laundry.

0	1	2	3	4	5	6
Never						Very often

18. Work on a needed house repair.

0	1	2	3	4	5	6
Never						Very often

Reprinted with permission of Dr. Robert Kerns, Dr. Dennis Turk, and Dr. Thomas Rudy.

MCGILL PAIN QUESTIONNAIRE, LONG-FORM AND SHORT-FORM

Purpose and Development

The McGill Pain Questionnaire is a four-part interview developed by Ronald Melzack (1975) to assess the subjective experience of pain. On the basis of the clinical literature, Melzack generated a large number of pain descriptors which he then asked patients to classify into the following qualities of pain: sensory, affective, and evaluative. The descriptors within each subclass were rated by medical personnel on intensity of pain described and the final descriptors were selected on the basis of these ratings. Although the results of early factor analytic studies provided only partial support for distinct sensory, affective, and evaluative dimensions of the Pain Rating Index portion of the questionnaire, later more statistically sophisticated factor analytic studies have found factors confirming the three dimensions (Lowe, Walker, & McCallum, 1991; Turk, Rudy, & Salovey, 1985).

The questionnaire is widely used and has become the standard in the field of pain assessment (e.g., Melzack & Katz, 1992; Culpepper, 1992). It has been translated into numerous languages including Arabic, Chinese, Flemish, Finnish, French, German, Italian, Japanese, Norwegian, Polish, Slovak, and Spanish (Melzack & Katz, 1992).

For the Short-Form McGill Pain Questionnaire, Melzack (1987) selected the 15 most frequently endorsed pain descriptors from the longer McGill Pain Questionnaire. The descriptors were the ones chosen by 33% or more of patients with a variety of pain syndromes. English, French, and Czech versions of the short form are available (Melzack, 1987; Melzack and Katz, 1992).

Administration and Scoring

The interviewer asks the patient to indicate where pain is located using an anatomical drawing, identify those pain descriptors that describe his or her present pain, describe the pattern of pain, and indicate the strength of the pain. If a word is not in a patient's vocabulary the interviewer defines it, and if a patient wishes, the interviewer rereads words. Melzack (1975) reports that beginners take 15–20 minutes to administer the questionnaire and those who are experienced in its use take 5–10 minutes.

Seven scores may be derived from the questionnaire (Melzack & Katz, 1992). Five scores may be obtained from the Pain Rating Index, which is based on the pain value of the words selected. The first word in a cluster has a value of "1," the second word a value of "2," and so on. The sum of these rank values for the 20 clusters is the total Pain Rating Index. Subscores may be derived by summing ratings for clusters 1–10 for the Sensory Pain Rating, clusters 11–15 for the Affective Pain Rating, cluster 16 for the Evaluative Pain Rating, and clusters 17–20 for a Miscellaneous Pain Rating. The total number of words chosen is a sixth way of quantifying pain. Finally, the 0 to 5 rating on the Present Pain Intensity question provides a seventh measure of pain. For all subscales higher scores indicate more pain.

For the short form the interviewer reads each pain descriptor to the respondent and asks the respondent to rate the intensity of that particular quality of pain on a 0–3 scale. Respondents are also asked to indicate their overall level of pain on a visual analog item and a 0–5 rating of present pain intensity. A total pain descriptor score may be obtained by summing the responses to the 15 descriptor items. Scores on this may range from 0 to 45. Items 1 through 11 tap the sensory dimension of pain and a Sensory subscale score may be derived by summing these items. Scores on the Sensory subscale may range from 0 to 33. Items 12–15 tap the affective dimension of pain and an Affective subscale score may be derived by summing these items. Scores on the Affective subscale may range from 0 to 12. The visual analog item and the present pain intensity item are used as single item subscales.

Sample Scores

Wilkie, Savedra, Holzemer, Tesler, and Paul (1990) established comprehensive norms for the long-form questionnaire on the basis of a meta-analysis of 51 studies using a total of 3,624 subjects with a variety of painful conditions. These included cancer, low back pain, chronic pain of various origins, postsurgical pain, labor pain, dental pain, and experimentally induced pain. The number of individuals in each type of pain ranged from 340 to 797. Table 1 shows the average scores.

Melzack (1987) gave the English-language version of the short form to 27 postsurgical patients, 20 women with labor pains, and 10 patients with musculoskeletal pain. He asked them to complete the questionnaire before and after they were given relief from pain through drugs or transcutaneous electrical nerve stimulation. Table 2 shows the average scores.

Reliability

Melzack (1975) gave patients the long-form questionnaire three times at intervals of 3 to 7 days and found that there was a consistency of 70.3% in the pain clusters chosen at different administrations. Another group of chronic pain patients, who completed the long-form questionnaire twice at

TABLE 1

Scores on the Long-Form McGill Pain Questionnaire for Medical Patients
with Different Types of Pain (Wilkie et al., 1990)

Type of pain	Total index M	Sensory M	Affective M	Evaluative M	Miscel- laneous M	Number of words M	Present pain M
Cancer	24.0	12.1	4.8	2.7	4.5	9.3	2.2
Low back	27.9	16.3	5.5	2.4	5.6	9.7	2.3
Chronic	25.4	15.2	3.8	2.7	5.4	11.0	2.6
Postsurgical	20.5	14.2	2.3	2.3	3.9	9.0	1.6
Labor	24.7	16.3	2.7	2.2	5.1	6.9	2.4
Dental	17.8	10.7	1.8	2.5	3.8	8.2	2.2
Induced	19.5	12.1	1.5	2.6	5.6	8.6	2.2

intervals of several days, had test–retest reliabilities of .83 for the total Pain Rating Index, .76 for the Sensory Pain Rating, .78 for the Affective Pain Rating, and .47 for the Evaluative Pain Rating (Love, Leboeuf, & Crisp, 1989).

Validity

Melzack and others have found that the long-form questionnaire is sensitive to changes in pain due to treatment (Melzack, 1975; Melzack &

TABLE 2

Scores on the Short-Form McGill Pain Questionnaire for Medical Patients
with Different Types of Pain before and after Pain Relief (Melzack, 1987)

Type of pain	Total M	Total SD	Sensory M	Sensory SD	Affective M	Affective SD	Present pain M	Present pain SD	Visual analog M	Visual analog SD
Posturgical										
before	15.4	9.6	11.7	7.2	3.7	3.5	2.6	.9	5.2	2.3
after	9.1	9.7	6.9	7.3	2.2	2.8	1.5	1.1	2.4	1.8
Labor										
before	17.2	11.0	13.4	7.8	3.9	3.9	2.5	1.1	5.0	2.3
after	1.1	2.4	1.0	2.0	.2	.5	.4	.6	.5	.9
Musculoskeletal										
before	15.7	11.9	11.1	8.7	4.6	3.7	2.3	1.0	4.1	1.6
after	4.3	4.9	3.3	3.3	1.0	1.7	1.3	1.0	2.0	1.3

Katz, 1992). Melzack and Katz (1992) reviewed a number of studies that found the long-form questionnaire is able to differentiate between different types of pain syndromes. For example, different response patterns distinguish patients who have clear physical causes of low back pain versus those who do not, patients who have reversible versus irreversible damage to nerve fibers in a tooth, patients who have leg pain caused by diabetic neuropathy versus leg pain from other causes, and patients with trigeminal neuralgia versus atypical facial pain.

Melzack (1987) found that each subscale score as well as total scores of the Short-Form McGill Pain Questionnaire were highly correlated with corresponding scale scores on the longer version of the questionnaire.

In samples of patients with different types of pain, Melzack (1987), Guieu, Tardy-Gervet, and Roll (1991), and Stelian, Gil, Habot, Rosenthal, Abramovici, Kutok, and Khahil (1992) found that each subscale score as well as total scores on the Short-Form McGill Pain Questionnaire decreased significantly when pain relief was provided to patients. In their review of the questionnaire Melzack and Katz (1992) conclude that the questionnaire can also distinguish between different pain syndromes.

MCGILL PAIN QUESTIONNAIRE

Summary Scores

Pain Rating Index:

Total _____
(1–20)

Sensory _____	Affective _____	Evaluative _____	Miscellaneous _____
(1–10)	(11–15)	(16)	(17–19)

Total Number of Words Chosen: _____
Present Pain Intensity: _____

Clusters

1. Flickering	_____	Scalding	_____	15. Wretched	_____
Quivering	_____	Searing	_____	Blinding	_____
Pulsing	_____	8. Tingling	_____	16. Annoying	_____
Throbbing	_____	Itchy	_____	Troublesome	
Beating	_____	Smarting	_____		_____
Pounding	_____	Stinging	_____	Miserable	_____
2. Jumping	_____	9. Dull	_____	Intense	_____
Flashing	_____	Sore	_____	Unbearable	_____
Shooting	_____	Hurting	_____	17. Spreading	_____
3. Pricking	_____	Aching	_____	Radiating	_____
Boring	_____	Heavy	_____	Penetrating	_____
Drilling	_____	10. Tender	_____	Piercing	_____
Stabbing	_____	Taut	_____	18. Tight	_____
Lancinating	_____	Rasping	_____	Numb	_____
4. Sharp	_____	Splitting	_____	Drawing	_____
Cutting	_____	11. Tiring	_____	Squeezing	_____
Lacerating	_____	Exhausting	_____	Tearing	_____
5. Pinching	_____	12. Sickening	_____	19. Cool	_____
Pressing	_____	Suffocating	_____	Cold	_____
Gnawing	_____	13. Fearful	_____	Freezing	_____
Cramping	_____	Frightful	_____	20. Nagging	_____
Crushing	_____	Terrifying	_____	Nauseating	_____
6. Tugging	_____	14. Punishing	_____	Agonizing	_____
Pulling	_____	Grueling	_____	Dreadful	_____
Wrenching	_____	Cruel	_____	Torturing	_____
7. Hot	_____	Vicious	_____		
Burning	_____	Killing	_____		

Present Pain Intensity	*Pattern of Pain*	*Anatomical Location of Pain*

0 = No pain   _____
1 = Mild   _____
2 = Discomforting   _____
3 = Distressing   _____
4 = Horrible   _____
5 = Excruciating   _____

Brief   _____
Periodic   _____
Constant   _____

Please mark, on the drawing below, the areas where you feel pain. Put E if external, or I if internal, near the areas which you mark.

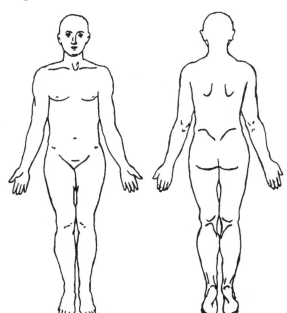

SHORT-FORM McGILL PAIN QUESTIONNAIRE

Please rate each of the following qualities of pain on the scale of "none," "mild," "moderate," or "severe."

	None	Mild	Moderate	Severe
1. Throbbing	0) ____	1) ____	2) ____	3) ____
2. Shooting	0) ____	1) ____	2) ____	3) ____
3. Stabbing	0) ____	1) ____	2) ____	3) ____
4. Sharp	0) ____	1) ____	2) ____	3) ____
5. Cramping	0) ____	1) ____	2) ____	3) ____
6. Gnawing	0) ____	1) ____	2) ____	3) ____
7. Hot–Burning	0) ____	1) ____	2) ____	3) ____
8. Aching	0) ____	1) ____	2) ____	3) ____
9. Heavy	0) ____	1) ____	2) ____	3) ____
10. Tender	0) ____	1) ____	2) ____	3) ____
11. Splitting	0) ____	1) ____	2) ____	3) ____
12. Tiring/Exhausting	0) ____	1) ____	2) ____	3) ____
13. Sickening	0) ____	1) ____	2) ____	3) ____
14. Fearful	0) ____	1) ____	2) ____	3) ____
15. Punishing/Cruel	0) ____	1) ____	2) ____	3) ____

Present Pain Index

0   No pain   ____
1   Mild   ____
2   Discomforting ____
3   Distressing   ____
4   Horrible   ____
5   Excruciating   ____

Visual Analog Scale

No pain   Worst possible pain

REFERENCES

Culpepper, L. (1992). Symptoms: Measures of the mind. In M. A. Stewart, F. Tudiver, M. J. Bass, E. V. Dunn, & P. G. Norton (Eds.) *Tools for Primary Care Research* (pp. 113–123). Newbury Park, CA: Sage.

Flor, H., Kerns, R. D., & Turk, D. C. (1987). The role of spouse reinforcement, perceived pain, and activity levels of chronic pain patients. *Journal of Psychosomatic Research, 31,* 251–259.

Guieu, R., Tardy-Gervet, M., & Roll, J. (1991). Analgesic effects of vibration and trans-cutaneous electrical nerve stimulation applied separately and simultaneously to patients with chronic pain. *Canadian Journal of Neurological Science, 18,* 113–119.

Kerns, R. D., & Jacob, M. C. (1992). Assessment of the psychosocial context of pain. In D. Turk & R. Melzack (Eds.), *Handbook of Pain Assessment* (pp. 235–253). New York: Guilford Press.

Kerns, R. D., & Haythornthwaite, J. (1988). Depression among chronic pain patients: Cognitive-behavioral analysis and rehabilitation outcome. *Journal of Consulting and Clinical Psychology, 56,* 870–876.

Kerns, R. D., Haythornthwaite, J., Southwick, S., & Giller, E. L. (1990). The role of marital interaction in chronic pain and depressive symptom severity. *Journal of Psychosomatic Research, 34,* 401–408.

Kerns, R. D., Southwick, S., Giller, E. L., Haythornthwaite, J. A., Jacob, M. C., & Rosenberg, R. (1991). The relationship between reports of pain-related social interactions and expressions of pain and affective distress. *Behavior Therapy, 22,* 101–111.

Kerns, R. D., Turk, D. C., & Rudy, T. E. (1985). The West Haven-Yale Multidimensional Pain Inventory (WHYMPI). *Pain, 23,* 345–356.

Lloyd, G. G. (1990). Adjustment to illness. In S. F. Peck & C. M. Shapiro (Eds.), *Measuring Human Problems* (pp. 177–192). New York: John Wiley & Sons.

Love, A., Leboeuf, C., & Crisp, T. C. (1989). Chiropractic chronic low back pain sufferers and self-report assessment methods. Part I. A reliability study of the Visual Analog Scale, the Pain Drawing, and the McGill Pain Questionnaire. *Journal of Manipulative and Physiological Therapeutics, 12,* 21–25.

Lowe, N. K., Walker, S. N., & McCallum, R. C. (1991). Confirming the theoretical structure of the McGill Pain Questionnaire in acute clinical pain. *Pain, 46,* 53–60.

Main, C. J., & Waddell, G. (1987). Psychometric construction and validity of the Pilowsky Illness Behavior Questionnaire in British patients with chronic low back pain. *Pain, 28,* 13–26.

Melzack, R. (1975). The McGill Pain Questionnaire: Major properties and scoring methods. *Pain, 1,* 275–299.

Melzack, R. (1987). The Short-Form McGill Pain Questionnaire. *Pain, 30,* 191–197.

Melzack, R., & Katz, J. (1992). The McGill Pain Questionnaire: Appraisal and current status. In D. Turk & R. Melzack (Eds.), *Handbook of Pain Assessment* (pp. 152–108). New York: Guilford Press.

Pilowsky, I. (1992). *Manual for the Illness Behavior Questionnaire (IBQ): Recent Normative Data on General Hospital Psychiatric Inpatients and Pain Clinic Patients.* Adelaide: University of Adelaide.

Pilowsky, I. (1993). Dimensions of illness behaviour as measured by the Illness Behaviour Questionnaire: A replication study. *Journal of Psychosomatic Research, 37,* 53–62.

Pilowsky, I., & Barrow, C. G. (1990). A controlled study of psychotherapy and amitriptyline used individually and in combination in the treatment of chronic intractable, 'psychogenic' pain. *Pain, 40,* 3–19.

Pilowsky, I., & Spence, N. D. (1975). Patterns of illness behavior in patients with intractable pain. *Journal of Psychosomatic Research, 19,* 279–287.

Pilowsky, I., & Spence, N. D. (1983). *Manual for the Illness Behavior Questionnaire (IBQ).* Adelaide: University of Adelaide.

Stelian, J., Gil, I., Habot, B., Rosenthal, M., Abramovici, I., Kutok, N., & Khahil, A. (1992). Improvement of pain and disability in elderly patients with degenerative osteoarthritis of the knee treated with narrow-band light therapy. *Journal of the American Geriatrics Society, 40,* 23–26.

Turk, D. C., & Rudy, T. E. (1988). Toward an empirically derived taxonomy of chronic pain patients: Integration of psychological assessment data. *Journal of Consulting and Clinical Psychology, 56,* 233–238.

Turk, D. C., & Rudy, T. E. (1990). The robustness of an empirically derived taxonomy of chronic pain patients. *Pain, 43,* 27-36.

Turk, D. C., Rudy, T. E., & Salovey, P. (1985). The McGill Pain Questionnaire reconsidered: Confirming the factor structures and examining appropriate uses. *Pain, 21,* 385–397.

Tyrer, S. P., Capon, M., Peterson, D. M., Charlton, J. E., & Thompson, J. W. (1989). The detection of psychiatric illness and psychological handicaps in a British pain clinic population. *Pain, 36,* 63–74.

Waddell, G., Pilowsky, I., & Bond, M. R. (1989). Clinical assessment and interpretation of abnormal illness behavior in low back pain. *Pain, 39,* 41–51.

Wilkie, D. J., Savedra, M. C., Holzemer, W. L., Tesler, M. D., & Paul, S. M. (1990). Use of the McGill Pain Questionnaire to measure pain: A meta-analysis. *Nursing Research, 39,* 36–41.

Wilson-Barnett, J., & Trimble, M. R. (1985). An investigation of hysteria using the Illness Behavior Questionnaire. *British Journal of Psychiatry, 146,* 601–608.

Zonderman, A. B., Heft, M. W., & Costa, P. T. (1985). Does the Illness Behavior Questionnaire measure abnormal illness behavior? *Health Psychology, 4,* 425–436.

CHAPTER 8

Dissociative Disorders

DISSOCIATIVE EXPERIENCES SCALE

Purpose and Development

The Dissociative Experiences Scale measures the extent and frequency of dissociative experiences. The scale is a 28-item self-report measure developed by Bernstein and Putnam (1986). Bernstein and Putnam (1986) generated items based on interviews with individuals who had been diagnosed as having a dissociative disorder and consultation with clinicians experienced in the treatment of dissociative disorders. Pilot testing and further consultation with clinicians shaped the final version of the scale. Carlson and Putnam (1993) reported that a factor analytic study of the responses of psychiatric patients and nonpatients identified three main factors they described as (a) amnestic dissociation, (b) absorption and imaginative involvement, and (c) depersonalization and derealization. They reported that two other factor analytic studies that examined only the responses of nonpatients found three somewhat different factors.

The scale has been translated into a number of languages, including French, Spanish, Italian, Hindi, Cambodian, Hebrew, Japanese, Swedish, Norwegian, Czech, and German (Carlson & Putnam, 1993).

Administration and Scoring

Respondents are asked to indicate how frequently they have each of the experiences described on the scale. They give frequency ratings using an 11-point scale which ranges from 0% to 100%. The total scale score is the average of all 28 items.

Carlson and Putnam (1993) suggested that, as well as looking at the total scale score, clinicians may wish to ask clients follow-up questions for those items rated 20% or greater. They pointed out that the scale is best used as a measure of the extent of dissociative experiences rather than as a definitive diagnostic tool for identifying multiple personality disorder.

Sample Scores and Cutoff Scores

Bernstein and Putnam (1986) gave the scale to eight different groups of subjects. The median scale scores were 4.38 for 34 adults with no psychiatric diagnosis, 4.72 for 14 alcoholics, 6.04 for 24 phobic-anxious clients, 7.41 for 29 agoraphobics, 14.11 for 31 college students, 20.63 for 20 schizophrenics, 31.25 for 10 posttraumatic stress disorder clients, and 57.06 for 20 clients with multiple personality disorder.

In a sample of 1,051 psychiatric patients Carlson, Putnam, Ross, To-rem, Coons, Dill, Loewenstein, and Braun (1993) selected 30 as a cutoff score to identify individuals who may have a dissociative disorder or another disorder with substantial dissociative symptoms. A cutoff score of 30 correctly identified 74% of individuals who had a diagnosis of multiple personality disorder and correctly identified 80% of those who did not have a diagnosis of multiple personality disorder. Of the individuals who scored over the cutoff of 30 but did not have a diagnosis of multiple personality disorder, 61% had a dissociative disorder other than multiple personality disorder or had posttraumatic stress disorder.

Reliability

Carlson and Putnam (1993) summarized the results of studies examining the reliability of the Dissociative Experiences Scale. A study that examined internal consistency found Cronbach's alpha was .95. The two studies that examined split-half reliability found correlations of .83 and .93. The findings of the three studies that examined test–retest reliability ranged from a one month test–retest reliability of .96 to a six-week to two-month test–retest reliability of .79.

Validity

Two studies found a significant correlation between scores on the Dissociative Experiences Scale and scores on measures of perceptual alteration and absorption, which are dissociative-like experiences (Nadon, Hoyt, Register, & Kihlstrom, 1991; Frischholz, Braun, Sachs, Schwartz, Lewis, Shaeffer, Westergaard, & Pasquotto, 1991). Another study found that individuals who scored higher on the scale were much more likely to have had traumatic childhood experiences (Saxe, van der Kolk, Berkowitz, Chinman, Hall, Lieberg, & Schwartz, 1993).

Frischholz, Braun, Sachs, Schwartz, Lewis, Shaeffer, Westergaard, and Pasquotto (1992) found that individuals with higher scale scores were more susceptible to hypnotism, and Frischholz et al. (1991) also found that, as they had predicted, individuals who scored high on the scale had low tolerance of ambiguity.

Bernstein and Putnam (1986) compared the scores of individuals drawn from eight populations and found that individuals with diagnosis of multiple personality disorder and posttraumatic stress disorder scored significantly higher than individuals from the other groups and that individuals with multiple personality disorder scored significantly higher than individuals with posttraumatic stress disorder. Carlson and Putnam (1993) summarized the findings of nine other studies. In these studies adults in the general population had the lowest scores, individuals with psychiatric problems had somewhat elevated scores, individuals with posttraumatic stress disorder and dissociative disorders other than multiple personality disorder had higher scores, and individuals with multiple personality disorder had the highest scores. Carlson et al. (1993) found that individuals who scored at or above the cutoff of 30 were much more likely to have a diagnosis of multiple personality disorder than individuals who scored below the cutoff.

Reading Level

Paolo, Ryan, Dunn, & van Fleet (1993) found that a tenth- to eleventh-grade reading level is required to complete the scale.

DISSOCIATIVE EXPERIENCES SCALE

Directions: This questionnaire consists of twenty-eight questions about experiences that you may have in your daily life. We are interested in how often you have these experiences. It is important, however, that your answers show how often these experiences happen to you when you *are not* under the influence of alcohol or drugs. To answer the questions, please determine to what degree the experience described in the question applies to you and circle the number to show what percentage of the time you have the experience.

1. Some people have the experience of driving or riding in a car or bus or subway and suddenly realize that they don't remember what has happened during all or part of the trip. Circle a number to show what percentage of the time this happens to you.

   0%   10   20   30   40   50   60   70   80   90   100%

2. Some people find that sometimes they are listening to someone talk and suddenly realize that they did not hear part or all of what was said. Circle a number to show what percentage of the time this happens to you.

   0%   10   20   30   40   50   60   70   80   90   100%

3. Some people have the experience of finding themselves in a place and having no idea how they got there. Circle a number to show what percentage of the time this happens to you.

   0%   10   20   30   40   50   60   70   80   90   100%

4. Some people have the experience of finding themselves dressed in clothes that they don't remember putting on. Circle a number to show what percentage of the time this happens to you.

   0%   10   20   30   40   50   60   70   80   90   100%

5. Some people have the experience of finding new things among their belongings that they do not remember buying. Circle a number to show what percentage of the time this happens to you.

   0%   10   20   30   40   50   60   70   80   90   100%

6. Some people sometimes find that they are approached by people who they do not know who call them by another name or insist that they have met them before. Circle a number to show what percentage of the time this happens to you.

0%   10   20   30   40   50   60   70   80   90   100%

7. Some people sometimes have the experience of feeling as though they are standing next to themselves or watching themselves do something and they actually see themselves as if they were looking at another person. Circle a number to show what percentage of the time this happens to you.

0%   10   20   30   40   50   60   70   80   90   100%

8. Some people are told that they sometimes do not recognize friends or family members. Circle a number to show what percentage of the time this happens to you.

0%   10   20   30   40   50   60   70   80   90   100%

9. Some people find that they have no memory for some important events in their lives (for example, a wedding or graduation). Circle a number to show what percentage of the time this happens to you.

0%   10   20   30   40   50   60   70   80   90   100%

10. Some people have the experience of being accused of lying when they do not think that they have lied. Circle a number to show what percentage of the time this happens to you.

0%   10   20   30   40   50   60   70   80   90   100%

11. Some people have the experience of looking in a mirror and not recognizing themselves. Circle a number to show what percentage of the time this happens to you.

0%   10   20   30   40   50   60   70   80   90   100%

12. Some people have the experience of feeling that other people, objects, and the world around them are not real. Circle a number to show what percentage of the time this happens to you.

0%   10   20   30   40   50   60   70   80   90   100%

➤

13. Some people have the experience of feeling that their body does not seem to belong to them. Circle a number to show what percentage of the time this happens to you.

0%   10   20   30   40   50   60   70   80   90   100%

14. Some people have the experience of sometimes remembering a past event so vividly that they feel as if they were reliving that event. Circle a number to show what percentage of the time this happens to you.

0%   10   20   30   40   50   60   70   80   90   100%

15. Some people have the experience of not being sure whether things that they remember happening really did happen or whether they just dreamed them. Circle a number to show what percentage of the time this happens to you.

0%   10   20   30   40   50   60   70   80   90   100%

16. Some people have the experience of being in a familiar place but finding it strange and unfamiliar. Circle a number to show what percentage of the time this happens to you.

0%   10   20   30   40   50   60   70   80   90   100%

17. Some people find that when they are watching television or a movie they become so absorbed in the story that they are unaware of other events happening around them. Circle a number to show what percentage of the time this happens to you.

0%   10   20   30   40   50   60   70   80   90   100%

18. Some people find that they become so involved in a fantasy or daydream that it feels as though it were really happening to them. Circle a number to show what percentage of the time this happens to you.

0%   10   20   30   40   50   60   70   80   90   100%

19. Some people find that they sometimes are able to ignore pain. Circle a number to show what percentage of the time this happens to you.

0%   10   20   30   40   50   60   70   80   90   100%

20. Some people find that they sometimes sit staring off into space, thinking of nothing, and are not aware of the passage of time. Circle a number to show what percentage of the time this happens to you.

0%   10   20   30   40   50   60   70   80   90   100%

21. Some people sometimes find that when they are alone they talk out loud to themselves. Circle a number to show what percentage of the time this happens to you.

0%   10   20   30   40   50   60   70   80   90   100%

22. Some people find that in one situation they may act so differently compared with another situation that they feel almost as if they were two different people. Circle a number to show what percentage of the time this happens to you.

0%   10   20   30   40   50   60   70   80   90   100%

23. Some people sometimes find that in certain situations they are able to do things with amazing ease and spontaneity that would usually be difficult for them (for example, sports, work, social situations, etc.). Circle a number to show what percentage of the time this happens to you.

0%   10   20   30   40   50   60   70   80   90   100%

24. Some people sometimes find that they cannot remember whether they have done something or have just thought about doing that thing (for example, not knowing whether they have mailed a letter or have just thought about mailing it). Circle a number to show what percentage of the time this happens to you.

0%   10   20   30   40   50   60   70   80   90   100%

25. Some people find evidence that they have done things that they do not remember doing. Circle a number to show what percentage of the time this happens to you.

0%   10   20   30   40   50   60   70   80   90   100%

26. Some people sometimes find writings, drawings, or notes among their belongings that they must have done but cannot remember doing. Circle a number to show what percentage of the time this happens to you.

0%   10   20   30   40   50   60   70   80   90   100%

27. Some people sometimes find that they hear voices inside their head that tell them to do things or comment on things that they are doing. Circle a number to show what percentage of the time this happens to you.

0%   10   20   30   40   50   60   70   80   90   100%

→

28. Some people sometimes feel as if they are looking at the world through a fog so that people and objects appear far away or unclear. Circle a number to show what percentage of the time this happens to you.

0%   10   20   30   40   50   60   70   80   90   100%

REFERENCES

Bernstein, E. M., & Putnam, F. W. (1986). Development, reliability, and validity of a dissociation scale. *Journal of Nervous and Mental Disease, 174,* 727–735.

Carlson, E. B., & Putnam, F. W. (1993). An update on the dissociative experiences scale. *Dissociation, 6,* 16–27.

Carlson, E. B., Putnam, F. W., Ross, C. A., Torem, M., Coons, P., Dill, D., Loewenstein, R. J., & Braun, B. G. (1993). Validity of the Dissociative Experiences Scale in screening for multiple personality disorder: A multicenter study. *American Journal of Psychiatry, 150,* 1030–1036.

Frischholz, E J., Braun, B. G., Sachs, R. G. Schwartz, D. R., Lewis, J., Shaeffer, D., Westergaard, C., & Pasquotto, J. (1991). The Dissociative Experiences Scale (DES): I. The relationship between the DES and other self-report measures of dissociation. *Dissociation, 4,* 151–153.

Frischholz, E J., Braun, B. G., Sachs, R. G. Schwartz, D. R., Lewis, J., Shaeffer, D., Westergaard, C., & Pasquotto, J. (1992). Construct validity of the Dissociative Experiences Scale: The relationship between the DES and hypnotizability. *American Journal of Clinical Hypnosis, 35,* 145–152.

Nadon, R., Hoyt, I. P., Register, P. A., & Kihlstrom, J. F. (1991). Absorption and hypnotizability: Context effects reexamined. *Journal of Personality and Social Psychology, 60,* 144–153.

Paolo, A. M., Ryan, J. J., Dunn, G. E., & van Fleet, J. (1993). Reading level of the Dissociative Experiences Scale. *Journal of Clinical Psychology, 49,* 209–211.

Saxe, G. N., van der Kolk, B. A., Berkowitz, R., Chinman, G., Hall, K., Lieberg, G., & Schwartz, J. (1993). Dissociative disorders in psychiatric patients. *American Journal of Psychiatry, 150,* 1037–1042.

CHAPTER 9

Sexual Disorders

SEXUAL INTERACTION INVENTORY

Purpose and Development

The Sexual Interaction Inventory assesses the sexual adjustment and sexual satisfaction of heterosexual couples. The scale is a self-report measure consisting of 17 behaviors, each of which is rated on six aspects of sexuality (LoPiccolo & Steger, 1974).

Administration and Scoring

Both partners separately rate each of the 17 items on the following six questions: (1) frequency, (2) wished for frequency, (3) pleasantness, (4) perceived pleasantness for the partner, (5) ideal pleasantness, and (6) perceived ideal pleasantness for the partner. Respondents use a 6-point scale to answer each question.

Responses are summed across all 17 behaviors and used to obtain scores on 11 subscales. Scale 1, the Male Frequency Dissatisfaction Scale, is the sum of differences between men's responses to the frequency question and the wished-for-frequency question. Scale 2, the Female Frequency Dissatisfaction Scale, is the sum of differences between women's responses to the frequency question and the wished-for-frequency question. Scores can range from 0 to 85 and high scores indicate dissatisfaction with the frequency or range of sexual behaviors.

Scale 3, the Male Self-Acceptance Scale, is the sum of differences between men's responses to the pleasantness question and the ideal pleasantness question. Scale 4, the Female Self-Acceptance Scale, is the sum of differences between women's responses to the pleasantness question and the ideal pleasantness question. Scores can range from 0 to 85 and high scores indicate that an individual would like to experience more pleasure from sexual activities.

Scales 5 and 6, the Male Pleasure Scale and the Female Pleasure Scale, are calculated by summing the individual's responses to the pleasantness question for all 17 items and then dividing by 17. Scores can range from 1 to 6 and higher scores indicate that greater pleasure is derived from sexual activities.

Scale 7, the Male Perceptual Accuracy Scale, is the sum of differences between the man's responses to the perceived pleasantness for partner question and his partner's actual pleasantness rating. Scale 8, the Female Perceptual Accuracy Scale, is the sum of differences between the woman's responses to the perceived pleasantness for partner question and her partner's actual pleasantness rating. Scores can range from 0 to 85 and high scores indicate that an individual has little insight into his or her partner's sexuality and suggest the couple has poor communication about sexual matters.

Scale 9, the Male Mate Acceptance Scale, is the sum of differences between the man's responses to the perceived pleasantness for the partner question and his responses to the ideal pleasantness for the partner question. Scale 10, the Female Mate Acceptance Scale, is the sum of differences between the woman's responses to the perceived pleasantness for the partner question and her responses to the ideal pleasantness for the partner question. Scores can range from 0 to 85. LoPiccolo and Steger (1974) pointed out that high scale scores, which tend to indicate dissatisfaction with a partner's unresponsiveness, should be interpreted in conjunction with scores on the other scales.

Scale 11 is a summary scale of the total of all other scale scores except for scales 5 and 6. Scores can range from 0 to 680 and high scores indicate disharmony and dissatisfaction in the sexual relationship.

Sample Scores

LoPiccolo and Steger (1974) gave the Sexual Interaction Inventory to 28 couples seeking treatment for sexual dysfunction, to 16 of these same couples after they had completed treatment, and to a community sample of 63 couples who were satisfied with their sexual relationship. Table 1 shows the scores for these groups.

Reliability

In a community sample of couples, LoPiccolo and Steger (1974) found the internal consistency of the 11 scales of the Sexual Interaction Inventory

TABLE 1
Scores on the Sexual Interaction Inventory
(LoPiccolo and Steger, 1974)

	Clients		Satisfied couples
	Pretreatment	Posttreatment	
Frequency dissatisfaction			
Male	21.11 ± 8.03	9.88 ± 8.73	10.87 ± 6.73
Female	20.07 ± 6.71	8.56 ± 7.05	10.46 ± 6.25
Self-acceptance			
Male	7.19 ± 7.48	2.00 ± 2.13	3.89 ± 4.27
Female	15.74 ± 9.15	7.56 ± 7.59	6.79 ± 5.09
Pleasure			
Male	5.16 ± .68	5.56 ± .33	5.28 ± .54
Female	4.69 ± .68	5.36 ± .43	5.11 ± .54
Perceptual accuracy			
Male	12.13 ± 6.59	6.88 ± 3.69	9.59 ± 6.08
Female	15.31 ± 5.75	8.38 ± 5.49	10.58 ± 5.65
Mate acceptance			
Male	21.25 ± 12.77	8.81 ± 8.81	10.00 ± 7.29
Female	8.98 ± 6.47	4.00 ± 4.98	8.56 ± 7.65
Total dissatisfaction	120.79 ± 30.08	56.07 ± 26.39	70.57 ± 29.26

Values are Mean ± SD.

ranged from .79 to .93 as determined by Cronbach's alpha. In another community sample of couples, LoPiccolo and Steger (1974) found that the two-week test–retest reliability of the scales ranged from .53 to .89. LoPiccolo and Steger (1974) point out that the low test–retest reliability of some of the scales may be in part due to reactivity to the first completion of the inventory. They mention that for some couples completing the inventory prompted their first open discussion about sexuality and that such discussions may have influenced responses the second time couples completed the inventory.

Validity

LoPiccolo and Steger (1974) found that couples' overall rating of sexual satisfaction was significantly associated with scores on all Sexual Interaction Inventory scales except for the Male Perceptual Accuracy Scale and the Female Mate Acceptance Scale. As one would expect the highest association was found with the Total Dissatisfaction Scale. McCann and Biaggio (1989) found that individuals who saw more meaning in life had lower Dissatisfaction Scale scores (indicating more harmony).

LoPiccolo and Steger (1974) compared couples seeking treatment for a sexual dysfunction with couples satisfied with their sexual relationship and found that nine of the 11 scales discriminated between these two groups. The two scales that did not were the Male Pleasure Scale and the Female Mate Acceptance Scale. Studying couples going through treatment for a sexual dysfunction, LoPiccolo and Steger (1974) found that scores on all 11 scales indicated improved sexual functioning from before to after treatment.

Reading Level

Using the Forbes and Cottle method, Jensen, Witcher, and Upton (1987) found that instructions for the inventory require sixth-grade reading skills and the items in the inventory require college-level reading skills.

SEXUAL INTERACTION INVENTORY

[*Note to the administrator*: All six questions should be answered by both partners for each of the 17 items. To save space the six questions are listed only once, with item 1 used as an example.]

Item 1. The male seeing the female when she is nude.
Item 2. The female seeing the male when he is nude.
Item 3. The male and female kissing for one minute continuously.
Item 4. The male giving the female a body massage, not touching her breasts or genitals.
Item 5. The female giving the male a body massage, not touching his genitals.
Item 6. The male caressing the female's breasts with his hands.
Item 7. The male caressing the female's breasts with his mouth (lips or tongue).
Item 8. The male caressing the female's genitals with his hands.
Item 9. The male caressing the female's genitals with his hands until she reaches orgasm (climax).
Item 10. The female caressing the male's genitals with her hands.
Item 11. The female caressing the male's genitals with her hands until he ejaculates (has climax).
Item 12. The male caressing the female's genitals with his mouth (lips or tongue).
Item 13. The male caressing the female's genitals with his mouth until she reaches orgasm (climax).
Item 14. The female caressing the male's genitals with her mouth (lips or tongue).
Item 15. The female caressing the male's genitals with her mouth until he ejaculates (has a climax).
Item 16. The male and female having intercourse.
Item 17. The male and female having intercourse with both of them having an orgasm (climax).

Please check the response that is most true for the behavior below for each of the six questions.

1. *The male seeing the female when she is nude.*

When you and your mate engage in sexual behavior, does this particular activity usually occur? How often would you like this activity to occur?

➤

1. Currently occurs:
   _____ 1. Never
   _____ 2. Rarely (10% of the time)
   _____ 3. Occasionally (25% of the time)
   _____ 4. Fairly often (50% of the time)
   _____ 5. Usually (75% of the time)
   _____ 6. Always

2. I would like it to occur:
   _____ 1. Never
   _____ 2. Rarely (10% of the time)
   _____ 3. Occasionally (25% of the time)
   _____ 4. Fairly often (50% of the time)
   _____ 5. Usually (75% of the time)
   _____ 6. Always

How pleasant do you currently find this activity to be? How pleasant do you think your mate finds this activity to be?

3. I find this activity:
   _____ 1. Extremely unpleasant
   _____ 2. Moderately unpleasant
   _____ 3. Slightly unpleasant
   _____ 4. Slightly pleasant
   _____ 5. Moderately pleasant
   _____ 6. Extremely pleasant

4. I think my mate finds this activity:
   _____ 1. Extremely unpleasant
   _____ 2. Moderately unpleasant
   _____ 3. Slightly unpleasant
   _____ 4. Slightly pleasant
   _____ 5. Moderately pleasant
   _____ 6. Extremely pleasant

How would you like to respond to this activity? How would you like your mate to respond? (In other words, how pleasant do you think this activity *ideally should be*, for you and for your mate?)

5. I would like to find this activity:
   _____ 1. Extremely unpleasant
   _____ 2. Moderately unpleasant
   _____ 3. Slightly unpleasant
   _____ 4. Slightly pleasant
   _____ 5. Moderately pleasant
   _____ 6. Extremely pleasant

6. I would like my mate to find this activity:
   _____ 1. Extremely unpleasant
   _____ 2. Moderately unpleasant
   _____ 3. Slightly unpleasant
   _____ 4. Slightly pleasant
   _____ 5. Moderately pleasant
   _____ 6. Extremely pleasant

Reprinted with permission of Plenum Press from LoPiccolo, J., & Steger, J. C. (1974). The Sexual Interaction Inventory: A new instrument for assessment of sexual dysfunction. *Archives of Sexual Behavior, 3*, 585–595.

SEXUAL AROUSABILITY INDEX

Purpose and Development

The Sexual Arousability Index assesses the sexual arousability, sexual anxiety, and sexual satisfaction of heterosexual or homosexual women. It is a 28-item self-report measure originally developed by Hoon, Hoon, and Wincze (1976) to measure sexual arousability. They asked a large group of women to rate an initial pool of 131 items on how sexually arousing each item was. They then selected items that correlated highly with each other, correlated highly with four criterion variables, and fell into the five most important dimensions identified in a factor analysis. The five factors were foreplay, erotic visual and verbal stimulation through various media forms, breast stimulation, intercourse, and genital stimulation. In a later study Chambless and Lifshitz (1983) found a similar factor structure.

Dr. Emily Hoon later expanded the inventory to include rating scales of anxiety and satisfaction for each of the items. Chambless and Lifshitz (1984) found a high correlation between the arousal and satisfaction scales and suggested that they may be redundant. The arousal and anxiety scales were not significantly associated. Thus the remainder of this review focuses only on the arousal and anxiety scales of the inventory.

Although the inventory was designed for women, the items are gender neutral. The arousal scale has been used with male respondents by Harris, Yulis, and Lacoste (1980), who found no significant difference between men's and women's scores, and by Hoon and Hoon (1982), who found gender differences on specific items but also found no gender differences on the scale as a whole.

Administration and Scoring

Respondents rate each item on 7-point scales of sexual arousal and sexual anxiety. Ratings are summed for each scale. Scores can range from -28 to 140 on each scale, with higher scores indicating more arousability or anxiety.

Sample Scores

Hoon et al. (1976) gave the Sexual Arousal scale of the inventory to 285 women who were undergraduate students, graduate students, and members of women's groups. The women were from a variety of backgrounds and had varying amounts of sexual experience. On the basis of their responses Hoon et al. (1976) constructed cumulative percentile based norms for the Sexual Arousal scale. Table 1 presents extracts of these

TABLE 1
Percentile Norms for the Sexual Arousal Scale of the Sexual
Arousability Inventory, Hoon et al., 1976

Cumulative percentile	Raw score	Cumulative percentile	Raw score
1	4	55	88
5	37	60	91
10	52	65	94
15	60	70	97
20	66	75	99
25	70	80	102
30	73	85	105
35	77	90	108
40	80	95	113
45	83	99	126
50	86		

norms. They found that the average raw score of women who were entering treatment for a sexual dysfunction was at the 5th percentile.

Chambless and Lifshitz (1984) gave the Arousal and Anxiety scales of the inventory to 252 female college students, from whose responses they calculated cumulative percentile norms for the Anxiety Scale of the inventory. See Table 2 for extracts of these norms. Chambless and Lifshitz (1984) also gave the inventory to 90 women recruited from the community. The

TABLE 2
Percentile Norms for the Sexual Anxiety Scale of the Sexual
Arousability Inventory, Chambless and Lifshitz (1984)

Cumulative percentile	Raw score	Cumulative percentile	Raw score
1	−28	55	33
5	−15	60	37
10	−5	65	42
15	0	70	49
20	4	75	56
25	9	80	63
30	14	85	72
35	17	90	85
40	20	95	98
45	24	100	117
50	28		

average scores obtained from these two samples of women are presented in Table 3.

Reliability

In two samples of women, Hoon et al. (1976) found the internal consistency of the Sexual Arousal scale as measured by Cronbach's alpha was .91 and .92. Chambless and Lifshitz (1983) found that split-half reliability as assessed by the Spearman–Brown formula was .92 for the Arousal scale and .94 for the Anxiety scale. Hoon et al. (1976) found a two-month test–retest reliability of .69 for the Arousal scale.

Validity

In their samples of women, Hoon et al. (1976) found that higher scores on the Sexual Arousal scale were associated with greater number of sexual partners, satisfaction with sexual responsivity, awareness of physiological changes during sexual arousal, frequency of intercourse, frequency of orgasm, and higher scores on a heterosexual experience scale. Harris et al. (1980) replicated the association between Sexual Arousal scores, frequency of intercourse, and frequency of orgasm in samples of women and men. They also reported that women and men who had better imagery abilities had higher Arousal scores and that extroverted women had higher Arousal scores.

Chambless and Lifshitz (1983) reported that women with greater sexual experience had higher Arousal scale scores and lower Anxiety scale scores. In one sample of women, higher frequency of orgasm was associated with higher Arousal scale scores and lower Anxiety scale scores, but in another sample of women frequency of orgasm was not significantly associated with either scale.

Hoon et al. (1976) found that women seeking treatment for a sexual

TABLE 3
Scores on the Sexual Arousability Inventory,
Chambless and Lifshitz, 1984

	Arousal		Anxiety	
Group	M	SD	M	SD
College women	78.93	24.84	34.34	33.14
Community women	99.14	17.27	6.36	16.11

dysfunction scored significantly lower on the Sexual Arousal scale than other women. The scale is sensitive to change as shown by Murphy, Coleman, Hoon, and Scott (1980), who found a significant increase in the Arousal scale scores of women participating in a sexual enhancement program and Trudel and Laurin (1988) who found that women who completed bibliotherapy for orgasmic dysfunction scored higher on the Arousal scale than women in a waiting list control group.

Reading Level

Using the Forbes and Cottle method, Jensen, Witcher, and Upton (1987) found that both the instructions and the items of the inventory required college-level reading skills.

SEXUAL AROUSABILITY INDEX

Instructions: The experiences in this inventory may or may not be sexually arousing to you. There are no right or wrong answers. Read each item carefully, and then circle the number which indicates how sexually aroused you feel when you have the described experience, or how sexually aroused you think you would feel if you actually experienced it. Be sure to answer every item. If you aren't certain about an item, circle the number that seems about right. The meaning of the numbers is given below:

-1   adversely affects arousal; unthinkable, repulsive, distracting
 0   doesn't affect sexual arousal
 1   possibly causes sexual arousal
 2   sometimes causes sexual arousal; slightly arousing
 3   usually causes sexual arousal; moderately arousing
 4   almost always sexually arousing; very arousing
 5   always causes sexual arousal; extremely arousing

	How you feel or think you would feel if you were actually involved in this experience
ANSWER EVERY ITEM	
1. When a loved one stimulates your genitals with mouth and tongue	−1 0 1 2 3 4 5
2. When a loved one fondles your breasts with his/her hands	−1 0 1 2 3 4 5
3. When you see a loved one nude	−1 0 1 2 3 4 5
4. When a loved one caresses you with his/her eyes	−1 0 1 2 3 4 5
5. When a loved one stimulates your genitals with his/her finger	−1 0 1 2 3 4 5
6. When you are touched or kissed on the inner thighs by a loved one	−1 0 1 2 3 4 5
7. When you caress a loved one's genitals with your fingers	−1 0 1 2 3 4 5
8. When you read a pornographic or "dirty" story	−1 0 1 2 3 4 5
9. When a loved one undresses you	−1 0 1 2 3 4 5

→

10. When you dance with a loved one   −1 0 1 2 3 4 5
11. When you have intercourse with a loved   −1 0 1 2 3 4 5
    one
12. When a loved one touches or kisses your   −1 0 1 2 3 4 5
    nipples
13. When you caress a loved one (other than   −1 0 1 2 3 4 5
    genitals)
14. When you see pornographic pictures or   −1 0 1 2 3 4 5
    slides
15. When you lie in bed with a loved one   −1 0 1 2 3 4 5
16. When a loved one kisses you passionately   −1 0 1 2 3 4 5
17. When you hear sounds of pleasure during   −1 0 1 2 3 4 5
    sex
18. When a loved one kisses you with an ex-   −1 0 1 2 3 4 5
    ploring tongue
19. When you read suggestive or porno-   −1 0 1 2 3 4 5
    graphic poetry
20. When you see a strip show   −1 0 1 2 3 4 5
21. When you stimulate you partner's geni-   −1 0 1 2 3 4 5
    tals with your mouth and tongue
22. When a loved one caresses you (other   −1 0 1 2 3 4 5
    than genitals)
23. When you see a pornographic movie (stag   −1 0 1 2 3 4 5
    film)
24. When you undress a loved one   −1 0 1 2 3 4 5
25. When a loved one fondles your breasts   −1 0 1 2 3 4 5
    with mouth and tongue
26. When you make love in a new or unusual   −1 0 1 2 3 4 5
    place
27. When you masturbate   −1 0 1 2 3 4 5
28. When your partner has an orgasm   −1 0 1 2 3 4 5

Now rate each of the items according to how anxious you feel when you
have the experience. The meaning of anxiety is extreme uneasiness and
distress. Rate feelings of anxiety according to the scale below.

    −1 = Relaxing, calming
     0 = No anxiety
     1 = Possibly causes some anxiety
     2 = Sometimes causes anxiety; slightly anxiety producing
     3 = Usually causes anxiety; moderately anxiety producing
     4 = Almost always causes anxiety; very anxiety producing
     5 = Always causes anxiety; extremely anxiety producing

How you feel or think
you would feel if you
were actually involved
in this experience

1. When a loved one stimulates your genitals with mouth and tongue   −1 0 1 2 3 4 5

2. When a loved one fondles your breasts with his/her hands   −1 0 1 2 3 4 5

3. When you see a loved one nude   −1 0 1 2 3 4 5

4. When a loved one caresses you with his/her eyes   −1 0 1 2 3 4 5

5. When a loved one stimulates your genitals with his/her finger   −1 0 1 2 3 4 5

6. When you are touched or kissed on the inner thighs by a loved one   −1 0 1 2 3 4 5

7. When you caress a loved one's genitals with your fingers   −1 0 1 2 3 4 5

8. When you read a pornographic or "dirty" story   −1 0 1 2 3 4 5

9. When a loved one undresses you   −1 0 1 2 3 4 5

10. When you dance with a loved one   −1 0 1 2 3 4 5

11. When you have intercourse with a loved one   −1 0 1 2 3 4 5

12. When a loved one touches or kisses your nipples   −1 0 1 2 3 4 5

13. When you caress a loved one (other than genitals)   −1 0 1 2 3 4 5

14. When you see pornographic pictures or slides   −1 0 1 2 3 4 5

15. When you lie in bed with a loved one   −1 0 1 2 3 4 5

16. When a loved one kisses you passionately   −1 0 1 2 3 4 5

17. When you hear sounds of pleasure during sex   −1 0 1 2 3 4 5

18. When a loved one kisses you with an exploring tongue   −1 0 1 2 3 4 5

19. When you read suggestive or pornographic poetry   −1 0 1 2 3 4 5

20. When you see a strip show   −1 0 1 2 3 4 5

21. When you stimulate you partner's genitals with your mouth and tongue   −1 0 1 2 3 4 5

22. When a loved one caresses you (other than genitals)   −1 0 1 2 3 4 5

→

23. When you see a pornographic movie (stag   −1 0 1 2 3 4 5
    film)
24. When you undress a loved one   −1 0 1 2 3 4 5
25. When a loved one fondles your breasts   −1 0 1 2 3 4 5
    with mouth and tongue
26. When you make love in a new or unusual   −1 0 1 2 3 4 5
    place
27. When you masturbate   −1 0 1 2 3 4 5
28. When your partner has an orgasm   −1 0 1 2 3 4 5

Reprinted with permission of Plenum Press and Dr. Emily Hoon from Hoon, E. F., Hoon, P. W., & Wincze, J. P. (1976). An inventory for the measurement of female sexual arousability: The SAI. *Archives of Sexual Behavior, 5,* 291–300.

REFERENCES

Chambless, D. L., & Lifshitz, J. L. (1984). Self-reported sexual anxiety and arousal; The Expanded Sexual Arousal Inventory. *Journal of Sex Research, 20,* 241–254.

Harris, R., Yulis, S., & Lacoste, D. (1980). Relationships among sexual arousability, imagery ability, and introversion-extraversion. *The Journal of Sex Research, 16,* 72–86.

Hoon, P. W., & Hoon E. F. (1982). Effects of experience in cohabitation on erotic arousability. *Psychological Reports, 50,* 255–258.

Hoon, E. F., Hoon, P. W., & Wincze, J. P. (1976). An inventory for the measurement of female sexual arousability: The SAI. *Archives of Sexual Behavior, 5,* 291–300.

Jensen, B. J., Witcher, D. B., & Upton, L. R. (1987). Readability assessment of questionnaires frequently used in sex and marital therapy. *Journal of Sex and Marital Therapy, 13,* 137–141.

LoPiccolo, J., & Steger, J. C. (1974). The Sexual Interaction Inventory: A new instrument for assessment of sexual dysfunction. *Archives of Sexual Behavior, 3,* 585–595.

McCann, J. T., & Biaggio, M. K. (1989). Sexual satisfaction in marriage as a function of life meaning. *Archives of Sexual Behavior, 18,* 59–72.

Murphy, W., Coleman, E., Hoon, E. F., & Scott, C. (1980). Sexual dysfunction and treatment in alcoholic women. *Sexuality and Disability, 3,* 240–255.

Trudel, G., & Laurin, F. (1988). The effects of bibliotherapy on orgasmic dysfunction and couple interactions: An experimental study. *Sexual and Marital Therapy, 3,* 223–228.

CHAPTER 10

Eating Disorders

SELF-REPORT QUESTIONNAIRE FOR SCREENING INDIVIDUALS AT RISK OF DEVELOPING AN EATING DISORDER

Purpose and Development

This 40-item self-report measure was developed by Slade and Dewey (1986) to detect individuals at risk for developing an eating disorder. The scale is based on Slade's Functional-Analytic model of anorexia nervosa. According to the model, eating disorders develop when individuals set conditions that create a strong need for bodily control and eating is used to achieve this bodily control. The items on the questionnaire were developed to assess the following five hypothetical aspects of setting conditions: dissatisfaction with life and oneself, perfectionistic tendencies, social and personal anxiety, adolescent problems, and weight control. Slade and Dewey (1986) did a factor analytic study to select the final items for the subscales that assess each of these aspects and confirmed the factor structure of the scale in a second study.

Administration and Scoring

Respondents answer each item using a 1–5 point scale. The General Dissatisfaction subscale is comprised of the sum of items 1, 2, 4, 6, 9, 17, and 28 and, after they are reverse coded, items 8, 12, 14, 18, 19, 26, and 32. Scores on this subscale can range from 14 to 70. The Social and Personal Anxiety subscale is comprised of items 3, 5, 11, 24, 28, 30, and 37 and, after they are reverse coded, items 15, 21, and 31. Scores on this subscale can range from 10 to 50. The Perfectionism subscale is comprised of items 7, 23, 35, and 38, and after they are reverse coded, items 20, 25, 29, and 33. Scores on this subscale can range from 8 to 40. The Adolescent Problems subscale is comprised of items 16, 27, and 36 after all are reverse coded. Scores on this subscale can range from 3 to 15. The Weight Control subscale is comprised of items 39 and 40 and scores can range from 2 to 10. On all scales higher scores indicate more disturbance.

Sample Scores and Cutoff Scores

Slade and Dewey (1986) gave the questionnaire to 245 adolescent girls, 141 female college students, 329 female and 25 male nursing students, 19 female clients and 1 male client with anorexia nervosa, and 20 female clients with bulimia nervosa. Table 1 shows the average scores of these groups.

Slade and Dewey (1986) suggested that a score of 42 or greater on the Dissatisfaction subscale and 22 or greater on the Perfectionism subscale be used to identify those at risk for developing eating disorders. In their samples they found that the combination of these cutoff scores resulted in 85% of the clients scoring at or above the cutoffs and 86% of the control individuals scoring below the cutoff. They point out that because the control individuals were not specifically screened for eating disorders before being included in the sample, a number of these individuals may have had eating disorders or been at risk for developing an eating disorder.

Reliability

In a sample of nursing students Slade and Dewey (1986) report the internal consistency as measured by Cronbach's alpha for each of the subscales as follows: .89 for the Dissatisfaction subscale, .81 for the Anxiety subscale, .66 for the Perfectionism subscale, .83 for the Adolescent Problems subscale, and .90 for the Weight Control subscale.

Validity

Slade, Butler, and Newton (1989) found that higher scores on the General Dissatisfaction subscale were associated with more neuroticism, introversion, and psychoticism while higher scores on the Perfectionism subscale were associated with lower psychoticism scores and more social desirability responding.

Slade and Dewey (1986) compared the questionnaire scores of clients with eating disorders to those of control subjects and found that anorexic and bulimic clients scored much higher on each of the five subscales. Two

TABLE 1

Scores on the Self-Report Questionnaire for Screening Individuals
at Risk of Developing an Eating Disorder (Slade and Dewey, 1986)

	Dissatisfaction		Anxiety		Perfectionism		Adolescent problems		Weight control	
	M	SD	M	SD	M	SD	M	SD	M	SD
Adolescent girls	36.01	7.41	23.97	5.37	23.04	3.97	3.11	2.52	7.85	2.06
College women	37.74	7.13	23.86	5.13	23.55	3.93	3.32	2.73	7.80	2.02
Nursing students	34.48	6.67	22.90	5.07	24.46	3.83	2.75	2.35	7.76	2.10
Anorexic clients	50.05	12.72	31.90	7.27	28.05	5.33	5.30	3.08	9.40	.94
Bulimic clients	52.55	6.19	31.65	6.19	27.65	3.98	5.20	2.97	9.80	.62

studies (Slade & Dewey, 1986; Kiemle, Slade, & Dewey, 1987) provided evidence for the classificatory power of the questionnaire. Both studies identified individuals at risk for developing eating disorders by using the cutoff scores established for the questionnaire. Comparisons of these at-risk individuals and the not-at-risk individuals on tests designed to measure existing eating disorders showed that the at-risk individuals scored much higher on these test than the not-at-risk individuals.

Self-Report Questionnaire for Screening Individuals at Risk of Developing an Eating Disorder

Instruction: Read each of the following questions carefully and then indicate your response by circling the appropriate statements beneath. Be sure to answer *all* questions.

1. In general how *satisfied* do you feel with your attainments to date (i.e., school, college, work, etc.)?

   Very satisfied; Somewhat satisfied; About average;
   Somewhat dissatisfied; Very dissatisfied

2. In general how *satisfied* do you feel with yourself?

   Very satisfied; Somewhat satisfied; About average;
   Somewhat dissatisfied; Very dissatisfied

3. In general if you had to compare yourself with the average person what *grade* would you give yourself?

   Excellent; Good; Average; Below average;
   A lot below average

4. In general how *satisfied* do you feel with your life at the moment?

   Very satisfied; Somewhat satisfied; About average;
   Somewhat dissatisfied; Very dissatisfied

5. Over the last couple of years how *often* have you felt confident?

   Very often; Fairly often; Sometimes; Almost never; Never

6. Over the last couple of years how *often* have you felt in control of your life?

   Very often; Fairly often; Sometimes; Almost never; Never

7. Over the last couple of years how *often* have you felt able to accept a below-par performance from yourself?

   Very often; Fairly often; Sometimes; Almost never; Never

8. Over the last couple of years how *often* have you felt generally fed-up?

   Very often; Fairly often; Sometimes; Almost never; Never

→

9. Over the last couple of years how *often* have you felt in total control of yourself?

Very often;   Fairly often;   Sometimes;   Almost never;   Never

10. Over the last couple of years how *often* have you got behind with the things you have to do?

Very often;   Fairly often;   Sometimes;   Almost never;   Never

11. Over the last couple of years how *often* have you found it easy to talk to someone of the opposite sex?

Very often;   Fairly often;   Sometimes;   Almost never;   Never

12. Over the last couple of years how *often* have you felt useless?

Very often;   Fairly often;   Sometimes;   Almost never;   Never

13. Over the last couple of years how *often* have you felt you were a mature and responsible adult?

Very often;   Fairly often;   Sometimes;   Almost never;   Never

14. Over the last couple of years how *often* have you wished you were really good at something or other?

Very often;   Fairly often;   Sometimes;   Almost never;   Never

15. Over the last couple of years how *often* have you been worried that you will say or do the wrong thing in company?

Very often;   Fairly often;   Sometimes;   Almost never;   Never

16. Over the last couple of years how *often* have you wished you were a child again?

Very often;   Fairly often;   Sometimes;   Almost never;   Never

17. Over the last couple of years how *often* have you felt happy with life?

Very often;   Fairly often;   Sometimes;   Almost never;   Never

18. Over the last couple of years how *often* have you wanted to have more control over some area of your life?

Very often;   Fairly often;   Sometimes;   Almost never;   Never

19. *Think of a person* who feels a failure in life. Is this person:

   Very much like you;   Much like you;   Somewhat like you;
   Very little like you;   Not at all like you

20. *Think of a person* who is a perfectionist. Is this person:

   Very much like you;   Much like you;   Somewhat like you;
   Very little like you;   Not at all like you

21. *Think of a person* who tries to avoid talking to strangers. Is this person:

   Very much like you;   Much like you;   Somewhat like you;
   Very little like you;   Not at all like you

22. *Think of a person* who would like to be treated in a more adult fashion. Is this person:

   Very much like you;   Much like you;   Somewhat like you;
   Very little like you;   Not at all like you

23. *Think of a person* who is not particularly concerned with standards. Is this person:

   Very much like you;   Much like you;   Somewhat like you;
   Very little like you;   Not at all like you

24. *Think of a person* who finds it easy to relax with other people. Is this person:

   Very much like you;   Much like you;   Somewhat like you;
   Very little like you;   Not at all like you

25. *Think of a person* who tries to be perfect in their work. Is this person:

   Very much like you;   Much like you;   Somewhat like you;
   Very little like you;   Not at all like you

26. *Think of a person* who would like to have more control over their body. Is this person:

   Very much like you;   Much like you;   Somewhat like you;
   Very little like you;   Not at all like you

→

27. *Think of a person* who would like to be a child again. Is this person:

    Very much like you;   Much like you;   Somewhat like you;
    Very little like you;   Not at all like you

28. *Think of a person* who feels they have much to be proud of. Is this
    person:

    Very much like you;   Much like you;   Somewhat like you;
    Very little like you;   Not at all like you

29. *Think of a person* who can (could) never do enough to please one or both
    of their parents. Is this person:

    Very much like you;   Much like you;   Somewhat like you;
    Very little like you;   Not at all like you

30. *Think of a person* who finds (found) adolescence (the teenage years) a
    very enjoyable time. Is this person:

    Very much like you;   Much like you;   somewhat like you;
    Very little like you;   Not at all like you

31. *Think of a person* who is worried about what others may think of them.
    Is this person:

    Very much like you;   Much like you;   Somewhat like you;
    Very little like you;   Not at all like you

32. *Think of a person* who would like to have more self-control. Is this
    person:

    Very much like you;   Much like you;   Somewhat like you;
    Very little like you;   Not at all like you

33. *Think of a person* who sets high standards for themself. Is this person:

    Very much like you;   Much like you;   Somewhat like you;
    Very little like you;   Not at all like you

34. *Think of a person* who is able to concentrate on a number of things at
    once. Is this person:

    Very much like you;   Much like you;   Somewhat like you;
    Very little like you;   Not at all like you

35. *Think of a person* who is generally *not* concerned about doing their best. Is this person:

Very much like you;   Much like you;   Somewhat like you;
Very little like you;   Not at all like you

36. *Think of a person* who is *not* sure whether they would prefer to be an adult of a child. Is this person:

Very much like you;   Much like you;   Somewhat like you;
Very little like you;   Not at all like you

37. *Think of a person* who is generally confident about the impression they create on others. Is this person:

Very much like you;   Much like you;   Somewhat like you;
Very little like you;   Not at all like you

38. *Think of a person* who is *not* usually concerned about their performance. Is this person:

Very much like you;   Much like you;   somewhat like you;
Very little like you;   Not at all like you

39. *Think of a person* who is *not at all* concerned about their weight. Is this person:

Very much like you;   Much like you;   Somewhat like you;
Very little like you;   Not at all like you

40. *Think of a person* who is *not at all* concerned about their body size and shape. Is this person:

Very much like you;   Much like you;   Somewhat like you;
Very little like you;   Not at all like you

EATING ATTITUDES TEST

Purpose and Development

The Eating Attitudes Test is a 40-item self-report measure developed by Garner and Garfinkel (1979) to assess symptoms associated with anorexia nervosa. They created items which asked about the range of symptoms associated with anorexia nervosa and gave these initial items to groups of anorexic and nonanorexic individuals. Then they selected those items that best differentiated between the two groups and added new items they thought would further differentiate between the two groups.

On the basis of a factor analytic study Garner, Olmstead, Bohr, and Garfinkel (1982) created a 26-item version of the Eating Attitudes Test which correlated very highly (.98) with the original version. This review focuses on the psychometric properties of the 40-item version. However, the items comprising the abbreviated version are mentioned in the scoring section.

Administration and Scoring

We believe that the written instructions may not be perfectly clear to all respondents and suggest that the test administrator emphasize that the respondent is to indicate how frequently each of the statements is true for her. Respondents rate each of the items on a 6-point scale of frequency. For each item a score of 3 is given for the most extreme response "always," a 2 is given for the next most extreme response "very often," a 1 is given for the response "often," and a 0 is given for the remaining three responses. Items 1, 18, 19, 23, 27, and 39 are reverse coded. The total scale score is the sum of responses to the 40 items and scores may range from 0 to 120. Higher scores indicate more disturbance.

The abbreviated, 26-item scale consists of items 4–10, 12–15, 22, 24–26, 29–34, 36–40. Scoring is the same as for the longer version.

Sample Scores and Cutoff Scores

Garner and Garfinkel (1979) gave the scale to 33 female clients with anorexia, 59 women who did not have anorexia, 49 men who did not have anorexia, and 16 obese women.

Eisler and Szmukler (1985) gave the scale to 1,331 teenage girls in private schools and 1,676 teenage girls in state schools. They found that 7% of the girls in the state schools and 5% of the girls in the public schools scored above the cutoff suggested by Garner and Garfinkel (1979). Interviews showed that of those who scored above the cutoff, 74% of the girls in the state schools did not have anorexia and 42% of the girls in the public schools did not have anorexia. Thus both the Garner and Garfinkel (1979) and Eisler and Szmukler (1985) studies indicate that a high percentage of individuals who do not have anorexia score above the cutoff score of 30.

Channon and DeSilva (1985) gave the scale to 45 female and three male anorexic inpatients at admission and again at discharge. Steinhausen (1985) gave the scale to 24 teenage anorexic girls at admission for inpatient treatment and again at discharge. Raciti and Norcross (1987) obtained scale scores from 238 female college freshmen and sophomores. Table 1 shows the average scores for these groups.

By examining scores of anorexic and nonanorexic individuals, Garner and Garfinkel (1979) arrived at a cutoff score of 30 or greater for identifying individuals with eating disturbances. All anorexic clients and 13% of the nonanorexic individuals in their sample scored at or above this cutoff score.

Garner et al. (1982) recommend a cutoff score of 20 or greater for the abbreviated 26-item version of the scale. Using a discriminant function analysis, they found that overall this cutoff correctly identified 83.6% of individuals who had eating disorders or did not have eating disorders.

Reliability

Garner and Garfinkel (1979) assessed the internal consistency of the scale and found an alpha of .79 for a sample of anorexic subjects and .94 for a combined sample of anorexic and nonanorexic subjects. In a sample of college women, Raciti and Norcross (1987) found an alpha of .86.

TABLE 1
Scores on the Eating Attitudes Test

	M	SD
Women with anorexia (Garner & Garfinkel, 1979)	58.9	13.3
Anorexic clients (Channon & DeSilva, 1985)		
At admission	60.8	24.3
At discharge	39.2	29.8
Teenage girls with anorexia (Steinhausen, 1985)		
At admission	37.1	
At discharge	12.7	
Women without anorexia (Garner & Garfinkel, 1979)	15.6	9.3
Men without anorexia (Garner & Garfinkel, 1979)	8.6	5.3
College women (Raciti & Norcross, 1987)	16.7	11.8
Teenage girls (Eisler & Szmukler, 1985)		
From private schools	10.7	9.4
From state schools	12.63	9.6
Obese women (Garner & Garfinkel, 1979)	16.5	9.6

Validity

In a sample of nonanorexic women, Garner and Garfinkel (1979) found that high scores on the Eating Attitudes Test were associated with high scores on a measure of eating restraint, and Raciti and Norcross (1987) found that individuals who scored high on the Eating Attitudes Test had high scores on another measure of eating disorders. High scores have also been found to be associated with higher levels of somatization, depression, obsessive-compulsive tendencies, anxiety, and interpersonal sensitivity (Garner & Garfinkel, 1980).

In a sample of nonanorexic subjects, Garner and Garfinkel (1979) found that the Eating Attitudes Test was not associated with weight fluctuations, indicating that it does not just assess weight difficulties. They also found that the test was not associated with extroversion or neuroticism, while Clarke and Palmer (1983) found that high scores were associated with more neuroticism.

Garner and Garfinkel (1979) found that the Eating Attitudes Test successfully differentiated between female anorexic clients and the following three control groups of individuals without anorexia: nonanorexic women, nonanorexic men, and obese women. They also examined the scores of a small number of recovered anorexic clients and found their scores to be similar to that of the nonanorexic women, suggesting that the scale is sensitive to change. Garner et al. (1982) found scale scores were much higher for a group of anorexic women than for a control group of women, but found that scores did not differ between bulimic and restricted-eating anorexic clients. Cooper, Waterman, and Fairburn (1984) found that women who considered themselves to have an eating problem had much higher scores than those who did not. Button and Whitehouse (1981) and Clarke and Palmer (1983) interviewed women in samples of university students who scored above the cutoff and found that even though few completely fulfilled the diagnostic criteria for anorexia, most showed eating disorders of varying degrees of severity, indicating that the scale may be sensitive to milder forms of eating disorders.

Both Steinhausen (1985) and Channon and DeSilva (1985) found that for anorexic clients scores on the Eating Attitudes Test were much higher before treatment than after treatment. Channon and DeSilva (1985) also found that anorexic individuals' scores predicted their weight gain during treatment and after treatment.

Eisler and Szmukler (1985) found a response bias related to social class. Teenage girls of higher social economic status apparently under-reported eating problems on the Eating Attitudes Test.

EATING ATTITUDES TEST

Please place an (X) under the column which applies best to each of the numbered statements. All of the results will be strictly confidential. Most of the questions directly relate to food or eating, although other types of questions have been included. Please answer each question carefully. Thank you.

	Always	Very often	Often	Some-times	Rarely	Never
1. Like eating with other people.	( )	( )	( )	( )	( )	( )
2. Prepare foods for others but do not eat what I cook.	( )	( )	( )	( )	( )	( )
3. Become anxious prior to eating.	( )	( )	( )	( )	( )	( )
4. Am terrified about being overweight.	( )	( )	( )	( )	( )	( )
5. Avoid eating when I am hungry.	( )	( )	( )	( )	( )	( )
6. Find myself pre-occupied with food.	( )	( )	( )	( )	( )	( )
7. Have gone on eating binges where I feel that I may not be able to stop.	( )	( )	( )	( )	( )	( )
8. Cut my food into small pieces.	( )	( )	( )	( )	( )	( )
9. Aware of the calorie content of foods that I eat.	( )	( )	( )	( )	( )	( )
10. Particularly avoid foods with a high carbohydrate content (e.g., bread, potatoes, rice, etc.).	( )	( )	( )	( )	( )	( )
11. Feel bloated after meals.	( )	( )	( )	( )	( )	( )

→

12. Feel that others would prefer if I ate more.	( )	( )	( )	( )	( )	( )
13. Vomit after I have eaten.	( )	( )	( )	( )	( )	( )
14. Feel extremely guilty after eating.	( )	( )	( )	( )	( )	( )
15. Am preoccupied with a desire to be thinner.	( )	( )	( )	( )	( )	( )
16. Exercise strenuously to burn off calories.	( )	( )	( )	( )	( )	( )
17. Weigh myself several times a day.	( )	( )	( )	( )	( )	( )
18. Like my clothes to fit tightly.	( )	( )	( )	( )	( )	( )
19. Enjoy eating meat.	( )	( )	( )	( )	( )	( )
20. Wake up early in the morning.	( )	( )	( )	( )	( )	( )
21. Eat the same foods day after day.	( )	( )	( )	( )	( )	( )
22. Think about burning up calories when I exercise.	( )	( )	( )	( )	( )	( )
23. Have regular menstrual periods.	( )	( )	( )	( )	( )	( )
24. Other people think that I am too thin.	( )	( )	( )	( )	( )	( )
25. Am preoccupied with the thought of having fat on my body.	( )	( )	( )	( )	( )	( )
26. Take longer than others to eat my meals.	( )	( )	( )	( )	( )	( )
27. Enjoy eating at restaurants.	( )	( )	( )	( )	( )	( )
28. Take laxatives.	( )	( )	( )	( )	( )	( )
29. Avoid foods with sugar in them.	( )	( )	( )	( )	( )	( )
30. Eat diet foods.	( )	( )	( )	( )	( )	( )

31. Feel that food con- ( ) ( ) ( ) ( ) ( ) ( )
    trols my life.
32. Display self-control ( ) ( ) ( ) ( ) ( ) ( )
    around food.
33. Feel that others ( ) ( ) ( ) ( ) ( ) ( )
    pressure me to eat.
34. Give too much time ( ) ( ) ( ) ( ) ( ) ( )
    and thought to
    food.
35. Suffer from con- ( ) ( ) ( ) ( ) ( ) ( )
    stipation.
36. Feel uncomfortable ( ) ( ) ( ) ( ) ( ) ( )
    after eating sweets.
37. Engage in dieting ( ) ( ) ( ) ( ) ( ) ( )
    behavior.
38. Like my stomach to ( ) ( ) ( ) ( ) ( ) ( )
    be empty.
39. Enjoy trying new ( ) ( ) ( ) ( ) ( ) ( )
    rich foods.
40. Have the impulse to ( ) ( ) ( ) ( ) ( ) ( )
    vomit after meals.

THREE-FACTOR EATING QUESTIONNAIRE

Purpose and Development

This questionnaire measures cognitive restraint in eating, disinhibition in eating, and susceptibility to hunger. The Three-Factor Eating Questionnaire is a 51-item self-report measure developed by Stunkard and Messick (1985), who created a pool of items in which some were based on a previous restrained eating questionnaire, some on a previous obesity questionnaire, and some on clinical experience. Several factor analyses of these items and identification of them that contributed most to the reliability of the scale led to the selection of the final items. Later factor analytic studies (Collins, Lapp, Helder, & Saltzberg, 1992; Ganley, 1988; Hyland, Irvine, Thacker, Dann & Dennis, 1989) found strong support for the Cognitive Restraint subscale but did not find that items consistently grouped into factors supporting the Disinhibition and Hunger subscales.

Administration and Scoring

Respondents indicate whether items 1 through 36 are true or false for them. Then they use a 4-point scale of frequency to answer items 37 to 49. Item 50 asks respondents to rate themselves on a 6-point scale of eating restraint and item 51 asks them to rate themselves on a 4-point scale of dieting behavior. Items 10, 16, 21, 25, 30, 31, and 47 are reverse coded. On the true and false items, respondents receive a 1 if they answer true and a 0 if they answer false. On the remaining items, respondents receive a score of 1 if they give a response of 3 or 4 (3 or more for item 50) and a 0 if they select a response of 1 or 2 (2 or less for item 50). Items 4, 6, 10, 14, 18, 21, 23, 28, 30, 32, 33, 35, 37, 38, 40, 42, 43, 44, 46, 48, and 50 are summed for the Cognitive Restraint subscale. Scores on this subscale may range from 0 to 21. Items 1, 2, 7, 9, 11, 13, 15, 16, 20, 25, 27, 31, 36, 45, 49, and 51 are summed for the Disinhibition subscale. Scores on this subscale may range from 0 to 16. Items 3, 5, 8, 12, 17, 19, 22, 24, 26, 29, 34, 39, 41, and 47 are summed for the Hunger subscale. Scores on this subscale may range from 0 to 14. Higher scores indicate more disturbance.

Sample Scores

Allison, Kalinsky, and Gorman (1992) asked 901 male and female college students to fill out the Cognitive Restraint subscale and found a mean score of 8.96 (SD = 5.75). We were not able to find other sample scores in our literature review.

Reliability

Stunkard and Messick (1985) found that internal consistency of the subscales for a combined sample of dieters and free eaters was .93 for the Cognitive Restraint subscale, .91 for the Disinhibition subscale, and .85 for the Hunger subscale as measured by coefficient alpha. Stunkard and Messick (1985) mentioned that in a personal communication to them Ganley reported that in a small sample of college students one-month test–retest reliability was .93 for the Cognitive Restraint subscale, .83 for the Disinhibition subscale, and .83 for the Hunger subscale.

Validity

In a sample of female college students, Collins et al. (1992) found that scores on the Cognitive Restraint subscale were associated with motivation to diet and scores on the combined Disinhibition and Hunger subscales were associated with a measure of negative emotions and a measure of responsiveness to food cues. Laessle, Tuschl, Kotthaus, and Pirke (1989) found a strong association between the Cognitive Restraint subscale scores and caloric intake.

Stunkard and Messick (1985) described two studies that support further the validity of the Three-Factor Eating Questionnaire. A study of obese women found that the severity of binge eating was related to scores on the Disinhibition subscale and the Hunger subscale but not to scores on the Cognitive Restraint subscale. Another study found that scores on the Disinhibition subscale but not on the other two subscales were related to overeating in a laboratory study of food intake.

THREE-FACTOR EATING QUESTIONNAIRE

PART I

Directions: Please answer the following questions by circling "T" for true or "F" for false depending on which response is most appropriate for you.

T   F   1. When I smell a sizzling steak or see a juicy piece of meat, I find it very difficult to keep from eating, even if I have just finished a meal.

T   F   2. I usually eat too much at social occasions, like parties and picnics.

T   F   3. I am usually so hungry that I eat more than three times a day.

T   F   4. When I have eaten my quota of calories, I am usually good about not eating any more.

T   F   5. Dieting is so hard for me because I just get too hungry.

T   F   6. I deliberately take small helpings as a means of controlling my weight.

T   F   7. Sometimes things just taste so good that I keep on eating even when I am no longer hungry.

T   F   8. Since I am often hungry, I sometimes wish that while I am eating, an expert would tell me that I have had enough or that I can have something more to eat.

T   F   9. When I feel anxious, I find myself eating.

T   F   10. Life is too short to worry about dieting.

T   F   11. Since my weight goes up and down, I have gone on reducing diets more than once.

T   F   12. I often feel so hungry that I just have to eat something.

T   F   13. When I am with someone who is overeating, I usually overeat too.

T   F   14. I have a pretty good idea of the number of calories in common food.

T   F   15. Sometimes when I start eating, I just can't seem to stop.

T   F   16. It is not difficult for me to leave something on my plate.

T   F   17. At certain times of the day, I get hungry because I have gotten used to eating then.

T   F   18. While on a diet, if I eat food that is not allowed, I consciously eat less for a period of time to make up for it.

T   F   19. Being with someone who is eating often makes me hungry enough to eat also.

T   F   20. When I feel blue, I often overeat.

T F 21. I enjoy eating too much to spoil it by counting calories or watching my weight.
T F 22. When I see a real delicacy, I often get so hungry that I have to eat right away.
T F 23. I often stop eating when I am not really full as a conscious means of limiting the amount that I eat.
T F 24. I get so hungry that my stomach often seems like a bottomless pit.
T F 25. My weight has hardly changed at all in the last ten years.
T F 26. I am always hungry so it is hard for me to stop eating before I finish the food on my plate.
T F 27. When I feel lonely, I console myself by eating.
T F 28. I consciously hold back at meals in order not to gain weight.
T F 29. I sometimes get very hungry late in the evening or at night.
T F 30. I eat anything I want, any time I want.
T F 31. Without even thinking about it, I take a long time to eat.
T F 32. I count calories as a conscious means of controlling my weight.
T F 33. I do not eat some foods because they make me fat.
T F 34. I am always hungry enough to eat at any time.
T F 35. I pay a great deal of attention to changes in my figure.
T F 36. While on a diet, if I eat a food that is not allowed, I often then splurge and eat other high calorie foods.

PART II

Directions: Please answer the following questions by circling the number above the response that is appropriate to you.

37. How often are you dieting in a conscious effort to control your weight?

1	2	3	4
rarely	sometimes	usually	always

38. Would a weight fluctuation of 5 lbs affect the way you live your life?

1	2	3	4
not at all	slightly	moderately	very much

39. How often do you feel hungry?

1	2	3	4
only at mealtimes	sometimes between meals	often between meals	almost always

➜

40. Do your feelings of guilt about overeating help you to control your food intake?

1	2	3	4
never	rarely	often	always

41. How difficult would it be for you to stop eating halfway through dinner and not eat for the next four hours?

1	2	3	4
easy	slightly difficult	moderately difficult	very difficult

42. How conscious are you of what you are eating?

1	2	3	4
not at all	slightly	moderately	extremely

43. How frequently do you avoid 'stocking up' on tempting foods?

1	2	3	4
almost never	seldom	usually	almost always

44. How likely are you to shop for low calorie foods?

1	2	3	4
unlikely	slightly unlikely	moderately likely	very likely

45. Do you eat sensibly in front of others and splurge alone?

1	2	3	4
never	rarely	often	always

46. How likely are you to consciously eat slowly in order to cut down on how much you eat?

1	2	3	4
unlikely	slightly likely	moderately likely	very likely

47. How frequently do you skip dessert because you are no longer hungry?

1	2	3	4
almost never	seldom	at least once a week	almost every day

48. How likely are you to consciously eat less than you want?

1	2	3	4
unlikely	slightly likely	moderately likely	very likely

49. Do you go on eating binges though you are not hungry?

1	2	3	4
never	rarely	sometimes	at least once a week

50. On a scale of 0 to 5, where 0 means no restraint in eating (eating whatever you want, whenever you want it) and 5 means total restraint (constantly limiting food intake and never 'giving in'), what number would you give yourself?

0

eat whatever you want, whenever you want it

1

usually eat whatever you want, whenever you want it

2

often eat whatever you want, whenever you want it

3

often limit food intake, but often 'give in'

4

usually limit food intake, rarely 'give in'

5

constantly limiting food intake, never 'giving in

51. To what extent does this statement describe your eating behavior? 'I
    start dieting in the morning, but because of any number of things that
    happen during the day, by evening I have given up and eat, what I
    want, promising myself to start dieting again tomorrow.'

1	2	3	4
not like me	little like me	pretty good description of me	describes me perfectly

Reprinted from *Journal of Psychosomatic Research*, 29, Stunkard, A,. & Messick, S., The Three-Factor Eating Questionnaire to measure dietary restraint, disinhibition, and hunger, Copyright 1985, 71–83, with kind permission from Elsevier Science Ltd., The Boulevard, Langford Lane, Kidlington OX5 1GB, UK.

BINGE EATING SCALE

Purpose and Development

The Binge Eating Scale is a 16-item self-report instrument developed by Gormally, Black, Daston, and Rardin (1982) to assess the behaviors, feelings, and cognitions relating to a binge episode in obese individuals. The items on the Binge Eating Scale were developed by Gormally et al. (1982) on the basis of their clinical experience.

Administration and Scoring

For each item respondents select the statement that is most true of them. Each statement has a different weight that reflects the severity of the problem indicated. The weights are as follows for each item's alternative statements: item 1 (1 = 0, 2 = 0, 3 = 1, 4 = 3), item 2 (1 = 0, 2 = 1, 3 = 2, 4 = 3), item 3 (1 = 0, 2 = 1, 3 = 3, 4 = 3), item 4 (1 = 0, 2 = 0, 3 = 0, 4 = 2), item 5 (1 = 0, 2 = 1, 3 = 2, 4 = 3), item 6 (1 = 0, 2 = 1, 3 = 3), item 7 (1 = 0, 2 = 2, 3 = 3, 4 = 3), item 8 (1 = 0, 2 = 1, 3 = 2, 4 = 3), item 9 (1 = 0, 2 = 1, 3 = 2, 4 = 3), item 10 (1 = 0, 2 = 1, 3 = 2, 4 = 3), item 11 (1 = 0, 2 = 1, 3 = 2, 4 = 3), item 12 (1 = 0, 2 = 1, 3 = 2, 4 = 2), item 13 (1 = 0, 2 = 0, 3 = 2, 4 = 3), item 14 (1 = 0, 2 = 1, 3 = 2, 4 = 3), item 15 (1 = 0, 2 = 1, 3 = 2, 4 = 3), item 16 (1 = 0, 2 = 1, 3 = 2). Scoring can be greatly simplified by numbering response options as they are scored (e.g., 0a, 0b, 1, 3 rather than 1–4 for item 1), but doing so might conceivably alter responses. The total scale score is the sum of all items and scores can range from 0 to 45, with higher scores indicating more problems with binge eating.

Sample Scores

Gormally et al. (1982) gave the scale to a group of 65 women seeking treatment for obesity and to a group of 32 women and 15 men seeking treatment for obesity. Interviewers rated each of these individuals on how severe a problem binge eating was for them. Table 1 shows the average scores for these groups. Marcus, Wing, and Hopkins (1988) suggest using 27 as the cutoff score for identifying individuals with serious binging problems.

Reliability

In a sample of obese women, Gormally et al. (1982) tested the internal consistency of the scale through a Kruskal–Wallis analysis of ranked data and found that all items were related to each other at the p < .01 level.

TABLE 1
Scores on the Binge Eating Scale
for Two Samples of Obese
Individuals Drawn by Gormally
et al. (1982)

	M	SD
Obese women	20.8	8.4
No binging	14.9	8.2
Moderate binging	19.6	6.7
Severe binging	28.9	7.5
Obese women and men	21.4	9.2
No binging	13.4	5.2
Moderate binging	21.1	7.0
Severe binging	31.3	6.6

Validity

In a sample of obese women seeking treatment, Marcus et al. (1988) found a 98% concordance rate between binge eating scores of 27 or greater and interview-based DSM-III diagnosed bulimia.

In samples of obese individuals, studies have found that those who scored higher on the Binge Eating Scale showed more unrealistic dieting and lower self-efficacy in dieting (Gormally et al., 1982), restricted food intake, disinhibition, hunger, and greater weight (Marcus, Wing, & Lamparski, 1985; Marcus et al., 1988), depression, anxiety, various neurotic symptoms, and maladaptive diet-related cognitions (LaPorte, 1992; Marcus et al., 1988).

Gormally et al. (1982) compared the scale scores of individuals who had been rated by interviewers as severe binge eaters, moderate binge eaters, or as having no problem with binge eating. As predicted, those who had been rated as having the most severe binge eating problems had significantly higher scale scores than those who had been rated as having moderate binge eating problems, and those who had been rated as moderate had significantly higher scale scores than those who had been rated as having no binge eating problems.

BINGE EATING SCALE

EATING HABITS CHECKLIST

Instructions: Below are groups of numbered statements. Read all of the statements in each group and circle the number of the one that best describes the way you feel about the problems you have controlling your eating behavior.

Group 1

1. I don't feel self-conscious about my weight or body size when I'm with others.
2. I feel concerned about how I look to others, but it normally does not make me feel disappointed with myself.
3. I do get self-conscious about my appearance and weight, which makes me feel disappointed in myself.
4. I feel very self-conscious about my weight and frequently I feel intense shame and disgust for myself. I try to avoid social contacts because of my self-consciousness.

Group 2

1. I don't have any difficulty eating slowly in the proper manner.
2. Although I seem to "gobble down" foods, I don't end up feeling stuffed because of eating too much.
3. At times, I tend to eat quickly and then I feel uncomfortably full afterward.
4. I have the habit of bolting down my food, without really chewing it. When this happens I usually feel uncomfortably stuffed because I've eaten too much.

Group 3

1. I feel able to control my eating urges when I want to.
2. I feel like I have failed to control my eating more than the average person.
3. I feel utterly helpless when it comes to feeling in control of my eating urges.
4. Because I feel so helpless about controlling my eating, I have become very desperate about trying to get in control.

➛

Group 4

1. I don't have the habit of eating when I'm bored.
2. I sometimes eat when I'm bored, but often I'm able to "get busy" and get my mind off food.
3. I have a regular habit of eating when I'm bored, but occasionally, I can use some other activity to get my mind off eating.
4. I have a strong habit of eating when I'm bored. Nothing seems to help me break the habit.

Group 5

1. I'm usually physically hungry when I eat something.
2. Occasionally, I eat something on impulse even though I really am not hungry.
3. I have the regular habit of eating foods that I might not really enjoy to satisfy a hungry feeling even though, physically, I don't need the food.
4. Even though I'm not physically hungry, I get a hungry feeling in my mouth that only seems to be satisfied when I eat a food, like a sandwich, that fills my mouth. Sometimes, when I eat the food to satisfy my mouth hunger, I then spit the food out so I won't gain weight.

Group 6

1. I don't feel any guilt or self-hate after I overeat.
2. After I overeat, occasionally I feel guilt or self-hate.
3. Almost all the time I experience strong guilt or self-hate after I overeat.

Group 7

1. I don't lose total control of my eating when dieting even after periods when I overeat.
2. Sometimes when I eat a "forbidden food" on a diet, I feel like I "blew it" and eat even more.
3. Frequently, I have the habit of saying to myself, "I've blown it now, why not go all the way" when I overeat on a diet. When that happens I eat even more.
4. I have a regular habit of starting strict diets for myself, but I break the diets by going on an eating binge. My life seems to be either a "feast" or "famine."

Group 8

1. I rarely eat so much food that I feel uncomfortably stuffed afterward.
2. Usually about once a month, I eat such a quantity of food, I end up feeling very stuffed.

3. I have regular periods during the month when I eat large amounts of food, either at mealtime or at snacks.
4. I eat so much food that I regularly feel quite uncomfortable after eating and sometimes a bit nauseous.

Group 9

1. My level of calorie intake does not go up very high or go down very low on a regular basis.
2. Sometimes after I overeat, I will try to reduce my caloric intake to almost nothing to compensate for the excess calories I've eaten.
3. I have a regular habit of overeating during the night. It seems that my routine is not to be hungry in the morning but overeat in the evening.
4. In my adult years, I have had week-long periods where I practically starve myself. This follows periods when I overeat. It seems I live a life of either "feast or famine."

Group 10

1. I usually am able to stop eating when I want to. I know when "enough is enough."
2. Every so often, I experience a compulsion to eat which I can't seem to control.
3. Frequently, I experience strong urges to eat which I seem unable to control, but at other times I can control my eating urges.
4. I feel incapable of controlling urges to eat. I have a fear of not being able to stop eating voluntarily.

Group 11

1. I don't have any problem stopping eating when I feel full.
2. I usually can stop eating when I feel full but occasionally overeat, leaving me feeling uncomfortably stuffed.
3. I have a problem stopping eating once I start and usually I feel uncomfortably stuffed after I eat a meal.
4. Because I have a problem not being able to stop eating when I want, I sometimes have to induce vomiting to relieve my stuffed feeling.

Group 12

1. I seem to eat just as much when I'm with others (family, social gatherings) as when I'm by myself.
2. Sometimes, when I'm with other persons, I don't eat as much as I want to eat because I'm self-conscious about my eating.
3. Frequently, I eat only a small amount of food when others are present, because I'm very embarrassed about my eating.

→

4. I feel so ashamed about overeating that I pick times to overeat when I know no one will see me. I feel like a "closet eater."

Group 13

1. I eat three meals a day with only an occasional between meal snack.
2. I eat 3 meals a day, but I also normally snack between meals.
3. When I am snacking heavily, I get in the habit of skipping regular meals.
4. There are regular periods when I seem to be continually eating, with no planned meals.

Group 14

1. I don't think much about trying to control unwanted eating urges.
2. At least some of the time, I feel my thoughts are preoccupied with trying to control my eating urges.
3. I feel that frequently I spend much time thinking about how much I ate or about trying not to eat anymore.
4. It seems to me that most of my waking hours are preoccupied by thoughts about eating or not eating. I feel like I'm constantly struggling not to eat.

Group 15

1. I don't think about food a great deal.
2. I have strong cravings for food but they last only for brief periods of time.
3. I have days when I can't seem to think about anything else but food.
4. Most of my days seem to be preoccupied with thoughts about food. I feel like I live to eat.

Group 16

1. I usually know whether or not I'm physically hungry. I take the right portion of food to satisfy me.
2. Occasionally, I feel uncertain about knowing whether or not I'm physically hungry. At these times it's hard to know how much food I should take to satisfy me.
3. Even though I might know how many calories I should eat, I don't have any idea what is a "normal" amount of food for me.

Reprinted from *Addictive Behaviors*, 7, Gormally, J., Black, S., Daston, S., & Rardin, D. The assessment of binge eating severity among obese persons, 47–55, Copyright 1982, with kind permission from Elsevier Science Ltd, The Boulevard, Langford Lane, Kidlington OX5 1GB, UK.

BODY SHAPE QUESTIONNAIRE

Purpose and Development

The Body Shape Questionnaire is a 34-item self-report measure developed by Cooper, Taylor, Cooper, and Fairburn (1987) to assess concerns about body shape in individuals with eating disorders such as bulimia. They interviewed some individuals with eating disorders and some without eating disorders and asked them to describe "feeling fat" and the emotional and behavioral consequences of such feelings. The resulting information was grouped into categories. Next items that reflected the categories were generated. From this pool of items, those items were selected that contributed most to the internal consistency of the questionnaire, distinguished most between groups of eating and noneating disordered individuals, and had adequate variance.

Administration and Scoring

Respondents are asked to reflect on how they felt about their appearance over the past four weeks and to rate each item on a 6-point scale of frequency for that time frame. The total score is the sum of all items and scores may range from 34 to 204, with higher scores indicating more distress.

Sample Scores

Cooper et al. (1987) gave the questionnaire to 38 female clients with bulimia nervosa and a community sample of 535 women recruited from among those attending a family planning clinic, occupational therapy students, and undergraduate students. On the basis of several screening questions given to women in the community sample, they identified 10 individuals who had bulimia nervosa and 316 individuals who did not have bulimia. They also divided a portion of their community sample into 95 women who indicated slimness was important to them and that they were dieting and 79 women who were not concerned about slimness. Table 1 shows the average scores for these women.

Reliability

Each item correlated at .60 or above with the total scale in a sample of patients and a sample of nonpatients (Cooper et al., 1987).

TABLE 1
Scores on the Body Shape Questionnaire
in Samples Drawn by Cooper et al. (1987)

	M	SD
Female clients with bulimia nervosa	136.9	22.5
Women from a community sample	81.5	28.4
Probable cases of bulimia nervosa	129.3	17.0
Non-cases of Bulimia nervosa	71.9	23.6
Women concerned with slimness	109.0	21.2
Women not concerned with slimness	55.9	14.4

Validity

Cooper et al. (1987) and Hadigan and Walsh (1991) found that higher scores on the Body Shape Questionnaire were associated with higher scores on several measures of eating disorders. Studies of bulimic clients have found higher scores were related to depression and lower self-esteem (Cooper & Fairburn, 1993, Hadigan & Walsh, 1991).

Cooper et al. (1987) found that bulimic clients scored much higher on the Body Shape Questionnaire than women in a community sample, and that in a community sample women who on the basis of screening questions were identified as probably having bulimia scored higher on the questionnaire than women who did not have bulimia. They also found that women who were concerned with slimness scored higher on the questionnaire than women not concerned with slimness. Hadigan and Walsh (1991) also found that female bulimic clients scored much higher on the questionnaire than other women.

BODY SHAPE QUESTIONNAIRE

We would like to know how you have been feeling about your appearance over the PAST FOUR WEEKS. Please read each question and mark the appropriate number to the left. Please answer all the questions.

OVER THE PAST FOUR WEEKS:

Never	Rarely	Sometimes	Often	Very often	Always
1	2	3	4	5	6

_____ 1. Has feeling bored made you brood about your shape?

_____ 2. Have you been so worried about your shape that you have been feeling that you ought to diet?

_____ 3. Have you thought that your thighs, hips, or bottom are too large for the rest of you?

_____ 4. Have you been afraid that you might become fat (or fatter)?

_____ 5. Have you worried about your flesh not being firm enough?

_____ 6. Has feeling full (e.g., after eating a large meal) made you feel fat?

_____ 7. Have you felt so bad about your shape that you have cried?

_____ 8. Have you avoided running because your flesh might wobble?

_____ 9. Has being with thin women made you feel self-conscious about your shape?

_____ 10. Have you worried about your thighs spreading out when sitting down?

_____ 11. Has eating even a small amount of food made you feel fat?

_____ 12. Have you noticed the shape of other women and felt that your own shape compared unfavorably?

_____ 13. Has thinking about your shape interfered with your ability to concentrate (e.g., while watching television, reading, listening to conversations)?

_____ 14. Has being naked, such as when taking a bath, made you feel fat?

_____ 15. Have you avoided wearing clothes which make you particularly aware of the shape of your body?

_____ 16. Have you imagined cutting off fleshy areas of your body?

_____ 17. Has eating sweets, cakes, or other high calorie food made you feel fat?

_____ 18. Have you not gone out to social occasions (e.g., parties) because you have felt bad about your shape?

→

_____ 19. Have you felt excessively large and rounded?

_____ 20. Have you felt ashamed of your body?

_____ 21. Has worry about your shape made you diet?

_____ 22. Have you felt happiest about your shape when your stomach has been empty (e.g., in the morning)?

_____ 23. Have you thought that you are the shape you are because you lack self-control?

_____ 24. Have you worried about other people seeing rolls of flesh around your waist or stomach?

_____ 25. Have you felt that it is not fair that other women are thinner than you?

_____ 26. Have you vomited in order to feel thinner?

_____ 27. When in company have you worried about taking up too much room (e.g., sitting on a sofa or a bus seat)?

_____ 28. Have you worried about your flesh being dimply?

_____ 29. Has seeing your reflection (e.g., in a mirror or shop window) made you feel bad about your shape?

_____ 30. Have you pinched areas of your body to see how much fat there is?

_____ 31. Have you avoided situations where people could see your body (e.g., communal changing rooms or swimming baths)?

_____ 32. Have you taken laxatives in order to feel thinner?

_____ 33. Have you been particularly self-conscious about your shape when in the company of other people?

_____ 34. Has worry about your shape made you feel you ought to exercise?

REFERENCES

Allison, D. B., Kalinsky, L. B., & Gorman, B. S. (1992). A comparison of the psychometric properties of three measures of dietary restraint. *Psychological Assessment, 4*, 391–398.

Button, E. J., & Whitehouse, A. (1981). Subclinical anorexia nervosa. *Psychological Medicine, 11*, 509–516.

Channon, S., & DeSilva, W. P. (1985). Psychological correlates of weight gain in patients with anorexia nervosa. *Journal of Psychiatric Research, 19*, 267–271.

Clarke, M. G., & Palmer, R. L. (1983). Eating attitudes and neurotic symptoms in university students. *British Journal of Psychiatry, 142*, 299–304.

Collins, R., Lapp, W., Helder, L., & Saltzberg, J. (1992). Cognitive restraint and impulsive eating: Insights from the Three-Factor Eating Questionnaire. *Psychology of Addictive Behaviors, 6*, 47–53.

Cooper, P. J., & Fairburn, C. G. (1993). Confusion over the core psychopathology of bulimia nervosa. *International Journal of Eating Disorders, 13*, 385–389.

Cooper, P. J., Taylor, M., Cooper, Z., & Fairburn, C. G. (1987). The development and validation of the Body Shape Questionnaire. *International Journal of Eating Disorders, 6*, 485–494.

Cooper, P. J., Waterman, G. C., & Fairburn, C. G. (1984). Women with eating problems: A community survey. *British Journal of Clinical Psychology, 23*, 45–52.

Eisler, I., & Szmukler, G. (1985). Social class as a confounding variable in the Eating Attitudes Test. *Journal of Psychiatric Research, 19*, 171–176.

Ganley, R. M. (1988). Emotional eating and how it relates to dietary restraint, disinhibition, and perceived hunger. *International Journal of Eating Disorders, 7*, 635–647.

Garner, D., & Garfinkel, P. (1979). The Eating Attitudes Test: An index of the symptoms of anorexia nervosa. *Psychological Medicine, 9*, 273–279.

Garner, D., & Garfinkel, P. (1980). Socio-cultural factors in the development of anorexia nervosa. *Psychological Medicine, 10*, 647–656.

Garner, D., Olmstead, M., Bohr, Y., & Garfinkel, P. (1982). The Eating Attitudes Test: Psychometric features and clinical correlates. *Psychological Medicine, 12*, 871–878.

Gormally, J., Black, S., Daston, S., & Rardin, D. (1982). The assessment of binge eating severity among obese persons. *Addictive Behaviors, 7*, 47–55.

Hadigan, C. M., & Walsh, B. T. (1991). Body shape concerns in bulimia nervosa. *International Journal of Eating Disorders, 10*, 323–331.

Heatherton, T., Herman, C., Polivy, J., King, G., & McGree, S. (1988). The (mis) measurement of restraint: An analysis of conceptual and psychometric issues. *Journal of Abnormal Psychology, 97*, 19–28.

Hyland, M. E., Irvine, S. H., Thacker, C., Dann. P. L., & Dennis, I. (1989). Psychometric analysis of the Stunkard–Messick Eating Questionnaire (SMEQ) and comparison with the Dutch Eating Behavior Questionnaire (DEBQ). *Current Psychology Research and Reviews, 8*, 228–233.

Kiemle, G., Slade, P., & Dewey M. (1987). Factors associated with abnormal eating attitudes and behaviors: Screening individuals at risk of developing an eating disorder. *International Journal of Eating Disorders, 6*, 713–724.

Laessle, R., Tuschl, R., Kotthaus, B., & Pirke, K. (1989). A comparison of the validity of three scales for the assessment of dietary restraint. *Journal of Abnormal Psychology, 98*, 504–507.

LaPorte, D. (1992). Treatment response in obese binge eaters: Preliminary results using a very low calorie diet (VLCD) and behavior therapy. *Addictive Behaviors, 17*, 247–257.

Marcus, M. D., Wing, R. R., & Hopkins, J. (1988). Obese binge eaters: Affect, cognitions, and response to behavioral weight control. *Journal of Consulting and Clinical Psychology, 56*, 433–439.

Marcus, M. D., Wing, R. R., & Lamparski, D. M. (1985). Binge eating and dietary restrain in obese patients. *Addictive Behaviors, 10,* 163–168.

Raciti, M., & Norcross, J. (1987). The EAT and EDI: Screening, Interrelationships, and Psychometrics. *International Journal of Eating Disorders, 6*(4), 579–586.

Slade, P., Butler, N., & Newton, T. (1989). A short note on the relationship between the Setting Conditions for Anorexia Nervosa Scale (SCANS) and the Eysenck Personality Questionnaire (EPQ). *Personality and Individual Differences, 10,* 801–802.

Slade, P., & Dewey, M. (1986). Development and preliminary validation of SCANS: A screening instrument for identifying individuals at risk of developing anorexia and bulimia nervosa. *International Journal of Eating Disorders, 5,* 517–538.

Steinhausen, H. C. (1985). Evaluation of inpatient treatment of adolescent anorexic patients. *Journal of Psychiatric Research, 19,* 371–375.

Stunkard, A., & Messick, S. (1985). The Three-Factor Eating Questionnaire to measure dietary restraint, disinhibition, and hunger. *Journal of Psychosomatic Research, 29,* 71–83.

CHAPTER 11

Sleep Disorders

POST-SLEEP INVENTORY

Purpose and Development

This scale assesses subjective evaluation of a preceding sleep period. The Post-Sleep Inventory is a 29-item self-report measure (Webb, Bonnet, & Blume, 1976). Thirty items were developed on the basis of 81 undergraduate and graduate students' descriptions of their sleep during the past night and their sleep in general. The items were grouped into the categories of pre-sleep, during sleep, and post-sleep. One of the 30 items did not correlate well with the other items and was eliminated from the scale. Webb et al. (1976) factor analyzed the responses of college students to the 29-item scale and found that the seven most important factors were mental activity, morning factors, sleep factors, evening/night ailments, dream amount, sleepiness in the evening, and dream emotion.

Administration and Scoring

Respondents are asked to respond to each item using a 13-point scale which has descriptors at bi-polar endpoints. They may also check the alternatives "Unimportant" or "Don't Know." Items 1, 3, 5, 6, 10, 11, 13, 16, 18, 20, 25, 28, and 29 are reverse coded. Webb et al. (1976) did not specify how to code "Unimportant" or "Don't Know" responses; we suggest that these responses be given the average of a respondent's other ratings and then be added into the total scale score. The total scale score is the sum of all items and scores may range from 29 to 377, with low scores indicating worse sleep. Blankstein, Flett, Watson, and Koledin (1990) suggested that

333

TABLE 1
Scores on the Post-Sleep
Inventory, Webb et al.
(1976)

	M	SD
College students		
Poor sleepers	183	34.5
Good sleepers	253	40.9

three subscale scores may be obtained by summing the items in the three subsections: pre-sleep, during sleep, and post-sleep.

Sample Scores

Webb et al. (1976) gave the scale to 92 college students who were also asked to judge whether their sleep had been good or poor. The number of individuals who had good or poor sleep was not reported. Table 1 shows the mean scale scores.

Reliability

Webb et al. (1976) reported that in a sample of college students all the scale items correlated significantly with each other at the $p < .001$ level, but did not report the actual magnitude of the correlation. Blankstein et al. (1990) reported the following alphas for the three subsections of the scale: .61 for pre-sleep, .71 for during sleep, and .66 for post-sleep.

Validity

Webb et al. (1976) found that college students who reported poor sleep had significantly lower scale scores than those who reported good sleep. The scale also differentiated between the sleep of elderly individuals, who are generally thought to have poorer sleep, and young individuals (Webb et al., 1976) and between earlier and late risers (Webb & Bonnet, 1978). Blankstein et al. (1990) found that students with greater test anxiety had poorer sleep as assessed by the scale.

POST-SLEEP INVENTORY

All of the following items ask about how you slept *last night*. The numbers below each item represent degrees to which the statement on the left versus the right is true. For each item please circle the number that best describes what was true for you. If you don't know or the item is unimportant, check that response.

GOING TO BED

1. Asleep quickly   Long time awake

1 2 3 4 5 6 7 8 9 10 11 12 13
Don't know or unimportant _____

2. Felt very physically tense   Felt very physically relaxed

1 2 3 4 5 6 7 8 9 10 11 12 13
Don't know or unimportant _____

3. No worries on my mind   Many worries on my mind

1 2 3 4 5 6 7 8 9 10 11 12 13
Don't know or unimportant _____

4. Many thoughts   No thoughts

1 2 3 4 5 6 7 8 9 10 11 12 13
Don't know or unimportant _____

5. Felt very sleepy   Felt very wide awake

1 2 3 4 5 6 7 8 9 10 11 12 13
Don't know or unimportant _____

6. Felt very exhausted   Not exhausted at all

1 2 3 4 5 6 7 8 9 10 11 12 13
Don't know or unimportant _____

7. Had many physical ailments   Had no physical ailments

1 2 3 4 5 6 7 8 9 10 11 12 13
Don't know or unimportant _____

→

8. Went to bed in a   Went to bed in a
   very bad mood   very good mood

       1 2 3 4 5 6 7 8 9 10 11 12 13
       Don't know or unimportant _____

DURING THE NIGHT

9. Frequently awakened   Uninterrupted sleep

       1 2 3 4 5 6 7 8 9 10 11 12 13
       Don't know or unimportant _____

10. No noises   Very noisy

       1 2 3 4 5 6 7 8 9 10 11 12 13
       Don't know or unimportant _____

11. Very comfortable room temperature   Extremely hot or cold

       1 2 3 4 5 6 7 8 9 10 11 12 13
       Don't know or unimportant _____

12. Very uncomfortable bed   Very comfortable bed

       1 2 3 4 5 6 7 8 9 10 11 12 13
       Don't know or unimportant _____

13. Little or no body movement   Tossed and turned all night

       1 2 3 4 5 6 7 8 9 10 11 12 13
       Don't know or unimportant _____

14. Awakened and took an extremely   Awakened but immediately
    long time to go back to sleep   went back to sleep

       1 2 3 4 5 6 7 8 9 10 11 12 13
       Don't know or unimportant _____

15. Lightest sleep possible   Deepest sleep possible

       1 2 3 4 5 6 7 8 9 10 11 12 13
       Don't know or unimportant _____

16. Adequate amount of sleep   Not enough sleep at all

         1 2 3 4 5 6 7 8 9 10 11 12 13

         Don't know or unimportant _____

17. Many thoughts   No thoughts

         1 2 3 4 5 6 7 8 9 10 11 12 13

         Don't know or unimportant _____

18. Felt very physically relaxed   Felt very physically tense

         1 2 3 4 5 6 7 8 9 10 11 12 13

         Don't know or unimportant _____

19. Had many physical ailments   Had no physical ailments

         1 2 3 4 5 6 7 8 9 10 11 12 13

         Don't know or unimportant _____

20. Extremely pleasant dreams   Extremely unpleasant dreams

         1 2 3 4 5 6 7 8 9 10 11 12 13

         Don't know or unimportant _____

21. Many dreams   No dreams

         1 2 3 4 5 6 7 8 9 10 11 12 13

         Don't know or unimportant _____

ON AWAKENING

22. Woke up long before or   Woke up exactly when
    after I expected to   I expected to

         1 2 3 4 5 6 7 8 9 10 11 12 13

         Don't know or unimportant _____

23. Woke up extremely tired   Woke up as rested as possible

         1 2 3 4 5 6 7 8 9 10 11 12 13

         Don't know or unimportant _____

24. Had a very hard time awakening   Woke up as easily as possible

     1 2 3 4 5 6 7 8 9 10 11 12 13
                Don't know or unimportant _____

25. Woke up in a very good mood   Woke up in a very bad mood

     1 2 3 4 5 6 7 8 9 10 11 12 13
                Don't know or unimportant _____

26. Remembered extremely   Remembered very
    unpleasant dreams   pleasant dreams

     1 2 3 4 5 6 7 8 9 10 11 12 13
                Don't know or unimportant _____

27. Woke up feeling as   Woke up feeling as
    physically poor as possible   physically good as possible

     1 2 3 4 5 6 7 8 9 10 11 12 13
                Don't know or unimportant _____

28. Woke up with no worries   Woke up with many worries
    on my mind

     1 2 3 4 5 6 7 8 9 10 11 12 13
                Don't know or unimportant _____

29. Woke up with no thoughts   Woke up with many thoughts
    on my mind

     1 2 3 4 5 6 7 8 9 10 11 12 13
                Don't know or unimportant _____

PRE-SLEEP AROUSAL SCALE

Purpose and Development

The 16-item self-report Pre-Sleep Arousal Scale measures the level of cognitive and somatic arousal an individual generally experiences before falling asleep (Nicassio, Mendlowitz, Fussell, and Petras, 1985). Nicassio et al. (1985) generated items on the basis of clinical observations and interviews with sleep-disturbed patients. Three judges then classified the items as reflecting cognitive or somatic arousal and showed 100% agreement in their classifications.

Administration and Scoring

Respondents rate each item on a 5-point scale of intensity. In the standard instructions respondents are asked to consider their general presleep time. However, in one study Nicassio et al. (1985) modified the instructions so that the focus was on the previous night's presleep time. The Somatic Arousal subscale score is the sum of items 1 through 8 and the Cognitive Arousal subscale score is the sum of items 9 through 16. Scores on each subscale can range from 8 to 40, with higher scores indicating more arousal.

Sample Scores

Nicassio et al. (1985) gave the scale to 16 male and 14 female insomniacs, 13 male and 17 female normal sleepers, and 85 male and 62 female college students. Table 1 shows the average scores for these groups.

Reliability

Nicassio et al. (1985) found the Cognitive Arousal subscale to have an internal consistency as measured by Cronbach's alpha of .88 for a group of college students, .67 for a group of normal sleepers, and .76 for a group of insomniacs. They found the Somatic Arousal subscale to have a Cronbach's alpha of .79 for the college students, .84 for normal sleepers, and .81 for insomniacs. They also found evidence that the items on each subscale correlated more with each other than with items on the other subscale, indicating that they tap two discrete dimensions of presleep arousal.

In a sample of college students, Nicassio et al. (1985) found a three-week test–retest reliability of .72 for the Cognitive Arousal subscale and .76 for the Somatic Arousal subscale.

TABLE 1
Scores on the Pre-Sleep Arousal Scale,
Nicassio (1985)

	Somatic arousal		Cognitive arousal	
	M	SD	M	SD
Insomniacs	17.67	6.45	25.50	6.57
Normal sleepers	11.17	3.99	12.80	2.75
College students	11.63	3.74	21.45	5.80

Validity

In a sample consisting of insomniacs, normal sleepers, and college students, Nicassio et al. (1985) found that higher scores on both the Somatic Arousal and the Cognitive Arousal subscales were significantly associated with longer sleep onset latency, less total sleep time, more awakening during the night, greater listlessness during the day, and a greater likelihood of being a self-described insomniac. Higher subscale scores were also significantly associated with more depression and more general anxiety. The Somatic Arousal subscale was more highly correlated with a measure of somatic anxiety than with a measure of cognitive anxiety, and the Cognitive Arousal subscale was significantly correlated with the measure of cognitive anxiety but not correlated with the measure of somatic anxiety.

Nicassio et al. (1985) compared the scores of insomniacs and normal sleepers and found that insomniacs scored much higher on both subscales than the normal sleepers.

Nicassio et al. (1985) also collected some validity data for the scale when it was used with reference to just the last night's presleep time. In a small group of college students they found a significant correlation between scores on the Cognitive Arousal and Somatic Arousal subscales and sleep-onset latency, but not between the subscales and number of awakenings or total sleep time.

PRE-SLEEP AROUSAL SCALE

Please describe how intensely you generally experience each of the following as you try to fall asleep in your own bedroom by marking a number next to each item. Use the following categories:

1	2	3	4	5
not at all	slightly	moderately	a lot	extremely

_____ 1. Heart racing, pounding, or beating irregularly
_____ 2. A jittery, nervous feeling in your body
_____ 3. Shortness of breath or labored breathing
_____ 4. A tight, tense feeling in your muscles
_____ 5. Cold feeling in your hands, feet, or your body in general
_____ 6. Have stomach upset (knot or nervous feeling in stomach, heartburn, nausea, gas, etc.)
_____ 7. Perspiration in palms of your hands or other parts of your body
_____ 8. Dry feeling in mouth or throat
_____ 9. Worry about falling asleep
_____ 10. Review or ponder events of the day
_____ 11. Depressing or anxious thoughts
_____ 12. Worry about problems other than sleep
_____ 13. Being mentally alert, active
_____ 14. Can't shut off your thoughts
_____ 15. Thoughts keep running through your head
_____ 16. Being distracted by sounds, noise in the environment (e.g., ticking of clock, house noises, traffic)

Reprinted with permission of Dr. Perry Nicassio.

ST. MARY'S HOSPITAL SLEEP QUESTIONNAIRE

Purpose and Development

The St. Mary's Hospital Sleep Questionnaire assesses individuals' previous night's sleep. The questionnaire is a 14-item self-report measure developed by Ellis, Johns, Lancaster, Raptopoulos, Angelopoulos, and Priest (1981). The straightforward items are based on an earlier questionnaire developed by Priest and Rizvi and were initially developed for use with hospital patients. In a factor analytic study of the items, Leigh, Bird, Hindmarch, Constable, and Wright (1988) found that the items grouped into factors they called sleep latency, sleep quality, amount of sleep, and sleep satisfaction.

Administration and Scoring

Respondents answer the items with reference to their previous night's sleep using time responses for some items and rating scales for other items. Each of the items is evaluated separately.

Sample Scores

Ellis et al. (1981) gave the questionnaire to a group of 32 psychiatric hospital patients, 16 surgical hospital patients, 21 medical hospital patients, and 24 nonpatients. Table 1 shows the average scores of this group.

Reliability

Ellis et al. (1981) asked groups of hospital patients and nonpatients to complete the questionnaire twice, with a four-hour interval, and found the test–retest reliability of items ranged from .70 to .96.

Validity

Snyder-Halpern and Verran (1987) found high correlations between items on the St. Mary's Hospital Questionnaire and similar items on another sleep scale. Reimer (1987) found significant differences on the questionnaire items between hospital and home sleeping patterns and Patel, Gura, Kurian, Lambert, Steinert, and Priest (1991) found that patients scored differently on some items of the questionnaire depending on which type of sleeping medication they received.

TABLE 1

Scores on the St. Mary's Hospital Sleep Questionnaire (Ellis et al., 1981)

Item	M	SE
1. Time settled for night (actual time)	22.81	.11
2. Time fell asleep (actual time)	23.83	.15
3. Time awoke (actual time)	6.44	.14
4. Time got up (actual time)	7.23	.13
5. Depth of sleep (higher scores indicate deeper sleep)	4.35	.18
6. Number of awakenings (actual number of awakenings)	1.89	.19
7. How much sleep during night (number of hours)	6.67	.18
8. How much sleep during previous day (number of hours)	.62	.12
9. How well slept (higher scores indicate better sleep)	4.22	.12
10. How clear-headed (higher numbers indicate greater alertness)	3.47	.12
11. How satisfied with sleep (higher numbers indicate more satisfaction)	3.69	.11
12. Troubled by waking ("no" is scored as 1 and "yes" as 2)	1.22	.04
13. Difficulty in going to sleep (higher numbers indicate more difficulty)	1.57	.08
14. How long it took to fall asleep (number of hours)	.71	.09

ST. MARY'S HOSPITAL SLEEP QUESTIONNAIRE

This questionnaire refers to your sleep over the past 24 hours. Please try and answer every question.

At what time did you:
1. Settle down for the night? _____ hrs. _____ mins.
2. Fall asleep last night? _____ hrs. _____ mins.
3. Finally wake this morning? _____ hrs. _____ mins.
4. Get up this morning? _____ hrs. _____ mins.
5. Was your sleep: (check one)
    1. Very light _____
    2. Light _____
    3. Fairly light _____
    4. Light average _____
    5. Deep average _____
    6. Fairly deep _____
    7. Deep _____
    8. Very deep _____
6. How many times did you wake up? (check one)
    0. Not at all _____
    1. Once _____
    2. Twice _____
    3. Three times _____
    4. Four times _____
    5. Five times _____
    6. Six times _____
    7. More than six times _____
How much sleep did you have?
7. Last night _____ hrs. _____ mins.
8. During the day, yesterday _____ hrs. _____ mins.
9. How well did you sleep last night? (check one)
    1. Very badly _____
    2. Badly _____
    3. Fairly badly _____
    4. Fairly well _____
    5. Well _____
    6. Very well _____
    If not well, what was the trouble? (e.g., restless, etc.)

    1. _____

2. _____

3. _____

10. How clear-headed did you feel after getting up this morning? (check one)
    1. Still very drowsy indeed   _____
    2. Still moderately drowsy   _____
    3. Still slightly drowsy   _____
    4. Fairly clear-headed   _____
    5. Alert   _____
    6. Very alert   _____

11. How satisfied were you with last night's sleep? (check one)
    1. Very unsatisfied   _____
    2. Moderately unsatisfied   _____
    3. Slightly unsatisfied   _____
    4. Fairly satisfied   _____
    5. Completely satisfied   _____

12. Were you troubled by waking early and being unable to get off to sleep again? (check one)
    1. No   _____
    2. Yes   _____

13. How much difficulty did you have in getting off to sleep last night? (check one)
    1. None or very little   _____
    2. Some   _____
    3. A lot   _____
    4. Extreme difficulty   _____

14. How long did it take you to fall asleep last night?
    _____ hrs.   _____ mins.

Reprinted from Ellis, B. W., Johns M. W., Lancaster, R., Raptopoulos, P., Angelopoulos, N., & Priest, R. G. (1981). The St. Mary's Hospital Sleep Questionnaire: A study of reliability. *Sleep, 4,* 93–97, with permission of the American Sleep Disorders Association. Thanks to Professor Priest for provided materials.

STANFORD SLEEPINESS SCALE

Purpose and Development

The Stanford Sleepiness Scale is a one-item self-report measure that assesses the degree of current sleepiness (Hoddes, Dement, & Zarcone, 1972; Hoddes, Zarcone, Smythe, Phillips, & Dement, 1973). The scale was based on the judgments of 95 individuals who rated 52 statements about sleepiness. The seven statements that best differentiated degrees of sleepiness were selected for the final scale. The scale has been used extensively to assess the effects of pharmaceutical interventions and the effects of sleep deprivation.

Administration and Scoring

Respondents are asked to select the scale value that best describes their state of sleepiness. Scores can range from 1 to 7, with higher scores indicating greater sleepiness.

Sample Scores

Hoddes et al. (1973) gave the scale to 5 male college students after they had normal sleep and after they had been deprived of sleep for one night. Carskadon and Dement (1981) gave the scale to 10 adult men and women after a full night's sleep and after the first, fourth, and seventh night of sleep restricted to five hours per night. Table 1 shows their average scores.

TABLE 1
Scores on the Stanford Sleepiness Scale

	M	SD
Male college students*		
After normal sleep	2.8	1.1
After 1 night Sleep Deprivation	4.6	1.4
Adult men and women**		
After normal sleep	2.4	.5
After 1 night partial deprivation	2.7	.4
After 4 nights partial deprivation	3.2	.3
After 7 nights partial deprivation	3.4	.3

*Hoddes et al. (1973), ** Carskadon and Dement (1981).

Reliability

Hoddes et al. (1972) reported an alternate form reliability of .88.

Validity

Several studies found strong relationships between Stanford Sleepiness Scale scores and scores on other subjective measures of sleepiness, but at the same time found inconsistent relationships between scale scores and objective measures of sleepiness (e.g. Johnson, Spinweber, Gomez, & Matteson, 1990; Johnson, Freeman, Spinweber, & Gomez, 1991). Higher scale scores have also been found to be associated with less alertness and more dysphoria (Spring, Maller, Wurtman, Digman, & Cozolino, 1983).

A number of studies found that the scale is sensitive to the effects of pharmacological interventions (e.g. Karacan, Orr, Roth, Kramer, Thornby, Bingham, & Kay, 1981; Johnson, Spinweber, & Gomez, 1990; Johnson et al. 1991) and sleep deprivation (e.g. Hoddes et al., 1973; Webb & Levy, 1982; Carskadon & Dement, 1981; Herscovitch & Broughton, 1981).

STANFORD SLEEPINESS SCALE

Please circle the scale value of the statement which best describes your state of sleepiness.

1 Feeling active and vital; alert; wide awake.
2 Functioning at a high level, but not at peak; able to concentrate.
3 Relaxed; awake; not at full alertness; responsive.
4 A little foggy; not at peak; let down.
5 Fogginess; beginning to lose interest in remaining awake; slowed down.
6 Sleepiness; prefer to be lying down; fighting sleep; woozy.
7 Almost in reverie; sleep onset soon; lost struggle to remain awake.

Reprinted with permission of Cambridge University Press from Hoddes, E., Zarcone, V., Smythe, H., Phillips, R., & Dement, W. C. (1973). Quantification of sleepiness: A new approach. *Psychophysiology*, *10*, 431–436.

PITTSBURGH SLEEP QUALITY INDEX

Purpose and Development

The Pittsburgh Sleep Quality Index assesses quality of sleep during the past month (Buysse, Reynolds, Monk, Berman, & Kupfer, 1989). The index consists of 19 self-report items which focus on the areas of subjective sleep quality, sleep latency, sleep duration, sleep efficiency, sleep disturbances, use of medications, and daytime dysfunction. The authors generated items on the basis of clinical experience with sleep disorder clients, previous sleep quality questionnaires, and pilot testing of initial items.

Administration and Scoring

Respondents are asked to think about their sleep habits during the past month and respond to items on a 0 to 3 scale. Seven components of sleep quality may be calculated from these scores. Higher scores indicate poorer sleep. Scale scores are calculated as follows.

The Pittsburgh Sleep Quality Index contains 19 self-rated questions and 5 questions rated by the bed partner or roommate (if one is available). Only self-rated questions are included in the scoring. The 19 self-rated items are combined to form seven "component" scores, each of which has a range of 0–3 points. In all cases, a score of "0" indicates no difficulty, while a score of "3" indicates severe difficulty. The seven component scores are then added to yield one "global" score, with a range of 0–21 points, "0" indicating no difficulty and "21" indicating severe difficulties in all areas.

Scoring proceeds as follows:

COMPONENT 1: SUBJECTIVE SLEEP QUALITY

Examine question #6 and assign scores as follows:

Response	Component 1 score
"Very good"	0
"Fairly good"	1
"Fairly bad"	2
"Very bad"	3

Component 1 score _____

COMPONENT 2: SLEEP LATENCY

1. Examine question #2 and assign scores as follows:

Response	Scores
≤ 15 minutes	0
16–30 minutes	1
31–60	2
> 60 minutes	3

Question #2 score _____

2. Examine question #5a and assign scores as follows:

Response	Scores
Not during the past month	0
Less than once a week	1
Once or twice a week	2
Three or more times a week	3

Question #5a score _____

3. Add #2 score and #5a score _____

4. Assign component 2 score as follows:

Sum of #2 and 5a score	Component 2 score
0	0
1–2	1
3–4	2
5–6	3

Component 2 score _____

COMPONENT 3: SLEEP DURATION

Examine question #4 and assign scores as follows:

Response	Component 3 score
> 7 hours	0
6–7 hours	1
5–6 hours	2
< 5 hours	3

Component 3 score _____

COMPONENT 4: HABITUAL SLEEP EFFICIENCY

(1) Write the number of hours slept (question #4) here: _____
(2) Calculate the number of hours spent in bed:

     Getting up time (question #3):   _____
     −Bedtime (question #1): _____   _____

     Number of hours spent in bed: _____

(3) Calculate habitual sleep efficiency as follows:

(Number of hours slept/Number of hours spent in bed) × 100 =
Habitual sleep efficiency (%)

          (_____/_____/ × 100 = _____ %

(4) Assign component 4 score as follows:

Habitual sleep efficiency %	Component 4 score
> 85%	0
75–84%	1
65–74%	2
< 65%	3

Component 4 score _____

COMPONENT 5: SLEEP DISTURBANCES

(1) Examine questions #5b–5j, and assign scores for *each* question as
     follows:

Response	Score
Not during the past month	0
Less than once a week	1
Once or twice a week	2
Three or more times a week	3

                                      #5b score _____
                                       c score _____
                                       d score _____
                                       e score _____
                                       f score _____
                                       g score _____
                                       h score _____
                                       i score _____
                                       j score _____

(2)   Add the scores for questions #5b–5j:

                                        Sum of #5b–5j: _____

(3)   Assign component 5 score as follows:

Sum of #5b–5j	Component 5 score
0	0
1–9	1
10–18	2
19–27	3

Component 5 score _____

COMPONENT 6: USE OF SLEEPING MEDICATION

Examine question #7 and assign scores as follows:

Response	Component 6 score
Not during the past month	0
Less than once a week	1
Once or twice a week	2
Three or more times a week	3

Component 6 score _____

Sample Scores

Buysse et al. (1989) gave the index to 45 individuals who were referred for assessment because of difficulties in initiating or maintaining sleep, 17 individuals who were referred for assessment because of excessive somnolence, 34 individuals with major depression, and 52 individuals with no sleep complaints and no psychiatric diagnosis. Table 1 shows their average scores.

Buysse et al. (1989) suggest a cutoff score of 5 or greater on the global score to identify individuals with sleep disturbances. Overall this cutoff identified correctly 88% of the sleep disturbed and not sleep disturbed individuals.

Reliability

In a sample of sleep disturbed individuals, depressed individuals, and individuals with no sleeping problems, Buysse et al. (1989) found that

TABLE 1
Scores on the Pittsburgh Sleep Quality Index (Buysse et al., 1989)

	Difficulty initiating or maintaining sleep	Excessive somnolence	Depressed	Control
Subjective sleep quality	1.96 ± .93	1.06 ± .75	1.88 ± .88	.35 ± .48
Sleep latency	1.42 ± 1.01	.59 ± .87	1.88 ± 1.15	.56 ± .73
Sleep duration	1.51 ± 1.20	.47 ± .80	1.71 ± 1.41	.29 ± .50
Habitual sleep efficiency	1.47 ± 1.24	.29 ± .77	1.59 ± 1.18	.10 ± .30
Sleep disturbance	1.40 ± .62	1.53 ± .72	1.47 ± .51	1.00 ± .40
Use of sleeping medication	1.20 ± 1.31	.35 ± 1.00	.76 ± 1.21	.04 ± .28
Daytime dysfunction	1.42 ± .94	2.24 ± .90	1.79 ± .69	.35 ± .48
Global score	10.38 ± 4.57	6.53 ± 2.98	11.09 ± 4.31	2.67 ± 1.70

Values are Mean ± SD.

both the overall internal consistency of the global scale and the average internal consistency of the subscales was .83 as measured by Cronbach's alpha. One month test–retest reliability was .85 for the global score and ranged from .65 to .84 for the subscales.

Validity

Buysse et al. (1989) correlated scores on the index with the results of polysomnography, but overall found no significant correlation between the two measures. In contrast, Buysse, Reynolds, Monk, Hoch, Yeager, and Kupfer (1991) did find that polysomnographic measures corresponded to a number of the scales on the index.

Buysse et al. (1989) found that as expected individuals who were referred because of sleep disturbances and depressed individuals scored higher on the global scale than control individuals. Those who had trouble initiating or maintaining sleep or were depressed also scored higher on the global scale than those who suffered from excessive somnolence. The subscales showed distinctive profiles for these different groups of individuals.

In a study comparing the sleep disturbances of Nazi Holocaust survivors, depressed individuals, and a comparison group, Rosen, Reynolds, Yeager, Houck, and Hurwitz (1991) found that both the group of depressed individuals and the group of Holocaust survivors had higher scores than the control group on the global scale and on all subscales. The depressed individuals also had higher scores than the Holocaust survivors on all scales but the Sleep Disturbance and Daytime Dysfunction scales. It is known that elderly individuals have poorer sleep than younger individuals. Studies by Buysse et al. (1991) and Monk, Reynolds, Machen, and Kupfer (1992) compared index scores of elderly and young individuals and found that the index was sensitive to their different sleep patterns.

Pittsburgh Sleep Quality Index

Instructions: The following questions relate to your usual sleep habits during the past month *only*. Your answers should indicate the most accurate reply for the *majority* of days and nights in the past month. Please answer all questions.

1. During the past month, when have you usually gone to bed at night?

    Usual bed time _____

2. During the past month, how long (in minutes) has it usually taken you to fall asleep each night?

    Number of minutes _____

3. During the past month, when have you usually gotten up in the morning?

    Usual getting-up time _____

4. During the past month, how many hours of *actual sleep* did you get at night? (This may be different than the number of hours you spend in bed.)

    Hours of sleep per night _____

For each of the remaining questions, check the one best response. Please answer *all* questions.

5. During the past month, how often have you had trouble sleeping because you ...

    (a) Cannot get to sleep within 30 minutes

    Not during the past month _____ Less than once a week _____
    Once or twice a week _____ Three or more times a week _____

    (b) Wake up in the middle of the night or early morning

    Not during the past month _____ Less than once a week _____
    Once or twice a week _____ Three or more times a week _____

➤

(c) Have to get up to use the bathroom

Not during the past month _____ Less than once a week _____
Once or twice a week _____ Three or more times a week _____

(d) Cannot breathe comfortably

Not during the past month _____ Less than once a week _____
Once or twice a week _____ Three or more times a week _____

(e) Cough or snore loudly

Not during the past month _____ Less than once a week _____
Once or twice a week _____ Three or more times a week _____

(f) Feel too cold

Not during the past month _____ Less than once a week _____
Once or twice a week _____ Three or more times a week _____

(g) Feel too hot

Not during the past month _____ Less than once a week _____
Once or twice a week _____ Three or more times a week _____

(h) Had bad dreams

Not during the past month _____ Less than once a week _____
Once or twice a week _____ Three or more times a week _____

(i) Have pain

Not during the past month _____ Less than once a week _____
Once or twice a week _____ Three or more times a week _____

(j) Other reason(s), please describe _____

_____

How often during the past month have you had trouble sleeping because of this?

Not during the past month _____ Less than once a week _____ Once or twice a week _____ Three or more times a week _____

6. During the past month, how would you rate your sleep quality overall?

   Very good   _____
   Fairly good _____
   Fairly bad   _____
   Very bad   _____

7. During the past month, how often have you taken medicine (prescribed or "over the counter") to help you sleep?

   Not during the past month _____ Less than once a week _____
   Once or twice a week _____ Three or more times a week _____

8. During the past month, how often have you had trouble stayingawake
   while driving, eating meals, or engaging in social activities?

   Not during the past month _____ Less than once a week _____
   Once or twice a week _____ Three or more times a week _____

9. During the past month, how much of a problem has it been for you to
   keep up enough enthusiasm to get things done?

   No problem at all   _____
   Only a slight problem   _____
   Somewhat of a problem   _____
   A very big problem   _____

10. Do you have a bed partner or roommate?

    No bed partner or roommate   _____
    Partner/roommate in other room   _____
    Partner in same room, but not same bed _____
    Partner in same bed   _____

If you have a roommate or bed partner, ask him/her how often in
the past month you have had

(a) Loud snoring

    Not during the past month _____ Less than once a week _____
    Once or twice a week _____ Three or more times a week _____

→

(b) Long pauses between breaths while asleep

Not during the past month _____ Less than once a week _____
Once or twice a week _____ Three or more times a week _____

(c) Legs twitching or jerking while you sleep

Not during the past month _____ Less than once a week _____
Once or twice a week _____ Three or more times a week _____

(d) Episodes of disorientation or confusion during sleep

Not during the past month _____ Less than once a week _____
Once or twice a week _____ Three or more times a week _____

(e) Other restlessness while you sleep; please describe _____

_____

The scale and the scoring instructions in the Administration and Scoring section are reprinted from Buysse, D. J., Reynolds, C. F., Monk, T. H., Berman, S. R., & Kupfer, T. H. (1989). The Pittsburgh Sleep Quality Index: A new instrument for psychiatric practice and research. *Psychiatry Research, 28*, 193–213, with permission of Elsevier Scientific Publishers Ireland Ltd.

References

Blankstein, K. R., Flett, G. L., Watson, M. S., & Koledin, S. (1990). Test anxiety, self-evaluative worry, and sleep disturbance in college students. *Anxiety Research, 3,* 193–204.

Buysse, D. J., Reynolds, C. F., Monk, T. H., Berman, S. R., & Kupfer, D. J. (1989). The Pittsburgh Sleep Quality Index: A new instrument for psychiatric practice and research. *Psychiatry Research, 28,* 193–213.

Buysse, D. J., Reynolds, C. F., Monk, T. H., Hoch, C. C., Yeager, A. L., & Kupfer, D. J. (1991). Quantification of subjective sleep quality in healthy elderly men and women using the Pittsburgh Sleep Quality Index (PSQI). *Sleep, 14,* 331–338.

Carskadon, M. A., & Dement, W. (1981). Cumulative effects of sleep restriction on daytime sleepiness. *Psychophysiology, 18*(2), 107–113.

Ellis, B. W., Johns M. W., Lancaster, R., Raptopoulos, P., Angelopoulos, N., & Priest, R. G. (1981). The St. Mary's Hospital Sleep Questionnaire: A study of reliability. *Sleep, 4,* 93–97.

Herscovitch, J., & Broughton, R. (1981). Performance deficits following short-term partial sleep deprivation and subsequent recovery oversleeping. *Canadian Journal of Psychology, 35,* 309–322.

Hoddes, E., Dement, W. & Zarcone, V. (1972). The history and use of the Stanford Sleepiness Scale. *Psychophysiology, 9,* 150.

Hoddes, E., Zarcone, V., Smythe, H., Phillips, R., & Dement, W. C. (1973). Quantification of sleepiness: A new approach. *Psychophysiology, 10,* 431–436.

Johnson, L. C., Freeman, C. R., Spinweber, C. L., & Gomez, S. A. (1991). Subjective and objective measures of sleepiness: Effect of benzodiazepine and caffeine on their relationship. *Psychophysiology, 28,* 65–71.

Johnson, L. C., Spinweber, C. L., & Gomez, S. A. (1990). Benzodiazepines and caffeine: Effect on daytime sleepiness, performance and mood. *Psychopharmacology, 101,* 160–167.

Johnson, L. C., Spinweber, C. L., Gomez, S. A., & Matteson, L. T. (1990). Daytime sleepiness, performance, mood, and nocturnal sleep: The effect of benzodiazepine and caffeine on their relationship. *Sleep, 13,* 121–135.

Karacan, I., Orr, W., Roth, T., Kramer, M., Thornby, J., Bingham, S., & Kay, D. (1981). Dose-related effects of flurazepam on human sleep-waking patterns. *Psychopharmacology, 73,* 332–339.

Leigh, T. J., Bird, H. A., Hindmarch, I., Constable, P. D. L., & Wright, V. (1988). Factor analysis of the St. Mary's Hospital Sleep questionnaire. *Sleep, 11,* 448–453.

Monk, T. H., Reynolds, C. F., Machen, M. A., & Kupfer, D. J. (1992). Daily social rhythms in the elderly and their relation to objectively recorded sleep. *Sleep, 15,* 322–329.

Nicassio, P. M., Mendlowitz, D. R., Fussell, J. J., & Petras, L. (1985). The phenomenology of the pre-sleep state: The development of the Pre-Sleep Arousal Scale. *Behaviour Research and Therapy, 23,* 263–271.

Patel, A. G., Gura, R., Kurian, T., Lambert, M. T., Steinert, J., & Priest, R. G. (1991). A comparison of the hypnotic effects of temazepam capsules and temazepam elixir. *International Clinical Psychopharmacology, 6,* 1–9.

Reimer, M. (1987). Sleep pattern disturbance: Nursing interventions perceived by patients and their nurses as facilitating nocturnal sleep in hospital. In A. M. McLane (Ed.) *Classification of Nursing Diagnosis: North American Nursing Diagnosis Association,* St. Louis: Mosby.

Rosen, J., Reynolds, C. F., Yeager, A. L., Houck, P. R., & Hurwitz, L. F. (1991). Sleep disturbances in survivors of the Nazi Holocaust. *The American Journal of Psychiatry, 148,* 62–66.

Snyder-Halpern, R., & Verran, J. A. (1987). Instrumentation to describe subjective sleep characteristics in healthy subjects. *Research in Nursing & Health, 10,* 155–163.

Spring, B., Maller, O., Wurtman, J., Digman, L. & Cozolino, L. (1983). Effects of protein and carbohydrate meals on mood and performance: Interactions with sex and age. *Journal of Psychiatric Research, 17*, 155–167.

Webb, W. B., & Bonnet, M. H. (1978). The sleep of 'morning' and 'evening' types. *Biological Psychology, 7*, 29–35.

Webb, W. B., Bonnet, M., & Blume, G. (1976). A post-sleep inventory. *Perceptual and Motor Skills, 43*, 987–993.

Webb, W. B., & Levy, C. M. (1982). Age, sleep deprivation, and performance. *Psychophysiology, 19*, 272–276.

CHAPTER 12

Impulse-Control Disorders

BARRATT IMPULSIVENESS SCALE

Purpose and Development

This scale measures the characteristic impulsiveness of individuals. The latest version of the Barratt Impulsiveness Scale is a 30-item self-report measure (Patton, Stanford, & Barratt, in press). Barratt developed the first version of the scale in 1959 (Barratt, 1959) and then revised and refined the scale over the years (Barratt, 1985; Barratt, 1993). The eleventh and latest version was created by eliminating from the previous version of the scale those items that did not contribute to the reliability or validity of the scale. Patton et al. (in press) factor analyzed the responses of undergraduate students, psychiatric inpatients, and prisoners in a maximum security facility and found three main second-order factors. These factors were motor impulsiveness, nonplanning impulsiveness, and attentional impulsiveness.

Administration and Scoring

Respondents rate each of the items on a 1–4 point scale of frequency. Items 1, 7, 8, 9, 10, 12, 13, 15, 20, 29, and 30 are reverse coded. The sum of all items is the total scale score. Scores can range from 30 to 120 and higher scores indicate more impulsiveness.

Sample Scores

Patton et al. (in press) gave the scale to 130 male and 279 female undergraduate students, 110 male and 54 female substance abuse in-

TABLE 1
Scores on the Barratt Impulsiveness
Scale (Patton et al., in press)

Group	M	SD
Students	63.82	10.17
Substance abuse clients	69.26	10.28
General psychiatry clients	71.37	12.61
Prisoners	76.30	11.86

patients, 39 male and 45 female general psychiatry inpatients, and 73 male inmates of a maximum security prison. There were no significant differences between the scores of men and women. Table 1 shows the average scores for each group.

Reliability

Patton et al. (in press) found that the internal consistency of the scale as measured by Cronbach's alpha ranged from .79 to .82 in samples of students, psychiatric clients, and prisoners.

Validity

Using a slightly different previous version of the scale, studies have found a strong association between scale scores and other measures of impulsivity and venturesomeness (Campbell, 1987; Luengo, Carrillo-de-la-Pena, & Otero, 1991; Carrillo-de-la-Pena, Otero, & Romero, 1993).

Patton et al. (in press) compared the scores of undergraduate students, substance abuse clients, general psychiatry clients, and prison inmates. As expected, the prison inmates had higher impulsivity scores than any of the other groups and the substance abuse and general psychiatry clients had higher impulsivity scores than the students. Royse and Wiehe (1988) gave the previous version of the scale to groups of felons and unwed mothers who they hypothesized would be more impulsive than a sample of individuals drawn from the general population and found that the scale scores of both the felons and the unwed mothers were higher.

BARRATT IMPULSIVENESS SCALE

Directions: People differ in the ways they act and think in different situations. This is a test to measure some of the ways in which you act and think. Read each statement and check the appropriate space on the right side of the page. Do not spend too much time on any statement. Answer quickly and honestly.

	Rarely/ never	Occasionally	Often	Almost always/ Always
1. I plan tasks carefully.	( )	( )	( )	( )
2. I do things without thinking.	( )	( )	( )	( )
3. I make up my mind quickly.	( )	( )	( )	( )
4. I am happy-go-lucky.	( )	( )	( )	( )
5. I don't "pay attention."	( )	( )	( )	( )
6. I have "racing" thoughts.	( )	( )	( )	( )
7. I plan trips well ahead of time.	( )	( )	( )	( )
8. I am self-controlled.	( )	( )	( )	( )
9. I concentrate easily.	( )	( )	( )	( )
10. I save regularly.	( )	( )	( )	( )
11. I "squirm" at plays or lectures.	( )	( )	( )	( )
12. I am a careful thinker.	( )	( )	( )	( )
13. I plan for job security.	( )	( )	( )	( )
14. I say things without thinking.	( )	( )	( )	( )
15. I like to think about complex problems.	( )	( )	( )	( )
16. I change jobs.	( )	( )	( )	( )
17. I act "on impulse."	( )	( )	( )	( )
18. I get easily bored when solving thought problems.	( )	( )	( )	( )
19. I act on the spur of the moment.	( )	( )	( )	( )
20. I am a steady thinker.	( )	( )	( )	( )
21. I change residences.	( )	( )	( )	( )
22. I buy things on impulse.	( )	( )	( )	( )

→

23. I can only think about one problem at a time.	( )	( )	( )	( )
24. I change hobbies.	( )	( )	( )	( )
25. I spend or charge more than I earn.	( )	( )	( )	( )
26. I often have extraneous thoughts when thinking.	( )	( )	( )	( )
27. I am more interested in the present than the future.	( )	( )	( )	( )
28. I am restless at the theater or lectures.	( )	( )	( )	( )
29. I like puzzles.	( )	( )	( )	( )
30. I am future oriented.	( )	( )	( )	( )

South Oaks Gambling Screen

Purpose and Development

The purpose of this scale is to assess pathological gambling. The South Oaks Gambling Screen is a 20-item instrument that can be used as a self-report measure or as an interview measure (Lesieur & Blume, 1987). An initial pool of 60 items was based on the DSM-III criteria for pathological gambling, interviews with clients and their family members, and counselors' clinical expertise. The final items selected from this pool were the ones that were frequently endorsed and best differentiated between clients. After the scale had been extensively used for several years, Lesieur and Blume (1993) made wording changes that clarified the meaning of several of the items. The scale has been translated into several languages and adapted for use in different cultures (Lesieur and Blume, 1993).

Administration and Scoring

Whether the scale is used as a self-report measure or an interview measure, respondents first indicate how often they engaged in different types of gambling behavior, the maximum amount of money they have gambled within a day, and how many relatives or close friends have had gambling problems. Responses to these first three questions are not a part of the total scale score and the first two questions may be modified to reflect local conditions (Lesieur & Blume, 1993). For example, if cockfights are a prevalent form of gambling locally, then cockfights may be added as a response category for the item assessing types of gambling behavior. Items 4 through 6 are rated on scales of frequency. A point is given on item 4 for the responses "most of the time I lose" or "every time I lose." A point is given on item 5 for the responses "yes, less than half the time I lost" or "yes, most of the time." A point is given on item 6 for the responses "yes, in the past but not now" and "yes." The remainder of the items ask for "yes" or "no" responses and a point is given for each "yes" response. The total scale score is the sum of items 4 through 11, and items 13 through 16i. Questions 1, 2, 3, 12, 16j, and 16k are not included in the total score. Total scores can range from 0 to 20, with higher scores indicating more gambling problems.

The South Oaks Gambling Screen asks about lifetime gambling behavior. Lesieur and Blume (1993) mention that some researchers interested in obtaining information about current gambling behavior adapted the scale to ask about different time frames such as the past six months or the past year.

Cutoff Scores

Lesieur and Blume (1987) recommend a cutoff score of 5 or greater to identify pathological gambling. They found this cutoff score identified 98% of 213 members of Gamblers Anonymous as pathological gamblers and identified 5% of a group of 384 university students and 1.3% of a group of 152 hospital employees as pathological gamblers. Lesieur and Blume (1987) further assessed the accuracy of the cutoff score by relating it to questionnaire items asking about DSM-III-R criteria for pathological gambling. They found that the cutoff score of 5 resulted in 1.9% total errors in classification in the Gamblers Anonymous group, 4.7% total errors for the students, and .7% total errors for the hospital employees. Volberg and Banks (1990) explored different techniques for assessing the accuracy of the South Oaks Gambling Screen and concluded that it has a high rate of detecting pathological gambling and a low rate of false detection.

Problem gambling is less severe than pathological gambling and several epidemiological studies have used cutoff scores of 3 and 4 on the scale to assess problem gambling (Volberg & Steadman, 1988; Volberg & Steadman, 1989; Lesieur, Cross, Frank, Welch, White, Rubenstein, Mosley, & Mark, 1991). As Lesieur and Blume (1993) point out, more research is needed to determine whether scores of 3 or 4 are sensitive indicators of problem gambling.

Reliability

In a sample of members of Gamblers Anonymous, university students, and hospital employees, Lesieur and Blume (1987) found that the internal consistency of the scale as measured by Cronbach's alpha was .97. Lesieur and Blume (1987) also asked groups of inpatients and outpatients being treated for alcoholism, other drug dependencies, and pathological gambling to complete the scale again a month or more after they first completed it. Test–retest reliability was 1.00 for the outpatients and .61 for the inpatients.

Validity

Lesieur and Blume (1987) asked counselors to assess whether inpatients with alcohol or drug abuse problems were pathological gamblers; they also gave these inpatients the South Oaks Gambling Screen and found a very high correlation between the counselors' assessments and the South Oaks Gambling Screen scores. Lesieur and Blume (1987) also compared family members' assessment of gambling problems in these inpatients to the inpatients' scale scores and found a significant correlation between family members' assessments and scale scores. Lesieur and Blume (1987) further found that assessment of gambling using DSM-III-R criteria and the South Oaks Gambling Screen were highly related. In a sample of prisoners, Templer, Kaiser, and Siscoe (1993) found higher scale scores were associated with greater psychopathology, including depression, sociopathy, and paranoia.

Lesieur and Blume (1987) found a large difference between samples drawn from Gamblers Anonymous, university students, and hospital employees in the percentage of individuals identified as pathological gamblers by the scale. As one would expect, a high percentage (98%) of the individuals who were members of Gamblers Anonymous had scale scores that identified them as pathological gamblers; relatively few individuals in the student group (5%) and hospital employee group (1%) had scale scores that identified them as pathological gamblers.

chines, or other gambling machines

j. ____ ____ ____ bowled, shot pool, played golf,
or some other game of skill for
money

k. ____ ____ ____ pull tabs or "paper" games
other than lotteries

l. ____ ____ ____ some form of gambling not
listed above (please specify) ____

2. What is the largest amount of money you have ever gambled with on any one day?

____ never have gambled   ____ more than $100 up to $1000

____ $1 or less   ____ more than $1,000 up to $10,000

____ more than $10 up to $100   ____ more than $10,000

3. Check which of the following people in your life has (or had) a gambling problem.

_____ father
_____ mother
_____ brother/sister
_____ grandparent
_____ my spouse/partner
_____ my child(ren)
_____ another relative
_____ a friend or someone else important in my life.

4. When you gamble, how often do you go back another day to win back money you lost?

_____ never
_____ some of the time (less than half the time I lost)
_____ most of the time I lost
_____ every time I lost

5. Have you ever claimed to be winning money gambling but weren't really? In fact you lost?

_____ never (or never gamble)
_____ yes, less than half the time I lost
_____ yes, most of the time

6. Do you feel you have had a problem with betting money or gambling?

_____ no
_____ yes, in the past but not now
_____ yes

7. Did you ever gamble more than you in-   yes _____   no _____
tended to?

8. Have people criticized your betting or told   yes _____   no _____
you that you had a gambling problem, re-
gardless of whether or not you thought it
was true?

9. Have you ever felt guilty about the way you   yes _____   no _____
gamble or what happens when you gamble?

→

10. Have you ever felt like you would like to   yes _____   no _____
    stop betting money or gambling but didn't
    think you could?

11. Have you ever hidden betting slips, lottery   yes _____   no _____
    tickets, gambling money, I.O.U.s, or other
    signs of betting or gambling from you
    spouse, children or other important people
    in your life?

12. Have you ever argued with people you live   yes _____   no _____
    with over how you handle money?

13. (If you answered yes to question 12): Have   yes _____   no _____
    money arguments ever centered on your
    gambling?

14. Have you ever borrowed from someone and   yes _____   no _____
    not paid them back as a result of your gam-
    bling?

15. Have you ever lost time from work (school)   yes _____   no _____
    due to betting money or gambling?

16. If you borrowed money to gamble or to pay gambling debts, who or
    where did you borrow from? (Check "yes" or "no" for each.)

		no	yes
a.	from household money	( )	( )
b.	from your spouse	( )	( )
c.	from other relatives or in-laws	( )	( )
d.	from banks, loan companies, or credit unions	( )	( )
e.	from credit cards	( )	( )
f.	from loan sharks	( )	( )
g.	you cashed in stocks, bonds, or other securities	( )	( )
h.	you sold personal or family property	( )	( )
i.	you borrowed on your checking account (passed bad checks)	( )	( )
j.	you have (had) a credit line with a bookie	( )	( )
k.	you have (had) a credit line with a casino	( )	( )

REFERENCES

Barratt, E. S. (1959). Anxiety and impulsiveness related to psychomotor efficiency. *Perceptual and Motor Skills, 9,* 191–198.

Barratt, E. S. (1985). Impulsiveness subtraits: Arousal and information processing. In J. T. Spence and C. E. Izard (Eds.), *Motivation, Emotion, and Personality* (pp. 137–146). North Holland: Elsevier Science Publishers.

Barratt, E. S. (1993). Impulsivity: Integrating cognitive, behavioral, biological, and environmental data. In W. B. McCown, J. L. Johnson and M. B. Shure (Eds.), *The Impulsive Client: Theory, Research, and Treatment* (pp. 39–56). Washington, DC: American Psychological Association.

Campbell, J. B. (1987). Measures of impulsivity. *Personality and Individual Differences, 8,* 451.

Carrillo-de-la-Pena, M. T., Otero, J. M., & Romero, E. (1993). Comparison among various methods of assessment of impulsiveness. *Perceptual and Motor Skills, 77,* 567–575.

Lesieur, H.R., & Blume, S. B. (1987). The South Oaks Gambling Screen (The SOGS): A new instrument for the identification of pathological gamblers. *American Journal of Psychiatry, 144,* 1184–1188.

Lesieur, H. R., & Blume, S. B. (1993). Revising the South Oaks Gambling Screen in different settings. *Journal of Gambling Studies, 9,* 213–223.

Lesieur, H. R., Cross, J., Frank, M., Welch, M., White, C. M., Rubenstein, G., Mosley, K., & Mark, M. (1991). Gambling and pathological gambling among university students. *Addictive Behavior: An International Journal, 16,* 517–527.

Luengo, M. A., Carrillo-de-la-Pena, M. T., & Otero, J. M. (1991). The components of impulsiveness: A comparison of the I.7 Impulsiveness Questionnaire and the Barratt Impulsiveness Scale. *Personality and Individual Differences, 12,* 657–667.

Patton, J H., Stanford, M. S., & Barratt, E. S. (in press). Factor Structure of the Barratt Impulsiveness Scale. *Journal of Clinical Psychology.*

Royse, D., & Wiehe, V. R. (1988). Impulsivity in felons and unwed mothers. *Psychological Reports, 62,* 335–336.

Templer, D. I., Kaiser, G., & Siscoe, K. (1993). Correlates of pathological gambling propensity in prison inmates. *Comprehensive Psychiatry, 34,* 347–351.

Volberg, R. A., & Banks, S. M. (1990). A review of two measures of pathological gambling in the United States. *Journal of Gambling Studies, 6,* 153–163.

Volberg, R. A., & Steadman, H. (1988). Refining prevalence estimates of pathological gambling. *American Journal of Psychiatry, 145,* 502–505.

Volberg, R. A., & Steadman, H. (1989). Prevalence estimates of pathological gambling in New Jersey and Maryland. *American Journal of Psychiatry, 146,* 1618–1619.

CHAPTER 13

Relationship Problems

LOCKE–WALLACE SHORT MARITAL ADJUSTMENT TEST

Purpose and Development

The Locke–Wallace Short Marital Adjustment Test assesses a couple's satisfaction with their marriage, their agreement on key marital issues, and their accommodation to each other. The test is a popular 15-item self-report measure developed by Locke and Wallace (1959), who selected items that had proven useful in previous studies and that spanned a range of marital issues. A factor analytic study by Cross and Sharpley (1981) found that the items group into one major factor.

Administration and Scoring

The test may be given to both partners or to just one partner. The respondent uses a scale with seven reference points to indicate marital happiness in item 1, a 6-point scale of agreement to respond to items 2 through 9, and scales tailored to each item for items 10 through 15. The scoring weights for item responses are given in the appendix; respondents do not see these weights. We suggest that because of changed societal conditions, both the first and second alternatives in item 10 be scored as 0. The item weights are summed for each individual. Scores can range from 2 to 158 and higher scores indicate greater marital satisfaction.

Sample and Cutoff Scores

From a sample of 118 husbands and 118 wives, Locke and Wallace (1959) identified 48 individuals who were in troubled marriages and 48 individuals, matched on gender and age with the troubled individuals, who were well-adjusted in their marriages. Those in troubled marriages were either currently seeking marital therapy, separated, or recently divorced. The well-adjusted individuals were rated by friends who knew them well as having an especially good marriage. Each of the two groups consisted of 22 men and 26 women.

The average score for those in troubled marriages was 71.7 and for those in good marriages was 135.9. Only 17% of the individuals in troubled marriages scored over 100 while 96% of the individuals in good marriages scored over 100.

Reliability

Locke and Wallace (1959) found the internal consistency of the test was .90 as measured by the Spearman–Brown formula for split-half reliability. Cross and Sharpley (1981) found an alpha of .83.

Validity

Schachter and O'Leary (1985) found that couples whose scale scores indicated less satisfaction showed more negative communication than those whose ratings indicated satisfaction. Examining the relationship between scale scores and self-role congruence, Chassin, Zeiss, Cooper, and Reaven (1985) found that those couples in which the wife and husband both experienced either congruence or incongruence had the highest level of marital satisfaction. In a sample of multiple-role women (working outside the home, mothers, and married), McLaughlin, Cormier, and Cormier (1988) found that those with scores indicating more satisfaction tended to use more time-management and self-care strategies.

Locke and Wallace (1959) reported that the 48 individuals who were in good marriages scored significantly higher on the test than 48 individuals in troubled marriages.

LOCKE–WALLACE SHORT MARITAL ADJUSTMENT TEST

1. Check the dot on the scale line below which best describes the degree of happiness, everything considered, of your present marriage. The middle point, "happy," represents the degree of happiness which most people get from marriage, and the scale gradually ranges on one side to those few who are very unhappy in marriage, and on the other, to those few who experience extreme joy or felicity in marriage.

0	2	7	15	20	25	35
·	·	·	·	·	·	·

Very unhappy   Happy   Perfectly happy

State the approximate extent of agreement or disagreement between you and your mate on the following items. Please place one check for each item.

	Almost agree	Almost always agree	Occa- sionally disagree	Fre- quently disagree	Almost always disagree	Always disagree
2. Handling family finances	5	4	3	2	1	0
3. Matters of recre- ations	5	4	3	2	1	0
4. Demonstration of affection	8	6	4	2	1	0
5. Friends	5	4	3	2	1	0
6. Sex relations	15	12	9	4	1	0
7. Conventionality (right good, or proper conduct)	5	4	3	2	1	0
8. Philosophy of life	5	4	3	2	1	0
9. Ways of dealing with in-laws	5	4	3	2	1	0

→

10. When disagreements arise, they usually result in:

    0   husband giving in
    2   wife giving in
    10 agreement by mutual give and take

11. Do you and your mate engage in outside interests together?

    10 all of them
    8   some of them
    3   very few of them
    0   none of them

12. In leisure time do you generally prefer: to be "on the go."   _____
                                                to stay at home?   _____

    Does your mate generally prefer: to be "on the go."   _____
                                                to stay at home?   _____

    (Stay at home for both, 10 points; "on the go" for both, 3 points; disagreement, 2 points)

13. Do you ever wish you had not married?

    0   frequently
    3   occasionally
    8   rarely
    15 never

14. If you had your life to live over, do you think you would?

    15 marry the same person
    0   marry a different person
    1   not marry at all

15. Do you confide in your mate?

    0   almost never
    2   rarely
    10 in most things
    10 in everything

McMaster Family Assessment Device

Purpose and Development

The McMaster Family Assessment Device is a 60-item self-report measure designed to assess family functioning in the following areas: problem solving, communication, roles, affective responsiveness, affective involvement, behavior control, and general functioning (Epstein, Baldwin, & Bishop, 1983; Kabacoff, Miller, Bishop, Epstein, & Keitner, 1990). Using the McMaster model of family functioning as a theoretical basis, Epstein et al. (1983) created an initial pool of 240 items consisting of 40 items for each of the first six dimensions mentioned above. They then gave these items to a large number of individuals and on the basis of their responses selected 41 items that were most representative of a single dimension and 12 items that were most highly related to all dimensions. Later this 53-item version was expanded to 60 items (Kabacoff et al., 1990). A factor analysis has confirmed the subscale structure of the measure (Kabacoff et al., 1990).

Administration and Scoring

Respondents answer each item as it applies to their family using a 1 to 4 scale with the descriptors strongly agree, agree, disagree, and strongly disagree. Items 1, 4, 5, 7, 8, 9, 11, 13, 14, 15, 17, 19, 21, 22, 23, 25, 27, 28, 31, 33, 34, 35, 37, 39, 41, 42, 44, 45, 47, 48, 51, 52, 53, 54, and 58 describe unhealthy functioning and are reverse scored. For all subscales items are summed and then divided by the number of items comprising the scale. Thus scores for each subscale may range from 1 to 4, with higher scores indicating more problems. The Problem Solving scale is the sum of items 2, 12, 24, 38, 50, and 60 divided by six; the Communication scale is the sum of items 3, 14, 18, 22, 29, 35, 43, 52 and 59, divided by nine; the Roles scale is the sum of items 4, 8, 10, 15, 23, 30, 34, 40, 45, 53, and 58, divided by 11; the Affective Responsiveness scale is the sum of items 9, 19, 28, 39, 49, and 57, divided by six; the Affective Involvement scale is the sum of items 5, 13, 25, 33, 37, 42, and 54, divided by seven; the Behavioral Control scale is the sum of items 7, 17, 20, 27, 32, 44, 47, 48, and 55, divided by nine; and the General Functioning Scale is the sum of items 1, 6, 11, 16, 21, 26, 31, 36, 41, 46, 51, and 56, divided by 12.

Sample Scores and Cutoff Scores

Table 1 shows the scores of 1,138 families undergoing psychiatric treatment, 298 families in which individuals were undergoing medical treatment, and 627 nonclinical families (Kabacoff et al., 1990).

TABLE 1
Scores on the McMaster Family Assessment Device (Kabacoff et al., 1990)

Group	Problem solving		Communication		Roles		Affective responsiveness		Affective involvement		Behavior control		General functioning	
	M	SD	M	SD	M	SD	M	SD	M	SD	M	SD	M	SD
Psychiatric	2.32	.53	2.37	.44	2.37	.40	2.36	.57	2.32	.55	2.14	.49	2.27	.51
Medical	1.95	.45	2.13	.43	2.22	.39	2.08	.53	2.02	.47	1.84	.42	1.89	.45
Nonclinical	1.91	.40	2.09	.40	2.16	.34	2.08	.53	2.00	.50	1.94	.44	1.84	.43

On the basis of several studies Miller, Epstein, Bishop, and Keitner (1985) suggested the following cutting scores to distinguish between healthy and unhealthy family functioning: Problem Solving, 2.2; Communication, 2.2; Roles, 2.3; Affective Responsiveness, 2.2; Affective Involvement, 2.1; Behavior Control, 1.9; and General Functioning, 2.0. These cutoff scores correctly identified 57% to 83% of troubled families and correctly identified 60% to 79% nontroubled families.

Reliability

Kabacoff et al. (1990) reported the internal consistency for three samples for each of the scales. Using this information we calculated the average consistency for the three samples and found internal consistency of the scales as measured by Cronbach's alpha ranged from .65 to .84.

Miller et al. (1985) reported the one-week test–retest reliability of the scales ranged from .66 to .76.

Validity

Scores on the scales have been found to correlate with clinicians' ratings of family functioning (Miller et al., 1985) and with other self-report measures of family functioning (Epstein et al., 1983; Miller et al., 1985; Perosa & Perosa, 1990). Miller et al. (1985) found that social desirability responding was quite low for all scales.

Two studies have found that individuals from troubled families scored significantly higher than other individuals on every scale (Epstein et al., 1983; Kabacoff et al., 1990).

McMaster Family Assessment Device

Instructions: Following are a number of statements about families. Please read each statement carefully, and decide how well it describes your own family. You should answer according to how you see your family. For each statement there are four (4) possible responses:

Strongly Agree (SA)	Check SA if you feel that the statement describes your family very accurately.
Agree (A)	Check A if you feel that the statement describes your family for the most part.
Disagree (D)	Check D if you feel that the statement does not describe your family for the most part.
Strongly Disagree (SD)	Check SD if you feel that the statement does not describe your family at all.

These four responses will appear below each statement like this:

41. We are not satisfied with anything short of perfection.

_____ SA _____ A _____ D _____ SD

Try not to spend too much time thinking about each statement, but respond as quickly and honestly as you can. If you have trouble with one, answer with your first reaction. Please be sure to answer *every* statement and mark all your answers in the *space provided below* each statement.

1. Planning family activities is difficult because we misunderstand each other.

_____ SA _____ A _____ D _____ SD

2. We resolve most everyday problems around the house.

_____ SA _____ A _____ D _____ SD

3. When someone is upset the others know why.

_____ SA _____ A _____ D _____ SD

4. When you ask someone to do something, you have to check that they did it.

_____ SA _____ A _____ D _____ SD

5. If someone is in trouble, the others become too involved.

_____ SA _____ A _____ D _____ SD

6. In times of crisis we can turn to each other for support.

_____ SA _____ A _____ D _____ SD

7. We don't know what to do when an emergency comes up.

_____ SA _____ A _____ D _____ SD

8. We sometimes run out of things that we need.

_____ SA _____ A _____ D _____ SD

9. We are reluctant to show our affection for each other.

_____ SA _____ A _____ D _____ SD

10. We make sure members meet their family responsibilities.

_____ SA _____ A _____ D _____ SD

11. We cannot talk to each other about the sadness we feel.

_____ SA _____ A _____ D _____ SD

12. We usually act on our decisions regarding problems.

_____ SA _____ A _____ D _____ SD

13. You only get the interest of others when something is important to them.

_____ SA _____ A _____ D _____ SD

14. You can't tell how a person is feeling from what they are saying.

_____ SA _____ A _____ D _____ SD

15. Family tasks don't get spread around enough.

_____ SA _____ A _____ D _____ SD

16. Individuals are accepted for what they are.

_____ SA _____ A _____ D _____ SD

➤

17. You can easily get away with breaking the rules.

_____ SA _____ A _____ D _____ SD

18. People come right out and say things instead of hinting at them.

_____ SA _____ A _____ D _____ SD

19. Some of us just don't respond emotionally.

_____ SA _____ A _____ D _____ SD

20. We know what to do in an emergency.

_____ SA _____ A _____ D _____ SD

21. We avoid discussing our fears and concerns.

_____ SA _____ A _____ D _____ SD

22. It is difficult to talk to each other about tender feelings.

_____ SA _____ A _____ D _____ SD

23. We have trouble meeting our bills.

_____ SA _____ A _____ D _____ SD

24. After our family tries to solve a problem, we usually discuss whether it worked or not.

_____ SA _____ A _____ D _____ SD

25. We are too self-centered.

_____ SA _____ A _____ D _____ SD

26. We can express feelings to each other.

_____ SA _____ A _____ D _____ SD

27. We have no clear expectations about toilet habits.

_____ SA _____ A _____ D _____ SD

28. We do not show our love for each other.

_____ SA _____ A _____ D _____ SD

29. We talk to people directly rather than through go-betweens.

_____ SA _____ A _____ D _____ SD

30. Each of us has particular duties and responsibilities.

_____ SA _____ A _____ D _____ SD

31. There are lots of bad feelings in the family.

_____ SA _____ A _____ D _____ SD

32. We have rules about hitting people.

_____ SA _____ A _____ D _____ SD

33. We get involved with each other only when something interests us.

_____ SA _____ A _____ D _____ SD

34. There's little time to explore personal interests.

_____ SA _____ A _____ D _____ SD

35. We often don't say what we mean.

_____ SA _____ A _____ D _____ SD

36. We feel accepted for what we are.

_____ SA _____ A _____ D _____ SD

37. We show interest in each other when we can get something out of it personally.

_____ SA _____ A _____ D _____ SD

38. We resolve most emotional upsets that come up.

_____ SA _____ A _____ D _____ SD

39. Tenderness takes second place to other things in our family.

_____ SA _____ A _____ D _____ SD

40. We discuss who is to do household jobs.

_____ SA _____ A _____ D _____ SD

➤

41. Making decisions is a problem for our family.

_____ SA _____ A _____ D _____ SD

42. Our family shows interest in each other only when they can get something out of it.

_____ SA _____ A _____ D _____ SD

43. We are frank with each other.

_____ SA _____ A _____ D _____ SD

44. We don't hold to any rules or standards.

_____ SA _____ A _____ D _____ SD

45. If people are asked to do something, they need reminding.

_____ SA _____ A _____ D _____ SD

46. We are able to make decisions about how to solve problems.

_____ SA _____ A _____ D _____ SD

47. If the rules are broken, we don't know what to expect.

_____ SA _____ A _____ D _____ SD

48. Anything goes in our family.

_____ SA _____ A _____ D _____ SD

49. We express tenderness.

_____ SA _____ A _____ D _____ SD

50. We confront problems involving feelings.

_____ SA _____ A _____ D _____ SD

51. We don't get along well together.

_____ SA _____ A _____ D _____ SD

52. We don't talk to each other when we are angry.

_____ SA _____ A _____ D _____ SD

53. We are generally dissatisfied with the family duties assigned to us.

_____ SA _____ A _____ D _____ SD

54. Even though we mean well, we intrude too much into each other's lives.

_____ SA _____ A _____ D _____ SD

55. There are rules about dangerous situations.

_____ SA _____ A _____ D _____ SD

56. We confide in each other.

_____ SA _____ A _____ D _____ SD

57. We cry openly.

_____ SA _____ A _____ D _____ SD

58. We don't have reasonable transport.

_____ SA _____ A _____ D _____ SD

59. When we don't like what someone has done, we tell them.

_____ SA _____ A _____ D _____ SD

60. We try to think of different ways to solve problems.

_____ SA _____ A _____ D _____ SD

CLINICAL RATING SCALE FOR THE CIRCUMPLEX MODEL OF
MARITAL AND FAMILY SYSTEMS

Purpose and Development

The Clinical Rating Scale measures family cohesion, family flexibility, and family communication. The scale is a 20-item interview measure developed by Olson (1993) to assess the dimensions of the Circumplex Model of Family systems (Olson, 1986; Olson, Russell, & Sprenkle, 1989). The scale is based on an earlier scale developed by Olson and Killorin and the items closely mirror the theoretical dimensions of the circumplex model.

Thomas and Olson (1993) factor analyzed responses to the scale and found an excellent fit between the factor structure of the scale and the three theoretical dimensions underlying the scale. Each item had the highest loading on the factor representing the theoretical dimension it was designed to tap. The three global ratings for each of the dimensions had the highest factor loading on the three corresponding factors.

Administration and Scoring

Olson (1993) suggests that the interview on which the evaluation is based may be semistructured, but that the interviewer should also encourage the couple or family to engage in dialogue with each other. The scale section shows sample questions designed by Olson (1993) for the semistructured portion of the interview. To encourage dialogue between family members, Olson (1993) suggests asking family members to describe their typical week and how they handle daily routines, decision-making, and conflict.

After the interview is over, the evaluator should first use the Coalitions scale, which records extreme emotional closeness and overinvolvement of a dyad within the family and a Disengaged Individuals scale, which records emotional separateness and low involvement of any individual family member. The evaluator then completes other scales by selecting a scale value that best describes the couple or family for each item that applies to that family. The three global ratings should be an overall evaluation of the dimension rather than just an average of the items ratings. The cohesion and flexibility items are rated on an 8-point scale and the communication items are rated on a 6-point scale. Each scale value has extensive descriptors.

Items 1 through 7 comprise the Family Cohesion scale. On this scale ratings of 1 or 2 indicate disengagement, ratings of 3 or 4 indicate separateness, ratings of 5 or 6 indicate connectedness, and ratings of 7 or 8 indicate enmeshedness. Items 8 through 13 comprise the Family Flexibility scale. On this scale, ratings of 1 or 2 indicate rigidity, ratings of 3 or 4 indicate structure, ratings of 5 or 6 indicate flexibility, and ratings of 7 or 8 indicate chaos. The Family Communication scale consists of items 14 through 20 and ratings of 1 indicate low levels of communication while ratings of 6 indicate high levels of communication.

The ratings may be used in different ways. First, the item scores themselves may provide useful insights. Second, the item averages for each of the three dimensions and the global ratings for each of the three dimensions provide measures of Family Cohesion, Family Flexibility, and Family Communication.

Third, the intersection of the Family Cohesion score and the Family Flexibility score shows where the family falls in the Circumplex Model. For example, families with a very low flexibility score and a very high cohesion score would fall in the rigidly enmeshed portion of the Circumplex Model. Families with a moderate flexibility score and a moderate cohesion score would fall in the flexibly connected portion of the Circumplex Model. According to the model, moderate scores on Cohesion and Flexibility tend to be more adaptive than extreme scores. The intersection of the scores on these two scales leads to the classification of three family types: Balanced (those with moderate scores on both dimensions), Midrange (those with moderate scores on one dimension but extreme scores on the other dimension), and Extreme (those with extreme scores on both dimensions).

Thomas and Olson (1993) point out that some of the items on the scale are directed at two-parent families and that in single-parent families different dynamics may underlie constructs tapped by the specific items. To remedy these problems, they suggest that the three global rating items be given more weight when a single-parent family is evaluated.

Sample Scores

Thomas and Olson (1993) obtained Clinical Rating Scale scores for 25 families that were going through family therapy, most of which had a troubled teenage family member; 35 families with a disturbed teenage family member and most of which were going through family therapy; 62 families that had a child with Down's syndrome, none of which were currently involved in therapy; and 60 families with at least one teenage child, none of which were currently involved in therapy. Table 1 shows the percentage of families from each of the four groups which fell into each of the four levels of cohesion and flexibility, each of the three levels of communication, and each of the three Circumplex Model family types.

TABLE 1
Percentage of Families Scoring at Different Levels
on the Clinical Rating Scale, Thomas and Olson (1993)

	Families in therapy	Families with troubled teenager	Families with Down's syndrome child	Control families
Family Cohesion				
Disengaged (%)	40	60	4	7
Separated (%)	26	20	25	34
Connected (%)	8	0	62	53
Enmeshed (%)	26	19	9	6
Family Flexibility				
Rigid (%)	30	27	5	8
Structured (%)	18	13	40	35
Flexible (%)	20	33	43	49
Chaotic (%)	32	27	12	8
Family Communication				
Poor (%)	44	60	10	9
Good (%)	56	37	48	57
Very good (%)	0	3	42	34
Circumplex Model Types				
Extreme (%)	40	49	8	8
Midrange (%)	48	35	14	12
Balanced (%)	12	16	78	80

Reliability

Thomas and Olson (1993) calculated the internal consistency and the interrater reliability of the scales in a sample consisting of families in therapy, families with a troubled teenager, families with a Down's syndrome child, and families who were not currently in therapy. Internal consistency as calculated by Cronbach's alpha was .95 for the Family Cohesion scale, .94 for the Family Flexibility scale, and .97 for the Family Communication scale. Interrater reliability was .83 for the Family Cohesion scale, .75 for the Family Flexibility scale, and .86 for the Family Communication scale.

Validity

Fristad (1989) found a strong association between scores on an earlier version of the scale and scores on another clinician rating scale of family functioning, but found no relationship between scores on the Cohesion scale and self-reported functioning and a negative relationship between the Adaptability scale and self-reported functioning.

Thomas and Olson (1993) compared the scores of troubled families that were involved in family therapy, or had a teenager who was emotionally or behaviorally disturbed, with those of control families not currently involved in therapy. They found that, as expected, significantly more of the troubled families had extremely high or low scores on the Family Cohesion and Family Flexibility scales and the troubled families had significantly lower scores on the Family Communication scale. The troubled families were also much more likely to fall into the extreme region of the Circumplex Model, while the great majority of the control families fell into the balanced region of the Circumplex Model.

CLINICAL RATING SCALE FOR THE CIRCUMPLEX MODEL OF MARITAL AND FAMILY SYSTEMS

INTERVIEW QUESTIONS FOR THE CLINICAL RATING SCALE

I. Questions for Assessing Family Cohesion

Emotional Bonding—How close do family members feel to each other?

Family Involvement—How actively involved are people in each other's lives?

Marital Relationship—How emotionally close are the parents?

Parent–Child Relationship—How close are the parent(s) and children? Are the generational boundaries age appropriate with the parents in control?

Internal Boundaries

Time—Do family members spend time together whenever possible?
Space—Do family members prefer more privacy and space apart than being together?

External Boundaries

Friends—Are most friends of the family or separate friends?
Interests—Do family members have both separate and joint interests?
Activities—Do people usually engage in activities alone or together?

Other Relevant Questions:

Does your family balance separateness and togetherness?
How does your family celebrate birthdays and holidays?
What is a typical evening and weekend like in your family?

II. Questions for Assessing Family Flexibility

Leadership—Is the leadership shared between parents?

Discipline—Is (was) the discipline strict in your your family?

Negotiation—How do you negotiate differences in your family?

Roles—Do the couple and family members perform certain tasks?

Rules—Are the rules stage appropriate and did they change over time?

Other Relevant Questions:

How open is your family to change?
Does your family seem disorganized?
Are the parent(s) in charge versus the child(ren)?

➤

FAMILY COHESION

Couple/Family Score	Disengaged		Separated		Connected		Enmeshed	
	1	2	3	4	5	6	7	8
1. Emotional Bonding	Extreme emotional separateness. Lack of family loyalty.		Emotional separateness. Limited closeness. Occasional family loyalty.		Emotional closeness. Some separateness. Loyalty to family expected.		Extreme emotional closeness. Little separateness. Loyalty to family demanded.	
2. Family Involvement	Very low involvement or interaction. Infrequent affective responsiveness.		Involvement acceptable. Personal distance preferred. Some affective responsiveness.		Involvement emphasized. Personal distance allowed. Affective interactions encouraged and preferred.		Very high involvement. Fusion, overdependency. High affective responsiveness and control.	
3. Marital Relationship	High emotional separateness. Limited closeness.		Emotional separateness. Some closeness.		Emotional closeness. Some separateness.		Extreme closeness, fusion. Limited separateness.	
4. Parent–Child Relationship	Rigid generational boundaries. Low p/c closeness.		Clear generational boundaries. Some p/c closeness.		Clear generational boundaries. High p/c closeness.		Lack of generational boundaries. Excessive p/c closeness.	

	Togetherness dominates.	More togetherness than separateness.	More separateness than togetherness.	Separateness dominates.
5. Internal Boundaries				
Time (physical and emotional)	Time together maximized. Little time alone permitted.	Time together important. Time alone preferred.	Time alone important. Some time together.	Time apart maximized. Rarely time together.
Space	Little private space permitted.	Sharing family space. Private space respected.	Separate space. Sharing of family space.	Separate space needed and preferred.
Decision-Making	Decisions subject to wishes of entire group.	Joint decisions preferred.	Individual decision-making, but joint possible.	Individual decision-making. (Oppositional)
6. External Boundaries	Mainly focused inside the family.	More focused inside than outside the family.	More focused inside the family.	Mainly focused outside the family.
Friends	Family friends preferred. Limited individual friendships.	Individual friendships shared with family.	Individual friendships seldom shared with family.	Individual friends seen alone.
Interests	Joint interests mandated.	Some joint interests.	Separate interests.	Disparate interests.
Activities	Separate activities seen as disloyal.	More shared than individual activities.	More separate than shared activities.	Mainly separate activities.

7. Global Cohesion Rating (1–8)	Very low	Low to moderate	Moderate to high	Very high

The global rating is based on your overall evaluation, not a sum score of the subscale.

FAMILY FLEXIBILITY

Couple/Family Score	Rigid		Structured		Flexible		Chaotic	
	1	2	3	4	5	6	7	8
8. Leadership (control)	Authoritarian leadership. Parent(s) highly controlling.		Primarily authoritarian but some equalitarian leadership.		Equalitarian leadership with fluid leadership.		Limited and/or erratic leadership. Parental control unsuccessful. Rebuffed.	
9. Discipline (for families only)	Autocratic "law & order." Strict, rigid consequences. Not lenient.		Somewhat democratic. Predictable consequences. Seldom lenient.		Usually democratic. Negotiated consequences. Somewhat lenient.		Laissez-faire and ineffective. Inconsistent consequences. Very lenient.	

10. Negotiation	Limited negotiations. Decisions imposed by parents.	Structured negotiations. Decisions made by parents.	Flexible negotiations. Agreed upon decisions.	Endless negotiations. Impulsive decisions.
11. Roles	Limited repertoire. Strictly defined roles. Unchanging routines.	Roles stable, but may be shared.	Role sharing and making. Fluid changes of roles.	Role shifts and role reversals for routines.
12. Rules	Unchanging rules. Rules strictly enforced.	Few rule changes. Rules firmly enforced.	Some rule changes. Rules flexibly enforced.	Frequent rule changes. Rules inconsistently enforced.
13. Global Flexibility (Rating 1–8)	Very low	Low to moderate	Moderate to high	Very high

The global rating is based on your overall evaluation, not a sum of the subscale.

FAMILY COMMUNICATION

Couple/Family Score	Low		Facilitating		High	
	1	2	3	4	5	6
14. Listener's skills						
Empathy	Seldom evident.		Sometimes evident.		Often evident.	
Attentive listening	Seldom evident.		Sometimes evident.		Often evident.	
15. Speaker's Skills						
Speaking for self	Seldom evident.		Sometimes evident.		Often evident.	
Speaking for others	Often evident.		Sometimes evident.		Seldom evident.	
*Note reverse scoring						
16. Self-Disclosure	Infrequent discussion of self, feelings, and relationships.		Some discussion of self, feelings, and relationships.		Open discussion of self, feelings, and relationships.	
17. Clarity	Inconsistent and/or unclear verbal messages.		Some degree of clarity, but not consistent across time or across all members.		Verbal messages very clear.	
	Frequent incongruences between verbal and nonverbal messages.		Some incongruent messages.		Generally congruent messages.	

18. Continuity/Tracking	Little continuity of content. Irrelevant/distracting nonverbals and asides frequently occur. Frequent/inappropriate topic changes.	Some continuity, but not consistent across time or across all members. Some irrelevant distracting nonverbals and asides. Topic changes not consistently appropriate.	Members consistently tracking. Few irrelevant/distracting nonverbals and asides. Facilitative nonverbals. Appropriate topic changes.
19. Respect and Regard	Lack of respect for feelings or message of others. Possibly overtly disrespectful or belittling attitude.	Somewhat respectful of others, but not consistent across time or across all members. Some incongruent messages.	Consistently appears respectful of other's feelings and messages.
20. Global Family Community Rating (1–6)			

The global rating is based on your overall evaluation, not a sum score of the subscale.

COALITIONS AND DISENGAGED INDIVIDUALS: COHESION SUBSCALE

Instructions: The functioning of some families can be adequately described through *global assessment* on the cohesion dimension of the Circumplex Model. However, many families include individuals or dyadic units whose functioning may be somewhat different from that of the family as a whole. A subsystem or individual's functioning may be markedly different from the family as a group. This rating scale provides a way of noting coalitions and disengaged individuals' patterns in family systems. After observing the family's interactions, the coalitions or disengaged individuals should be noted by checking the relevant categories below.

Coalition: An enmeshed subsystem is typified by extreme emotional closeness and over involvement with each other. During family interaction, the dyad is very connected to each other, often to the exclusion of other family members.

Disengaged Individual(s): These individuals are emotionally separated from the rest of the family. There is low involvement and interaction.

Coalitions	*Disengaged Individual(s)*
_____ Mother–Son	_____ Disengaged Mother
_____ Mother–Daughter	_____ Disengaged Father
_____ Father–Son	_____ Disengaged Child(ren)
_____ Father–Daughter	
_____ Son–Daughter	
_____ Same Sex Siblings	

REFERENCES

Chassin, L., Zeiss, A., Cooper, K., & Reaven, J. (1985). Role perceptions, self-role congruence, and marital satisfaction in dual-worker couples with preschool children. *Social Psychology Quarterly, 48*, 301–311.

Cross, D. G., & Sharpley, C. F. (1981). The Locke–Wallace Marital Adjustment Test reconsidered: Some psychometric findings in regard to its reliability and factorial validity. *Educational and Psychological Measurement, 41*, 1303–1306.

Epstein, N. B., Baldwin, L. M., & Bishop, D. S. (1983). The McMaster Family Assessment Device. *Journal of Marital and Family Therapy, 9*, 171–180.

Fristad, M.A. (1989). A comparison of the McMaster and Circumplex family assessment instruments. *Journal of Marital and Family Therapy, 15*, 259–269.

Kabacoff, R. I., Miller, I. W., Bishop, D. S., Epstein, N. B, & Keitner, G. I. (1990). A psychometric study of the McMaster Family Assessment Device in psychiatric, medical, and nonclinical samples. *Journal of Family Psychology, 3*, 431–439.

Locke, H. J., & Wallace, K. M. (1959). Short Marital-Adjustment and Prediction Tests: Their reliability and validity. *Marriage and Family Living, 21*, 251–255.

McLaughlin, M., Cormier, L. S., & Cormier, W. H. (1988). Relationship between coping strategies and distress, stress, and marital adjustment of multiple-role women. *Journal of Counseling Psychology, 35*, 187–193.

Miller, E. W., Epstein, N. B., Bishop, D. S., & Keitner, G. I, (1985). The McMaster Family Assessment Device: Reliability and validity. *Journal of Marital and Family Therapy, 11*, 345–356.

Olson, D. H. (1986). Circumplex Model VII: Validation studies and FACES III. *Family Process, 25*, 337–351.

Olson D. H. (1993). *Clinical Rating Scale (CRS) for the Circumplex Model of Marital and Family Systems.* St.Paul: University of Minnesota, Department of Social Science.

Olson, D. H., Russell, C., & Sprenkle, D. (1989). *Circumplex Model: Systematic Assessment and Treatment of Families.* New York: Haworth.

Perosa, L. M., & Perosa, S. L. (1990). Convergent and discriminant validity for family self-report measures. *Educational and Psychological Measurement, 50*, 855–868.

Thomas, V., & Olson, D. H. (1993). Problem families and the circumplex model: Observational assessment using the Clinical Rating Scale (CRS). *Journal of Marital and Family Therapy, 19*, 159–175.

Chapter 14

Other Conditions of Clinical Interest

RATHUS ASSERTIVENESS SCHEDULE

Purpose and Development

Rathus (1973) developed this 30-item self-report measure of assertiveness to measure changes produced by assertiveness training, which is now a common part of psychological interventions for chronic mental illness (Benton & Schroeder, 1990), as well as a type of training provided to individuals who have no psychological disorder. Rathus based the items on assertiveness items from multitrait scales, on assertion situations described by Wolpe and Lazarus, and on behaviors described in assertion diaries of college students.

The scale has been translated into Brazilian Portuguese (Pasquali & Goveia, 1990), French (Bouvard, Cottraux, Mollard, & Messy, 1986), Italian (Galeazzi, 1989), Spanish (Flores-Galaz, Diaz-Loving, & Rivera-Aragon, 1987), and Swedish (Gustafson, 1992).

Andrasik, Heimberg, Edlund, & Blankenberg (1981) reported that a tenth- to twelfth-grade reading level is needed for the scale instructions and an eighth- to ninth-grade level is needed for the items. In response, McCormick (1985) developed a more easily read version of the scale, but it has been little used in research.

Administration and Scoring

Respondents use a continuum of -3 to $+3$ to respond to each of 30 items. The scale score is the sum of all the responses, after reversing the sign (− or +) of responses on items 1, 2, 4, 5, 9, 11–17, 19, 23, 24, 26, and 30. Scores can range from −90 to +90, with higher scores indicating more assertiveness.

Sample Scores

Several studies of the scale have produced scores for a total of almost 2,000 college students. The mean scores have ranged from −1 to 12, $SD = 22$ to 28 (Chandler, Cook, & Dugovics, 1978; Hollandsworth, 1976; Hull & Hull, 1978; Morgan, 1974; Nevid & Rathus, 1978). For groups with a total of 35 inpatient or outpatient schizophrenics, Rathus and Nevid (1977) reported means of −23 to −12, $SD = 4$ to 35. For 71 assertion training participants from the community, Mann & Flowers (1978) reported an initial mean score of about −4 (no SD).

Reliability

Beck and Heimberg (1983), in a comprehensive review of assertiveness scales, reported Rathus Assertiveness Schedule internal consistency coefficients from several studies. These ranged from .59 to .86, with a median of about .76. The review also reported test–retest reliability in two studies of .78 and .80 for periods of 5 weeks and 11–15 days respectively.

Validity

Beck and Heimberg (1983) noted that studies have repeatedly found high correlations between scales scores and other assertiveness measures. Rathus (1973) found correlations between scale scores and both peer ratings of assertiveness and oral descriptions by the subjects of what they would do in certain assertion situations.

In the decade since Beck and Heimberg (1983) published their review of the scale, studies have found correlations between high scale scores and (a) observed assertiveness (Starke, 1987); (b) observed quantity and volume of speech during role-playing (Kimble & Musgrove, 1988); (c) low communication apprehension (Beatty, Plax, & Kearney, 1984); and low depression (Nezu, Nezu, & Nezu, 1986).

Studies have repeatedly found significant decreases in scores produced by assertion training (Beck and Heimberg, 1983; Brown & Carmichael, 1992; McIntyre, Jeffrey, & McIntyre, 1984; Starke, 1987).

Beck and Heimberg (1983) noted that some scale items do not on their face distinguish between assertiveness and aggression. However, there appears to be no evidence that these items harm the validity of the scale.

RATHUS ASSERTIVENESS SCHEDULE

Directions: Indicate how characteristic or descriptive each of the following statements is of you by using the code given below.

+3 very characteristic of me, extremely descriptive
+2 rather characteristic of me, quite descriptive
+1 somewhat characteristic of me, slightly descriptive
−1 somewhat uncharacteristic of me, slightly nondescriptive
−2 rather uncharacteristic of me, quite nondescriptive
−3 very uncharacteristic of me, extremely nondescriptive

_____ 1. Most people seem to be more aggressive and assertive than I am.
_____ 2. I have hesitated to make or accept dates because of "shyness."
_____ 3. When the food served at a restaurant is not done to my satisfaction, I complain about it to the waiter or waitress.
_____ 4. I am careful to avoid hurting other people's feelings, even when I feel that I have been injured.
_____ 5. If a salesman has gone to considerable trouble to show me merchandise which is not quite suitable, I have a difficult time in saying "no."
_____ 6. When I am asked to do something, I insist upon knowing why.
_____ 7. There are times when I look for a good, vigorous argument.
_____ 8. I strive to get ahead as well as most people in my position.
_____ 9. To be honest, people often take advantage of me.
_____ 10. I enjoy starting conversations with new acquaintances and strangers.
_____ 11. I often don't know what to say to attractive persons of the opposite sex.
_____ 12. I will hesitate to make phone calls to business establishments and institutions.
_____ 13. I would rather apply for a job or for admission to a college by writing letters than by going through with personal interviews.
_____ 14. I find it embarrassing to return merchandise.
_____ 15. If a close and respected relative were annoying me, I would smother my feelings rather than express my annoyance.
_____ 16. I have avoided asking questions for fear of sounding stupid.

➔

_____ 17. During an argument I am sometimes afraid that I will get so upset that I will shake all over.

_____ 18. If a famed and respected lecturer makes a statement which I think is incorrect, I will have the audience hear my point of view as well.

_____ 19. I avoid arguing over prices with clerks and salesmen.

_____ 20. When I have done something important or worthwhile, I manage to let others know about it.

_____ 21. I am open and frank about my feelings.

_____ 22. If someone has been spreading false and bad stories about me, I see him (her) as soon as possible to "have a talk" about it.

_____ 23. I often have a hard time saying "no."

_____ 24. I tend to bottle up my emotions rather than make a scene.

_____ 25. I complain about poor service in a restaurant and elsewhere.

_____ 26. When I am given a compliment, I sometimes just don't know what to say.

_____ 27. If a couple near me in a theater or at a lecture were conversing rather loudly, I would ask them to be quiet or to take their conversation elsewhere.

_____ 28. Anyone attempting to push ahead of me in a line is in for a good battle.

_____ 29. I am quick to express an opinion.

_____ 30. There are times when I just can't say anything.

Reprinted from Rathus (1973) with the permission of Academic Press.

AGGRESSION QUESTIONNAIRE

Purpose and Development

The Aggression Questionnaire measures four aspects of aggression: physical aggression, verbal aggression, anger, and hostility. The questionnaire is a 29-item self-report measure developed by Buss and Perry (1992) to improve on the original Buss–Durkee Hostility Scale. Their initial pool of items was a combination of some items from Buss and Durkee's (1957) widely used scale and new items. A factor analysis of the initial pool of items identified the four main factors of physical aggression, verbal aggression, anger (irritability and short-temperedness), and hostility (distrust and bitterness). The items that loaded highest on the four factors were retained for the scale. Factor analyses of the responses of two further large groups of subjects confirmed the factor structure of the scale and suggested that a general aggression factor underlies all the items.

Administration and Scoring

Respondents indicate how characteristic of them each item is using a 5-point scale. Items 12 and 19 are reverse scored. Items 2, 13–16, 18, 19, 24, and 25 are summed for the Physical Aggression subscale. Scores on this subscale can range from 9 to 45 with higher scores indicating more physical aggression. Items 1, 7–9, and 26 are summed for the Verbal Aggression subscale. Scores on this subscale can range from 5 to 25 with higher scores indicating more verbal aggression. Items 3, 10–12, 20, 27, and 28 are summed for the Anger subscale. Scores on this subscale can range from 7 to 35 with higher scores indicating more anger. Items 4–6, 17, 21–23, and 29 are summed for the Hostility subscale. Scores on this subscale can range from 8 to 40 with higher scores indicating more hostility. The 29 items may also be summed for a total scale score which can range from 29 to 145 on which higher scores indicate more overall aggression.

Sample Scores

Buss and Perry (1992) gave the questionnaire to 612 male and 641 female college students. Table 1 shows their mean scores.

Reliability

In a large sample of college students, Buss and Perry (1992) found that internal consistency as assessed by Cronbach's alpha was .85 for the

TABLE 1
College Students' Scores on the Aggression Questionnaire
(Buss and Perry, 1992)

Group	Physical		Verbal		Anger		Hostility		Total score	
	M	SD	M	SD	M	SD	M	SD	M	SD
Men	24.3	7.7	15.2	3.9	17.0	5.6	21.3	5.5	77.8	16.5
Women	17.9	6.6	13.5	3.9	16.7	5.8	20.2	6.3	68.2	17.0

Physical Aggression scale, .72 for the Verbal Aggression scale, .83 for the Anger scale, .77 for the Hostility scale, and .89 for the total score. In a sample of college students they also found nine-week test–retest reliability of .80 for the Physical Aggression scale, .76 for the Verbal Aggression scale, .72 for the Anger scale, .72 for the Hostility scale, and .80 for the total score.

Validity

Buss and Perry (1992) correlated scale scores with a number of personality traits to obtain validity information for the subscales. Higher Physical and Verbal Aggression scale scores were associated with greater impulsiveness, activity, assertiveness, and competitiveness. Higher Anger scale scores were associated with greater emotionality, activity, impulsiveness, assertiveness, competitiveness, and lower self-esteem. Higher Hostility scale scores were associated with greater emotionality, impulsiveness, assertiveness, competitiveness, public and private self-consciousness, and lower self-esteem. The total scale scores were associated with all the above mentioned traits. The strongest correlations were with impulsiveness, assertiveness, and competitiveness.

In a second study Buss and Perry (1992) asked members of college fraternities to rate each other on physical and verbal aggression, anger, and trust (in lieu of asking about the socially undesirable trait of hostility) and also asked them to fill out the Aggression Questionnaire. They found a significant association between peer ratings and self-reports for each of the subscales and the total score, with the highest congruence for physical aggression and the lowest congruence for verbal aggression.

Buss and Perry (1992) found that all four subscales were significantly correlated with each other. The Anger subscale was most strongly associated with the other scales and Buss and Perry suggest that anger may serve as a link between the cognitive construct of hostility and the behavioral constructs of verbal and physical aggression.

AGGRESSION QUESTIONNAIRE

Please indicate how well each of the following statements characterizes you. Give your response for each item by writing next to the item a number from the scale below.

1	2	3	4	5
extremely				extremely
uncharacteristic				characteristic
of me				of me

_____ 1. I tell my friends openly when I disagree with them.
_____ 2. Once in a while I can't control the urge to strike another person.
_____ 3. I flare up quickly but get over it quickly.
_____ 4. I am sometimes eaten up with jealousy.
_____ 5. At times I feel I have gotten a raw deal out of life.
_____ 6. Other people always seem to get the breaks.
_____ 7. I often find myself disagreeing with people.
_____ 8. When people annoy me, I may tell them what I think of them.
_____ 9. I can't help getting into arguments when people disagree with me.
_____ 10. When frustrated, I let my irritation show.
_____ 11. I sometimes feel like a powder keg ready to explode.
_____ 12. I am an even tempered person.
_____ 13. Given enough provocation, I may hit another person.
_____ 14. If somebody hits me, I hit back.
_____ 15. I get into fights a little more than the average person.
_____ 16. If I have to resort to violence to protect my rights, I will.
_____ 17. I wonder why sometimes I feel so bitter about things.
_____ 18. There are people who pushed me so far that we came to blows.
_____ 19. I can think of no good reason for ever hitting a person.
_____ 20. Some of my friends think I am a hothead.
_____ 21. I know that "friends" talk about me behind my back.
_____ 22. I am suspicious of overly friendly strangers.
_____ 23. I sometimes feel that people are laughing at me behind my back.
_____ 24. I have threatened people I know.
_____ 25. I have become so mad that I have broken things.
_____ 26. My friends say that I am somewhat argumentative.
_____ 27. Sometimes I fly off the handle for no good reason.
_____ 28. I have trouble controlling my temper.
_____ 29. When people are especially nice, I wonder what they want.

REACTION INVENTORY

Purpose and Development

The Reaction Inventory measures individuals' propensity for anger arousal (Biaggio and Maiuro, 1985). Evans and Stangeland (1971) developed the 76-item self-report measure to assess which situations arouse anger and subsequent aggression. Each of the authors created 100 items and they then selected items similar in both pools for the final scale. A factor analytic study found that the items grouped into ten separate factors (Evans & Stangeland, 1971).

Administration and Scoring

Respondents rate each item on a 5-point scale of how much anger they experience in the situation described. These ratings are summed for a total scale score which can range from 76 to 380. Higher scores indicate a greater propensity for anger.

Sample Scores

Biaggio (1980) found that the average scale score was 229.99 (SD = 40.38) for 72 male and 78 female college students. There were no sex differences.

Reliability

Evans and Stangeland (1971) reported that in a sample of college students and individuals drawn from the community the internal consistency of the scale was .95. In a sample of college students Biaggio, Supplee, and Curtis (1981) found a .70 two-week test–retest reliability for the scale.

Validity

Several studies found that higher scores on the Reaction Inventory were associated with higher scores on other measures of anger and hostility (Evans & Stangeland, 1971; Biaggio, 1980). Biaggio (1980) also found a low but significant correlation between scores on the Reaction Inventory and scores on a social desirability inventory.

An intervention aimed at reducing anger resulted in lowered scores (Hearn & Evans, 1972; Evans & Hearn, 1973).

REACTION INVENTORY

The items in this questionnaire refer to things and experiences that may cause anger or other unpleasant feelings. Please use numbers from the scale below to indicate how much you are angered by each of the situations described. Place a number that best expresses how you feel next to each item.

1 = Not at all
2 = A little
3 = A fair amount
4 = Much
5 = Very much

_____ 1. People pushing into line.
_____ 2. People being cruel to children.
_____ 3. People who destroy borrowed things.
_____ 4. Locking your keys in the car.
_____ 5. Waiting for someone who is late or doesn't show up.
_____ 6. People who are loud and obnoxious.
_____ 7. Injuring yourself.
_____ 8. Getting halfway to your destination and having forgot something.
_____ 9. Having things spilled on new clothes.
_____ 10. People asking personal questions.
_____ 11. Someone breaking something you value.
_____ 12. Running out of gas.
_____ 13. Being stuck in traffic when you're late.
_____ 14. People acting as though you are stupid.
_____ 15. Rude sales clerks.
_____ 16. People gossiping.
_____ 17. Losing money or valuables.
_____ 18. Waiting for a parking spot and having someone take it.
_____ 19. T.V. breaking down in the midst of a favorite program.
_____ 20. People making loud noises when you are trying to sleep.
_____ 21. Finding someone has lied to you.
_____ 22. Running out of something you need at the moment.
_____ 23. The telephone or doorbell ringing when you are busy at something.
_____ 24. Not having enough money to buy something.

→

_____ 25. Not having the right change for the telephone or parking meter.

_____ 26. Guests who arrive around meal time.

_____ 27. Someone driving carelessly.

_____ 28. Having to do something in a way which you know is inefficient.

_____ 29. Missing an activity that you really wanted to attend.

_____ 30. Finding out about something you would have liked to have seen after leaving a place.

_____ 31. People who don't control their children in public.

_____ 32. Destructive people.

_____ 33. Loud noises such as cars or motorcycles with no mufflers.

_____ 34. People who litter public areas.

_____ 35. People taking advantage of you.

_____ 36. Outdoor events being spoiled by bad weather.

_____ 37. Having your movements restricted.

_____ 38. Long waits for service in a restaurant.

_____ 39. Lazy people who won't do their share.

_____ 40. People complaining about things.

_____ 41. Windows that won't open.

_____ 42. Buying something, using it and seeing it cheaper elsewhere.

_____ 43. Being cheated in a business transaction.

_____ 44. Being forced to do something you don't want to do.

_____ 45. Missing a bus, train or plane.

_____ 46. People who brag about things.

_____ 47. Inaccurate newspaper articles.

_____ 48. Prejudiced people.

_____ 49. People who don't understand something you're trying to explain.

_____ 50. Being forced to repeat something several times.

_____ 51. Being interrupted.

_____ 52. Having to do something else when you're in a hurry.

_____ 53. Criticism.

_____ 54. Having to take orders.

_____ 55. People who think they know it all.

_____ 56. People being sarcastic toward you.

_____ 57. People trying to better you.

_____ 58. Unclean, smelly people.

_____ 59. People who can't follow your orders.

_____ 60. Breaking a tool in the midst of a job.

_____ 61. Servicemen failing to repair things.

_____ 62. People who are constantly fidgeting.

_____ 63. People who expect things done in their time not yours.
_____ 64. Being underpaid in a job.
_____ 65. Seeing people's rights violated by authorities.
_____ 66. Having to redo work.
_____ 67. Ill-mannered people.
_____ 68. People who speak on subjects they know nothing about.
_____ 69. People who think they are always right.
_____ 70. Phony people.
_____ 71. Stores that fail to back their merchandise.
_____ 72. Self-righteous people.
_____ 73. People who interfere in others' affairs.
_____ 74. Finding that someone has overcharged for services.
_____ 75. Being ignored by someone.
_____ 76. Being teased about your faults.

PLEASANT EVENTS SCHEDULE

Purpose and Development

The concept of the 320-item self-report Pleasant Events Schedule (MacPhillamy & Lewinsohn, 1982) is derived from Lewinsohn's model of depression, which focuses on the causal role of insufficient pleasant events. To create scale items, MacPhillamy and Lewinsohn (1982) asked 136 individuals to write lists of pleasurable events. After the elimination of items that were redundant, low in variance, or hard to rate, 320 items remained.

The schedule asks respondents to rate how often they have experienced each of 320 events in the past month and how much they enjoyed the event. Scale users can then calculate the cross-product for each item for obtained-pleasure ratings. A commonly used subscale, MR (mood-related) includes the 49 items that have been found to most highly correlate with mood.

Clinicians can use the scale to assess whether clients have a low frequency of pleasant events, and if so, use the frequency and enjoyability ratings to guide the client into increasing the rate of enjoyable events. Clinicians can also ask clients to use the scale for daily self-monitoring, which might by itself lead to increases in pleasant events. Usually, the clinician promotes this improvement by helping the client schedule enjoyable events (Hoberman, 1990).

Administration and Scoring

Respondents use a 3-point continuum to indicate how often a pleasant event has happened in the past 30 days and another 3-point continuum to indicate how pleasant the event was. Scale users multiply each frequency score by the corresponding enjoyability score to obtain an obtained-pleasure score, which can range from 1 to 9. Total scores are the mean of the individual scores, with higher means indicating more obtained pleasure.

Scale users may seek frequency ratings, enjoyability ratings, and/or obtained-pleasure (cross-product) scores. Researchers generally use either the frequency ratings or the obtained-pleasure scores.

Almost all published studies involving the scale have used either the full scale, which MacPhillamy and Lewinsohn (1982) called the "G" scale, or the mood-related ("MR") scale, which consists of 49 items found to correlate at least .30 with a daily mood measure. We will provide all 320 items and mark with an asterisk those that comprise the mood-related subscale.

Scale users may want to omit items that involve unhealthful activities (items 28, 229, and 280), illegal acts (97 and 110), or socially undesirable behaviors (222) or that are unlikely to have treatment value (87 and 162).

Sample Scores

For a sample of 464 normal adults living in the United States, Mac-Phillamy and Lewinsohn (1976) reported the mean scores listed in Table 1. The differences between males and females were negligible, but individuals over 55 years old had lower scores than the younger respondents (MacPhillamy & Lewinsohn, 1976).

Reliability

In one sample, internal consistency as measured by Cronbach's alpha ranged from .96 to .98 for frequency, enjoyability, and obtained-pleasure scores. (MacPhillamy & Lewinsohn, 1976). We were unable to find data on the internal consistency of the mood-related subscale.

Average one-month test–retest reliability was .71 for all three components of the full scale and .69 for components of the mood-related subscale.

Validity

To assess the validity of the frequency ratings, MacPhillamy and Lewinsohn (1982) had trained observers follow five individuals for five consecutive days and record immediately the frequency of events on the scale. The researchers also collected self-ratings from the subjects and ratings from a peer at the end of the five days. Intercorrelations of the three

TABLE 1
Pleasant Event Scale Scores
of 464 Normal Adults Living
in the United States
(MacPhillamy & Lewinsohn, 1976)

Scale	M	SD
Full scale		
Frequency	.78	.18
Enjoyability	1.03	.26
Obtained pleasure	1.04	.12
Mood-related subscale		
Frequency	1.31	.26
Enjoyability	1.51	.27
Obtained pleasure	2.13	.61

sets of ratings as measured by the gamma statistic ranged from .78 to .87 for the full scale.

To assess the validity of enjoyability ratings, MacPhillamy and Lewinsohn (1982) asked subjects to complete the scale, and a few weeks later asked them to choose among possible prizes as reward for participation in other research. The study found a significant correlation between their choices and their prior enjoyability ratings on the 10 items of the scale that could be evaluated in this way.

In a very positive review of the scale, Rehm (1987) noted that studies have found correlations between scale scores and depression. Rehm (1987) also noted that when the scale is used as a checklist for daily recording, studies have found a correlation with daily mood ratings.

MacPhillamy and Lewinsohn (1982) asked the spouse or roommate of 66 individuals to rate them on the scale. Correlations between self- and peer ratings were similar across frequency, enjoyability, and pleasure ratings. On average, self and peer scores correlated significantly at about .22 for the full scale and about .21 for the mood-related scores.

Because of these low correlations, MacPhillamy and Lewinsohn (1982) created a "moderator subscale" of the Pleasant Events Schedule to help increase the correlation between the two sources of information. However, there is little conceptual support for this subscale and no evidence that researchers have used it.

MacPhillamy and Lewinsohn (1982) found that scale scores were significantly lower for depressed clients than for other psychiatric clients or normals. Other studies have found that in depressed clients scale scores decreased with treatment (Rehm, 1987).

Dobson and Joffe (1986) applied various interventions to groups of normal college students and found that pleasant events scheduling led to increased scale frequency scores and to improvements in mood on one of two measures of depression. Baker and Wilson (1985) used a "100-item" version of the Pleasant Events Schedule with depressed outpatients and found that pleasant events scheduling led to a significant increase in enjoyability scores and cross-products and a nearly significant increase in frequency.

With regard to the mood-related subscale, studies by Bouman and Luteijn (1986), Wierzbicki and Rexford (1989), and Rose and Staats (1988) found a correlation (for frequency, enjoyability, and obtained pleasure) with depression. MacPhillamy and Lewinsohn (1982) found that subscale scores were significantly lower for depressed clients than for other psychiatric clients or normals and were significantly higher for depressed clients who had shown the most clinical improvement than for other depressed clients.

Pleasant Events Schedule

Form III-S

This schedule is designed to find out about the things you have enjoyed during the past month. The schedule contains a list of events or activities which people sometimes enjoy. You will be asked to go over the list twice, the first time rating each event on how many times it has happened in the past month and the second time rating each event on how pleasant it has been for you. There are no right or wrong answers. Please rate every event. Work quickly; there are many items and you will not be asked to make fine distinctions on your ratings. The schedule should take about an hour to complete. Please make your ratings in the columns next to the items. You will find two columns. Use the column labeled "A" to answer Question A; use the column labeled "B" to answer Question B.

DIRECTIONS—QUESTION A

On the following pages you will find a list of activities, events, and experiences. HOW OFTEN HAVE THESE EVENTS HAPPENED IN YOUR LIFE IN THE PAST MONTH? Please answer this question by rating each item on the following scale:

0 = This has *not* happened in the past 30 days.
1 = This has happened *a few times* (1 to 6) in the past 30 days.
2 = This has happened *often* (7 or more) in the past 30 days.

Place your rating for each item in the column labeled "A." Here is an example:

Item number 1 is "Being in the country." Suppose you have been in the country three times during the past 30 days. Then you would mark a "1" in the column under "A" next to item number 1.

Important: Some items will list *more than one event*; for these items, mark how often you have done *any* of the listed events. For example, item number 12 is "Doing art work (painting, sculpture, drawing, movie-making. etc.)." You should rate item 12 on how often you have done *any* form of art work in the past month.

➤

Since this list contains events that might happen to a wide variety of people, you may find that many of the events have not happened to you in the past 30 days. It is not expected that anyone will have done all of these things in one month. Now begin.

A   B

1. Being in the country*
2. Wearing expensive or formal clothes
3. Making contributions to religious, charitable, or other groups
4. Talking about sports
5. Meeting someone new of the same sex*
6. Taking tests when well prepared
7. Going to a rock concert
8. Playing baseball or softball
9. Planning trips or vacations*
10. Buying things for myself
11. Being at the beach
12. Doing art work (painting, sculpture, drawing, movie-making, etc.)
13. Rock climbing or mountaineering
14. Reading the Scriptures or other sacred work
15. Playing golf
16. Taking part in military activities
17. Rearranging or redecorating my room or house
18. Going naked
19. Going to a sports event
20. Reading a "How to Do It" book or article
21. Going to the races (horse, car, boat, etc.)
22. Reading stories, novels, poems, or plays*
23. Going to a bar, tavern, club, etc.
24. Going to lectures or hearing speakers
25. Driving skillfully*
26. Breathing clean air*
27. Thinking up or arranging songs or music
28. Getting drunk
29. Saying something clearly*
30. Boating (canoeing, kayaking, motor boating, sailing, etc.)
31. Pleasing my parents
32. Restoring antiques, refinishing furniture, etc.
33. Watching TV

_____ _____ 34. Talking to myself
_____ _____ 35. Camping
_____ _____ 36. Working in politics
_____ _____ 37. Working on machines (cars, bikes, motorcycles, tractors, etc.)
_____ _____ 38. Thinking about something good in the future*
_____ _____ 39. Playing cards
_____ _____ 40. Completing a difficult task
_____ _____ 41. Laughing*
_____ _____ 42. Solving a problem, puzzle, crossword, etc.
_____ _____ 43. Being at weddings, baptisms, confirmations, etc.
_____ _____ 44. Criticizing someone
_____ _____ 45. Shaving
_____ _____ 46. Having lunch with friends or associates
_____ _____ 47. Taking powerful drugs
_____ _____ 48. Playing tennis
_____ _____ 49. Taking a shower
_____ _____ 50. Driving long distances
_____ _____ 51. Woodworking, carpentry
_____ _____ 52. Writing stories, novels, plays, or poetry
_____ _____ 53. Being with animals*
_____ _____ 54. Riding in an airplane
_____ _____ 55. Exploring (hiking away from known routes, spelunking, etc.)
_____ _____ 56. Having a frank and open conversation*
_____ _____ 57. Singing in a group
_____ _____ 58. Thinking about myself or my problems
_____ _____ 59. Working on my job
_____ _____ 60. Going to a party*
_____ _____ 61. Going to church functions (socials, classes, bazaars, etc.)
_____ _____ 62. Speaking a foreign language
_____ _____ 63. Going to service, civic, or social club meetings
_____ _____ 64. Going to a business meeting or convention
_____ _____ 65. Being in a sporty or expensive car
_____ _____ 66. Playing a musical instrument
_____ _____ 67. Making snacks
_____ _____ 68. Snow skiing
_____ _____ 69. Being helped
_____ _____ 70. Wearing informal clothes*
_____ _____ 71. Combing or brushing my hair
_____ _____ 72. Acting

➤

            73. Taking a nap
            74. Being with friends*
            75. Canning, freezing, making preserves, etc.
            76. Driving fast
            77. Solving a personal problem
            78. Being in a city
            79. Taking a bath
            80. Singing to myself
            81. Making food or crafts to sell or give away
            82. Playing pool or billiards
            83. Being with my grandchildren
            84. Playing chess or checkers
            85. Doing craft work (pottery, jewelry, leather, beads, weaving, etc.)
            86. Weighing myself
            87. Scratching myself
            88. Putting on make-up, fixing my hair, etc.
            89. Designing or drafting
            90. Visiting people who are sick, shut in, or in trouble
            91. Cheering, rooting
            92. Bowling
            93. Being popular at a gathering*
            94. Watching wild animals*
            95. Having an original idea
            96. Gardening, landscaping, or doing yard work
            97. Shoplifting
            98. Reading essays or technical, academic, or professional literature
            99. Wearing new clothes
            100. Dancing
            101. Sitting in the sun*
            102. Riding a motorcycle
            103. Just sitting and thinking
            104. Social drinking
            105. Seeing good things happen to my family or friends*
            106. Going to a fair, carnival, circus, zoo, or amusement park
            107. Talking about philosophy or religion
            108. Gambling
            109. Planning or organizing something*
            110. Smoking marijuana
            111. Having a drink by myself

_____ _____ 112. Listening to the sounds of nature
_____ _____ 113. Dating, courting, etc.
_____ _____ 114. Having a lively talk*
_____ _____ 115. Racing in a car, motorcycle, boat, etc.
_____ _____ 116. Listening to the radio
_____ _____ 117. Having friends come to visit*
_____ _____ 118. Playing in a sporting competition
_____ _____ 119. Introducing people who I think would like each other
_____ _____ 120. Giving gifts
_____ _____ 121. Going to school or government meetings, court sessions, etc.
_____ _____ 122. Getting massages or back rubs
_____ _____ 123. Getting letters, cards, or notes
_____ _____ 124. Watching the sky, clouds, or a storm
_____ _____ 125. Going on outings (to the park, a picnic, or a barbecue, etc.)
_____ _____ 126. Playing basketball
_____ _____ 127. Buying something for my family
_____ _____ 128. Photography
_____ _____ 129. Giving a speech or lecture
_____ _____ 130. Reading maps
_____ _____ 131. Gathering natural objects (wild foods or fruit, rocks, driftwood, etc.)
_____ _____ 132. Working on my finances
_____ _____ 133. Wearing clean clothes*
_____ _____ 134. Making a major purchase or investment (car, appliance, house, stocks, etc.)
_____ _____ 135. Helping someone
_____ _____ 136. Being in the mountains
_____ _____ 137. Getting a job advancement (being promoted, given a raise, or offered a better job, accepted into a better school, etc.)
_____ _____ 138. Hearing jokes
_____ _____ 139. Winning a bet
_____ _____ 140. Talking about my children or grandchildren
_____ _____ 141. Meeting someone new of the opposite sex
_____ _____ 142. Going to a revival or crusade
_____ _____ 143. Talking about my health
_____ _____ 144. Seeing beautiful scenery*
_____ _____ 145. Eating good meals*
_____ _____ 146. Improving my health (having my teeth fixed, getting new glasses, changing my diet, etc.)

➤

——	——	147. Being downtown
——	——	148. Wrestling or boxing
——	——	149. Hunting or shooting
——	——	150. Playing in a musical group
——	——	151. Hiking
——	——	152. Going to a museum or exhibit
——	——	153. Writing papers, essays, articles, reports, memos, etc.
——	——	154. Doing a job well*
——	——	155. Having spare time*
——	——	156. Fishing
——	——	157. Loaning something
——	——	158. Being noticed as sexually attractive*
——	——	159. Pleasing employers, teachers, etc.
——	——	160. Counseling someone
——	——	161. Going to a health club, sauna bath, etc.
——	——	162. Having someone criticize me
——	——	163. Learning to do something new*
——	——	164. Going to a "drive-in" (Dairy Queen, MacDonald's, etc.)
——	——	165. Complimenting or praising someone*
——	——	166. Thinking about people I like*
——	——	167. Being at a fraternity or sorority
——	——	168. Taking revenge on someone
——	——	169. Being with my parents
——	——	170. Horseback riding
——	——	171. Protesting social, political, or environmental conditions
——	——	172. Talking on the telephone
——	——	173. Having daydreams
——	——	174. Kicking leaves, sand, pebbles, etc.
——	——	175. Playing lawn sports (badminton, croquet, shuffleboard, horseshoes, etc.)
——	——	176. Going to school reunions, alumni meetings, etc.
——	——	177. Seeing famous people
——	——	178. Going to the movies
——	——	179. Kissing*
——	——	180. Being alone
——	——	181. Budgeting my time
——	——	182. Cooking meals
——	——	183. Being praised by people I admire
——	——	184. Outwitting a "superior"
——	——	185. Feeling the presence of the Lord in my life*

_____ _____ 186. Doing a project in my own way*

_____ _____ 187. Doing "odd jobs" around the house

_____ _____ 188. Crying

_____ _____ 189. Being told I am needed

_____ _____ 190. Being at a family reunion or get-together

_____ _____ 191. Giving a party or get-together

_____ _____ 192. Washing my hair

_____ _____ 193. Coaching someone

_____ _____ 194. Going to a restaurant

_____ _____ 195. Seeing or smelling a flower or plant

_____ _____ 196. Being invited out

_____ _____ 197. Receiving honors (civic, military, etc.)

_____ _____ 198. Using cologne, perfume, or aftershave

_____ _____ 199. Having someone agree with me

_____ _____ 200. Reminiscing, talking about old times

_____ _____ 201. Getting up early in the morning

_____ _____ 202. Having peace and quiet*

_____ _____ 203. Doing experiments or other scientific work

_____ _____ 204. Visiting friends

_____ _____ 205. Writing in a diary

_____ _____ 206. Playing football

_____ _____ 207. Being counseled

_____ _____ 208. Saying prayers

_____ _____ 209. Giving massages or back rubs

_____ _____ 210. Hitchhiking

_____ _____ 211. Meditating or doing yoga

_____ _____ 212. Seeing a fight

_____ _____ 213. Doing favors for people

_____ _____ 214. Talking with people on the job or in class

_____ _____ 215. Being relaxed*

_____ _____ 216. Being asked for my help or advice

_____ _____ 217. Thinking about other people's problems

_____ _____ 218. Playing board games (Monopoly, Scrabble, etc.)

_____ _____ 219. Sleeping soundly at night*

_____ _____ 220. Doing heavy outdoor work (cutting or chop wood, clearing land, farm work, etc.)

_____ _____ 221. Reading the newspaper

_____ _____ 222. Shocking people, swearing, making obscene gestures, etc.

_____ _____ 223. Snowmobiling or dune-buggy riding

_____ _____ 224. Being in a body-awareness, sensitivity, encounter therapy, or "rap" group

→

_____ _____ 225. Dreaming at night
_____ _____ 226. Playing ping pong
_____ _____ 227. Brushing my teeth
_____ _____ 228. Swimming
_____ _____ 229. Being in a fight
_____ _____ 230. Running, jogging, or doing gymnastic, fitness, field exercises
_____ _____ 231. Walking barefoot
_____ _____ 232. Playing frisbee or catch
_____ _____ 233. Doing housework or laundry; cleaning things
_____ _____ 234. Being with my roommate
_____ _____ 235. Listening to music
_____ _____ 236. Arguing
_____ _____ 237. Knitting, crocheting, embroidery. or fancy needlework
_____ _____ 238. Petting, necking*
_____ _____ 239. Amusing people*
_____ _____ 240. Talking about sex
_____ _____ 241. Going to a barber or beautician
_____ _____ 242. Having house guests
_____ _____ 243. Being with someone I love*
_____ _____ 244. Reading magazines
_____ _____ 245. Sleeping late
_____ _____ 246. Starting a new project
_____ _____ 247. Being stubborn
_____ _____ 248. Having sexual relations with a partner of the opposite sex*
_____ _____ 249. Having other sexual satisfactions
_____ _____ 250. Going to the library
_____ _____ 251. Playing soccer, rugby, hockey, lacrosse, etc.
_____ _____ 252. Preparing a new or special food
_____ _____ 253. Birdwatching
_____ _____ 254. Shopping
_____ _____ 255. Watching people*
_____ _____ 256. Building or watching a fire
_____ _____ 257. Winning an argument
_____ _____ 258. Selling or trading something
_____ _____ 259. Finishing a project or task
_____ _____ 260. Confessing or apologizing
_____ _____ 261. Repairing things
_____ _____ 262. Working with others as a team
_____ _____ 263. Bicycling
_____ _____ 264. Telling people what to do

_____ _____ 265. Being with happy people*
_____ _____ 266. Playing party games
_____ _____ 267. Writing letters, cards, or notes
_____ _____ 268. Talking about politics or public affairs
_____ _____ 269. Asking for help or advice
_____ _____ 270. Going to banquets, luncheons, pot lucks, etc.
_____ _____ 271. Talking about my hobby or special interest
_____ _____ 272. Watching attractive women or men
_____ _____ 273. Smiling at people*
_____ _____ 274. Playing in sand, a stream, the grass, etc.
_____ _____ 275. Talking about other people
_____ _____ 276. Being with my husband or wife*
_____ _____ 277. Having people show interest in what I have said*
_____ _____ 278. Going on field trips, nature walks, etc.
_____ _____ 279. Expressing my love to someone
_____ _____ 280. Smoking tobacco
_____ _____ 281. Caring for house plants
_____ _____ 282. Having coffee, tea, a Coke, etc., with friends*
_____ _____ 283. Taking a walk
_____ _____ 284. Collecting things
_____ _____ 285. Playing handball, paddleball, squash, etc.
_____ _____ 286. Sewing
_____ _____ 287. Suffering for a good cause
_____ _____ 288. Remembering a departed friend or loved one, visiting the cemetery
_____ _____ 289. Doing things with children
_____ _____ 290. Beach combing
_____ _____ 291. Being complimented or told I have done well*
_____ _____ 292. Being told I am loved*
_____ _____ 293. Eating snacks
_____ _____ 294. Staying up late
_____ _____ 295. Having family members or friends do something that makes me proud of them
_____ _____ 296. Being with my children
_____ _____ 297. Going to auctions, garage sales, etc.
_____ _____ 298. Thinking about an interesting question
_____ _____ 299. Doing volunteer work; working on community service projects
_____ _____ 300. Water skiing, surfing, scuba diving
_____ _____ 301. Receiving money
_____ _____ 302. Defending or protecting someone; stopping fraud or abuse

➤

```
_____  _____  303.  Hearing a good sermon
_____  _____  304.  Picking up a hitchhiker
_____  _____  305.  Winning a competition
_____  _____  306.  Making a new friend
_____  _____  307.  Talking about my job or school
_____  _____  308.  Reading cartoons, comic strips, or comic books
_____  _____  309.  Borrowing something
_____  _____  310.  Traveling with a group
_____  _____  311.  Seeing old friends*
_____  _____  312.  Teaching someone
_____  _____  313.  Using my strength
_____  _____  314.  Traveling
_____  _____  315.  Going to office parties or departmental get-togethers
_____  _____  316.  Attending a concert, opera, or ballet
_____  _____  317.  Playing with pets
_____  _____  318.  Going to a play
_____  _____  319.  Looking at the stars or moon
_____  _____  320.  Being coached
```

STOP

If you have just gone through the list for the first time, next follow the directions for Question B.

If you have just finished answering Question B, you have completed the test.

DIRECTIONS—QUESTION B

Now please go over the list once again. This time the question is: HOW PLEASANT, ENJOYABLE, OR REWARDING WAS EACH EVENT DURING THE PAST MONTH? Please answer this question by rating each event on the following scale:

0 = This was *not* pleasant. (Use this rating for events which were either neutral or unpleasant.)

1 = This was *somewhat* pleasant. (Use this rating for events which were mildly or moderately pleasant.)

2 = This was *very* pleasant. (Use this rating for events which were strongly or extremely pleasant.)

Important: If an event has happened to you *more than once* in the past month, try to rate roughly how pleasant it was *on the average. If an event has not happened to you during the past month, then rate it according to how much fun you think it would have been.* When an item lists more than one event rate it on the events *you have actually done.* (If you haven't done any of the events in such an item, give it the average rating of the events in that item which you would like to have done.)

Place your rating for each event next to it in the column labeled "B". Here is an example:

Event number 1 is "Being in the country." Suppose that each time you were in the country in the past 30 days you enjoyed it a great deal. Then you would rate this event "2", since it was "very pleasant."

The list of items may have some events which you would not enjoy. The list was made for a wide variety of people, and it is not expected that one person would enjoy all of them.

Now go back to the list of events, start with item 1, and go through the entire list, rating each event on *roughly how pleasant it was (or would have been) during the past 30 days.* Please be sure that you rate each item.

Reprinted with permission of Dr. Peter Lewinsohn.

REASONS FOR LIVING INVENTORY

Purpose and Development

Linehan, Goodstein, Neilsen, and Chiles (1983) developed the 48-item self-report Reasons for Living Inventory to assess beliefs that play a role in suicide. The developers initially generated 72 different reasons by having a large group of students, workers, and senior citizens generate reasons for not committing suicide. Linehan et al. (1983) asked a different large group of adults from the community to indicate which of these reasons applied to them and then factor analyzed the responses. Six identifiable factors, with a total of 48 items, emerged. The scale developers labeled the factors Survival and Coping Beliefs, Responsibility to Family, Child-Related Concerns, Fear of Suicide, Fear of Social Disapproval, and Moral Objections. Subsequent factor analyses of responses from other groups have essentially confirmed the factor pattern (Kralik & Danforth, 1992; Osman, Gifford, Jones, Lickiss, Osman, & Wenzel, 1993; Osman, Gregg, & Osman, 1992).

Some researchers have used the full scale and some (e.g., Strosahl, Chiles, & Linehan, 1992) have used just the Survival and Coping Beliefs subscale, which has the best reliability and validity data of the subscales. Clinicians may prefer to use the full 48 items in the hope that completing and discussing the scale will help a suicidal client find new reasons to stay alive.

The scale has been translated into Chinese (Chiles, Strosahl, Ping, Michael, Hall, Jomelka, Senn, & Reto, 1989).

Administration and Scoring

Respondents use a 6-point continuum to indicate how important each idea is currently to him or her as a reason not to commit suicide. The scale score and subscale scores are mean scores. Typically, researchers and clinicians work with subscale scores rather than total scores. For the subscales, the items are Survival and Coping Beliefs—24 items (2–4, 8, 10, 12–14, 17, 19, 20, 22, 24, 25, 29, 32, 35–37, 39, 40, 42, 44, 45); Responsibility to Family—7 items (1, 7, 9, 16, 30, 47, 48); Child-Related Concerns—3 items (11, 21, 28); Fear of Suicide—7 items (6, 15, 18, 26, 33, 38, 46); Fear of Social Disapproval—3 items (31, 41, 43); and Moral Objections—4 items (5, 23, 27, 34).

Sample Scores

Table 1 shows subscale scores for groups of 19 and 51 psychiatric inpatients admitted because of suicidal behavior and for 82 adult shoppers

TABLE 1
Sample Scores on Reasons for Living Inventory Groups

| | Suicidal groups | | | | Nonsuicidal group[c] | |
| | Sample 1[a] | | Sample 2[b] | | | |
	Mean	SD	Mean	SD	Mean	SD
Suicide and coping beliefs	3.3	2.2	3.5	—	4.9	—
Responsibility to family	3.3	2.3	3.3	—	4.2	—
Child-related concerns	2.2	2.6	2.6	—	4.0	—
Fear of suicide	2.0	1.8	2.9	—	2.1	—
Fear of social disapproval	2.0	2.1	2.6	—	2.4	—
Moral objections	1.5	1.7	2.8	—	3.2	—

[a]19 psychiatric inpatient suicide attmempters (Chiles et al., 1989).
[b]51 psychiatric inpatient suicide attempters (Linehan et al., 1983).
[c]82 normal adults, never suicidal (Linehan et al., 1983).

who had never considered suicide. Strosahl, Chiles, and Linehan (1992) reported a Survival and Coping Beliefs mean of 3.6 for 51 general psychiatric inpatients with various degrees of suicide intention.

Reliability

Internal consistency, as measured by Cronbach's alpha, for the subscales has ranged from .61 to .91 in various studies (Kralik & Danforth, 1992; Linehan et al., 1983; Osman, et al., 1992; Range, Hall, & Meyers, 1993). When individual subscale alphas were reported, the Survival and Coping Beliefs subscale always had the highest internal consistency. Osman et al. (1992) reported an alpha of .89 for the total scale.

Validity

The validity findings for the Survival and Coping Beliefs subscale have been substantially stronger than for the other subscales. For instance, Connell and Meyer (1991) and Neyra, Range, and Goggin (1990) found that the Survival and Coping Beliefs, Family Responsibility, and Moral subscales correlated significantly with suicidal ideation. Neyra et al. (1990) also found a correlation with Child concerns. The other subscales were not associated with suicidal ideation.

Strosahl et al. (1992) found that Survival and Coping Beliefs scores correlated inversely with depression and hopelessness and had a higher correlation with suicidal intent than did either depression or hopelessness.

Further, depression and hopelessness added no significant explanatory power to the Beliefs score. Osman et al. (1993) found that Survival and Coping Beliefs scores correlated inversely with hopelessness, hostility, depression, psychoticism, psychological distress, negative self-evaluation, and suicidal ideation.

Two studies found correlations between total scale scores and self-predicted future suicide probability (Bonner & Rich 1987; Rich & Bonner, 1987). Ellis and Smith (1991) found that Moral Objections scores correlated with religiosity.

Linehan et al. (1983) divided shoppers into groups who had made a prior suicide attempt or thought seriously about one and others. Suicide attempters/ideators had significantly lower scores on all subscales except Social Disapproval and Moral Objections. The biggest differences were with regard to Survival and Coping Beliefs. Kralik and Danforth (1992) likewise found that Survival and Coping Beliefs discriminated between college-student groups with different levels of suicide ideation better than the other subscales did.

Linehan et al. (1983) found significant correlations between social desirability responding and two subscales: Survival and Coping Beliefs and Responsibility to Family. Hence, individuals may respond to these subscale items more positively than the truth warrants.

Because of the low base rates of attempted suicide it is very difficult for any scale to predict attempts more accurately than one can do by merely predicting that no one will commit suicide (Meehl & Rosen, 1955). Hence, it is not surprising that no findings exist showing that the Reasons for Living Inventory has this type of predictive validity. Instead, the scale has validity as a measure of beliefs relevant to suicide.

REASONS FOR LIVING INVENTORY

Instructions: A survey was conducted to learn more about the reasons why people do *not* kill themselves. The statements on the following pages represent the wide range of reasons that people gave.

Many people have thought of suicide at least once, others nave never considered it. Whether you have considered it or not, we are interested in the reasons you would have for *not* committing suicide *If* the thought were to occur to you or *If* someone were to suggest it to you.

We would like to know how important each of these statements would be to you at this time in your life as a reason for you to *not* kill yourself. Please rate this in the space at the left on each question.

Each reason can be rated from 1 (Not At All Important) to 6 (Extremely Important). If a reason does not apply to you or if you do not believe the statement is true, then it is not likely important and you should put a 1. Please use the whole range of choices so as not to rate only at the middle (2, 3, 4, 5) or only at the extremes (1, 6).

In each space put a number to indicate the importance to you of each reason for *not* killing yourself.

> 1 = Not at all important (as a reason to *not* kill myself, *or* does not apply to me, I don't believe this at all)
> 2 = Quite unimportant
> 3 = Somewhat *unimportant*
> 4 = Somewhat *important*
> 5 = Quite important
> 6 = Extremely important (as a reason for *not* killing myself, I believe this very much and it is very important)

Even if you never have or firmly believe you never would seriously consider killing yourself, it is still important that you rate each reason. In this case, rate on the basis of *why killing yourself is not or would never be an alternative for you.*

Regardless of whether you agree or disagree with these statements, please try to think of them as possible reasons for not killing yourself and rate their importance to you from 1 to 6 on this basis.

_____ 1. I have a responsibility and commitment to my family.
_____ 2. I believe I can learn to adjust or cope with my problems.
_____ 3. I believe I have control over my life and destiny.
_____ 4. I have a desire to live.

→

_____   5. I believe only God has the right to end a life.

_____   6. I am afraid of death.

_____   7. My family might believe I did not love them.

_____   8. I do not believe that things get miserable or hopeless enough that I would rather be dead.

_____   9. My family depends upon me and needs me.

_____ 10. I do not want to die.

_____ 11. I want to watch my children as they grow.

_____ 12. Life is all we have and is better than nothing.

_____ 13. I have future plans I am looking forward to carrying out.

_____ 14. No matter how badly I feel, I know that it will not last.

_____ 15. I am afraid of the unknown.

_____ 16. I love and enjoy my family too much and could not leave them.

_____ 17. I want to experience all that life has to offer and there are many experiences I haven't had yet which I want to have.

_____ 18. I am afraid that my method of killing myself would fail.

_____ 19. I care enough about myself to live.

_____ 20. Life is too beautiful and precious to end it.

_____ 21. It would not be fair to leave the children for others to take care of.

_____ 22. I believe I can find other solutions to my problems.

_____ 23. I am afraid of going to hell.

_____ 24. I have a love of life.

_____ 25. I am too stable to kill myself.

_____ 26. I am a coward and do not have the guts to do it.

_____ 27. My religious beliefs forbid it.

_____ 28. The effect on my children could be harmful.

_____ 29. I am curious about what will happen in the future.

_____ 30. It would hurt my family too much and I would not want them to suffer.

_____ 31. I am concerned about what others would think of me.

_____ 32. I believe everything has a way of working out for the best.

_____ 33. I could not decide where, when, and how to do it.

_____ 34. I consider it morally wrong.

_____ 35. I still have many things left to do.

_____ 36. I have the courage to face life.

_____ 37. I am happy and content with my life.

_____ 38. I am afraid of the actual "act" of killing myself (the pain, blood, violence).

_____ 39. I believe killing myself would not really accomplish or solve anything.

_____ 40. I have hope that things will improve and the future will be happier.
_____ 41. Other people would think I am weak and selfish.
_____ 42. I have an inner drive to survive.
_____ 43. I would not want people to think I did not have control over my life.
_____ 44. I believe I can find a purpose in life, a reason to live.
_____ 45. I see no reason to hurry death along.
_____ 46. I am so inept that my method would not work.
_____ 47. I would not want my family to feel guilty afterwards.
_____ 48. I would not want my family to think I was selfish or a coward.

Reprinted with the permission of Dr. Marsha M. Linehan.

IRRATIONAL BELIEF SCALE

Purpose and Development

The scale is a 20-item self-report measure developed by Malouff and Schutte (1986) to assess irrational beliefs which are thought to underlie depression and anxiety. An initial pool of 50 items was based on Ellis' Rational Emotive Theory. Five items represented each of the main 10 irrational beliefs in the model and all items tapped cognitions rather than affective or behavioral reactions. A sample of students responded to the items and the two items that had the highest item-total correlation were selected from each of the 10 five item clusters.

Administration and Scoring

Respondents use a 1 to 5 scale of agreement to answer each of the items. Ratings for the 20 items are summed for a total scale score. Scores can range from 20 to 100, with higher scales scores indicating more irrational beliefs. Clinicians may also examine which specific beliefs a client strongly agrees with and discuss these with the client.

Sample Scores

Warren and Zgourides (1989) found the following average scores: 55.59 ($SD = 14.70$) for 22 students in a stress management class, 59.44 ($SD = 12.36$) for 124 community college students, and 51.65 ($SD = 12.24$) for 51 school teachers. Templeman (1990) gave the scale to 36 female patients with depression or anxiety disorders and found a mean score of 66.97 ($SD = 12.92$).

Reliability

Malouff and Schutte (1986) found the internal consistency of the scale as assessed by Cronbach's alpha was .80 and two-week test–retest reliability was .89.

Validity

Three studies have found that scale scores are associated with scores on other measures of irrational beliefs (Malouff & Schutte, 1986; Malouff, Valdenegro, & Schutte, 1987; Wertheim & Poulakis, 1992). Because strong irrational beliefs theoretically result in maladjustment, a valid measure of irrational beliefs should be associated with scores on various measures of maladjustment. Scale scores have been found to be associated with depression (Malouff & Schutte, 1986; Templeman, 1990; Warren & Zgourides, 1989; Wertheim & Poulakis, 1992), anxiety (Malouff et al., 1987; Templeman, 1990), social phobias (Berotti, Heimberg, Holt, & Liebowitz, 1990), hostility (Malouff et al., 1987), neuroticism (Warren & Zgourides, 1989), and eating disorders (Mayhew & Edelman, 1989).

Three studies have found that scale scores decrease as clients go through treatment (Malouff & Schutte, 1986; Templeman, 1990; Nottingham & Neimeyer, 1992).

IRRATIONAL BELIEF SCALE

Please use the scale below to express how much you agree with each of the following statements. Write your response next to the statement number.

1. Strongly disagree
2. Disagree somewhat
3. Neither agree nor disagree
4. Agree somewhat
5. Strongly agree

_____ 1. To be a worthwhile person, I must be thoroughly competent in everything I do.

_____ 2. My negative emotions are the result of external pressures.

_____ 3. To be happy, I must maintain the approval of all the persons I consider significant.

_____ 4. Most people who have been unfair to me are generally bad individuals.

_____ 5. Some of my ways of acting are so ingrained that I could never change them.

_____ 6. When it looks as if something might go wrong, it is reasonable to be quite concerned.

_____ 7. Life should be easier than it is.

_____ 8. It is awful when something I want to happen does not occur.

_____ 9. It makes more sense to wait than to try to improve a bad life situation.

_____ 10. I hate it when I cannot eliminate an uncertainty.

_____ 11. Many events from my past so strongly influence me that it is impossible to change.

_____ 12. Individuals who take unfair advantage of me should be punished.

_____ 13. If there is a risk that something bad will happen, it makes sense to be upset.

_____ 14. It is terrible when things do not go the way I would like.

_____ 15. I must keep achieving in order to be satisfied with myself.

_____ 16. Things should turn out better than they usually do.

_____ 17. I cannot help how I feel when everything is going wrong.

_____ 18. To be happy I must be loved by the persons who are important to me.

_____ 19. It is better to ignore personal problems than to try to solve them.

_____ 20. I dislike having any uncertainty about my future.

Reprinted with permission of Plenum Publishing Corp. from Malouff, J. M., Valdenegro, J., Schutte, N. S. (1987). Further validation of a measure of irrational belief. *Journal of Rational-Emotive & Cognitive-Behavior Therapy*, 5, 189–193.

AUTOMATIC THOUGHTS QUESTIONNAIRE

Purpose and Development

Hollon and Kendall (1980) developed the Automatic Thoughts Questionnaire to identify thoughts reported by individuals when they are depressed. To create the scale items the authors asked 788 undergraduates to write thoughts they had during a depressing experience. After putting the thoughts into 100 nonredundant items, the authors determined which items discriminated between groups of students with normal and elevated scores on the MMPI–Depression Scale and the Beck Depression Inventory. The resulting 30 items comprise the final questionnaire. Recently, a Turkish version of the scale has been developed and evaluated (Sahin & Sahin, 1992).

Administration and Scoring

Respondents use a 5-point scale to state the frequency of each thought in the past week. Scale scores can range from 30 to 150, with high scores indicating more depressed thoughts.

Sample Scores

Hollon, Kendall, and Lumry (1986) reported mean scores of 85 to 96, $SD = 24$ to 37, in three groups of inpatients and outpatients diagnosed as depressed. DeRubeis, Evans, Hollon, Garvey, Grove, and Tuason (1990), Simons, Garfield, and Murphy (1984), and Hill, Oei, and Hill (1989) reported mean scores of 94 to 108, $SD = 18$ to 30, for groups of 62, 28, and 11 outpatients diagnosed as having major depression.

Kwon and Oei (1992) and Hill et al. (1989) reported mean scores of 52 and 56, $SD =$ about 18, in groups of 355 and 159 Australian college students. For a total of 97 individuals including normals and nondepressed psychiatric, substance abuse, and medical patients, Hollon et al. (1986) reported mean scores of 41 to 60, $SD = 10$ to 23.

Reliability

In two samples, internal consistency as measured by Cronbach's alpha ranged from .97 to .98 (Hollon & Kendall, 1980; Harrell & Ryon, 1983). Kwon and Oei (1992) found a three-month stability correlation of .67.

Validity

Scale scores have been found to correlate highly with the Beck Depression Inventory (Harrell & Ryan, 1983; Hollon & Kendall, 1980; Hollon et al. 1986; Kauth & Zettle, 1990; Kwon & Oei, 1992) and the MMPI–Depression scale (Hollon & Kendall, 1980). Master and Miller (1991) found that scale scores were higher in individuals exposed to irrational self-statements.

Scale scores also have been found to discriminate between depressed and both nondepressed psychiatric patients and normals (Ingram, Atkinson, Slater, Sacuzzi, & Garfin, 1990; Kauth & Zettle, 1990; McNamara, 1992, citing several studies).

Simons et al. (1984) found that scale scores decreased substantially with either cognitive or drug treatment. DeRubeis et al. (1990) found that scores decreased proportionately to decreases in depression during treatment.

However, in the initial validation research (Hollon & Kendall, 1980), the correlation between scale scores and anxiety was as high as the correlation between scale scores and depression, suggesting that the Automatic Thoughts Questionnaire is not specific to depression. Also, Hill et al. (1989) found that small groups of inpatient substance abusers and inpatients with personality disorders scored about as high as individuals diagnosed as depressed.

AUTOMATIC THOUGHTS QUESTIONNAIRE

Listed below are a variety of thoughts that pop into people's heads. Please read each thought and indicate how frequently, if at all, the thought occurred to you *over the last week*. Please read each item carefully and write the appropriate number next to each item using the following rating scale:

1 = "not at all"
2 = "sometimes"
3 = "moderately often"
4 = "often"
5 = "all the time"

_____   1. I feel like I'm up against the world.
_____   2. I'm no good.
_____   3. Why can't I ever succeed?
_____   4. No one understands me.
_____   5. I've let people down.
_____   6. I don't think I can go on.
_____   7. I wish I were a better person.
_____   8. I'm so weak.
_____   9. My life's not going the way I want it to.
_____   10. I'm so disappointed in myself.
_____   11. Nothing feels good anymore.
_____   12. I can't stand this anymore.
_____   13. I can't get started.
_____   14. What's wrong with me?
_____   15. I wish I were somewhere else.
_____   16. I can't get things together.
_____   17. I hate myself.
_____   18. I'm worthless.
_____   19. Wish I could just disappear.
_____   20. What's the matter with me?
_____   21. I'm a loser.
_____   22. My life is a mess.
_____   23. I'm a failure.
_____   24. I'll never make it.
_____   25. I feel so helpless.
_____   26. Something has to change.
_____   27. There must be something wrong with me.

_____ 28. My future is bleak.
_____ 29. It's just not worth it.
_____ 30. I can't finish anything.

Reprinted with permission of Dr. Steven D. Hollon.

COGNITIVE ERROR QUESTIONNAIRE

Purpose and Uses

Lefebvre (1981) developed the self-report Cognitive Error Questionnaire to measure the types of cognitive distortions that Aaron Beck theorized lead to depression. Lefebvre tried initially to create items for seven types of distortion but was able to develop nonoverlapping items for only four: catastrophizing, overgeneralizing, personalizing, and selective abstraction.

Each item includes a vignette about some event that might happen, followed by a distorted thought the respondent might have about it. Respondents rate how to what extent the thought is typical of them.

Lefebvre (1981) developed items for two very similar 24-item scales, one to measure cognitive distortion in general and one to measure cognitive distortion with regard to low-back pain. Because the general form has broader applicability, and because the low-back pain form showed no substantial value over the general form even with low-back pain sufferers in the initial validation study (Lefebvre, 1981), we will include and discuss only the general form. Unfortunately, some research reports do not make clear whether researchers used the general questionnaire or the general plus the low-back pain questionnaire.

Administration and Scoring

For each item respondents mark one of five responses that are scored on a 0–4 point scale. Each of the four subscales has six items, and item responses are summed for a subscale score, which can range from 0 to 24, with higher scores indicating greater cognitive error. Catastrophizing subscale items include numbers 2, 7, 12, 14, 17, and 24; overgeneralization: 4, 5, 8, 15, 18, and 19; personalization: 1, 6, 11, 13, 20, and 21; and selective abstraction: 3, 9, 10, 16, 22, and 23. Total scale scores, which are the sum of subscale scores, can range from 0 to 96, with higher scores indicating greater cognitive distortion.

Sample Scores

Table 1 shows sample scores for four groups: college students, anxious or depressed outpatients, depressed outpatients, and depressed inpatients.

TABLE 1
General Cognitive Error Questionnaire Sample Scores

Group	Scores									
	Catastrophizing		Overgeneralization		Personalization		Selective abstraction		Total	
	M	SD	M	SD	M	SD	M	SD	M	SD
College students (N = 40)[a]	5.0	4.1	3.0	3.4	3.5	3.0	5.0	3.5	16.6	11.8
Depressed or anxious outpatients (N = 24)[a]	6.6	5.5	4.8	5.5	4.9	5.2	7.4	5.5	23.8	19.3
Depressed outpatients (N = 71)[b]	8.1	4.5	8.1	5.8	5.8	6.3	8.6	6.9	30.7	17.7
Depressed inpatients (N = 18)[c]	6.8	4.5	6.4	4.8	3.9	2.9	6.4	3.8	22.7	12.7

[a]Poulakis & Wertheim (1993).
[b]Neimeyer & Feixas (1992).
[c]Levebvre (1981).

Reliability

Lefebvre (1981) reported that the general scale had internal consistency in the range of .89 to .92. Smith, Peck, Milano, and Ward (1988) found that internal consistency as measured by Cronbach's alpha was .90 for the total general scale and varied from .72 to .78 for the subscales. Total scores on the general questionnaire and the low-back version correlated about .87, providing an estimate of the parallel forms reliability of the general scale (Lefebvre, 1981).

Validity

High total scale scores have been found to correlate significantly with several other measures of dysfunctional thinking and irrational beliefs (Neimeyer & Feixas, 1992; Wertheim & Poulakis, 1992). Total scores have also been found to correlate with self-reported and interviewer-rated depression (Dankberg, 1991; Smith, Peck, Milano, & Ward, 1988), although Neimeyer and Feixas (1992) found no significant association with measures of depression in their study. Prezant and Neimeyer (1988) found in a group of depressed individuals that scores on two of the four subscales—overgeneralization and selective abstraction—correlated with lethality of current suicidal ideation when depression was partialed out.

High scale scores have also been found to discriminate significantly between groups of normals and diagnosed depressives (Lefebvre, 1981; Muran & Motta, 1993) and between groups of normals and diagnosed depressed or anxious outpatients (Wertheim & Poulakis, 1992).

No factor analysis has been reported, so there is no empirical support for viewing the subscales as measuring different constructs. Levebvre (1981) concluded that the high internal consistency of the scale suggests that it measures a single construct (Lefebvre, 1981). The high intercorrelations among subscales (from .64 to .85) found in a study by Neimeyer and Feixas (1992) provide further support for this view.

COGNITIVE ERROR QUESTIONNAIRE

This questionnaire describes a number of situations that might occur in daily life, each followed by a thought in "quotation marks" that a person in the situation might have. Underneath this is a group of statements that describes how similar the thought is to how *you* would think in that situation.

Please read each situation and *imagine* that it is happening to you. Then, read the thought (which is in "quotation marks") following that situation. Circle the statement underneath each thought that best describes how similar that thought is to how you would think in that situation.

Because you may not have had the experiences described in some of the situations, it is important that you *imagine* that it is happening to you. Be sure that you don't rate the situation, just rate how much the thought (which is in "quotation marks") is like the way you would think.

As an example, read the following:

You have just come our of the store and notice a dent in your car that wasn't there before you went in. You think to yourself, "Oh no, the car is wrecked."
    This thought is:

| almost exactly like I would think | a lot like I would think | somewhat like I would think | a little like I would think | not at all like I would think |

If that thought ("Oh no, the car is wrecked.") was *somewhat* like the way you would think in that situation you would circle:

somewhat like
I would think

Please start and rate every thought.

1. Your boss just told you that because of a general slowdown in the industry, he has to lay off all of the people who do your job, including you. You think to yourself, "I must be doing a lousy job or else he wouldn't have laid me off."
    This thought is:

| almost exactly like I would think | a lot like I would think | somewhat like I would think | a little like I would think | not at all like I would think |

→

2. You are a manager in a small business firm. You have to fire one of your
   employees who has been doing a terrible job. You have been putting
   off this decision for days and you think to yourself, "I just know that
   when I fire her, she is going to raise hell and will sue the company."
   This thought is:

almost exactly like I would think	a lot like I would think	somewhat like I would think	a little like I would think	not at all like I would think

3. Last week you painted the living room and your spouse said it really
   looked great. When you were cleaning up you found that you had got
   paint on the rug and thought, "Boy, this wasn't a very good painting
   job."
   This thought is:

almost exactly like I would think	a lot like I would think	somewhat like I would think	a little like I would think	not at all like I would think

4. You noticed recently that a lot of your friends are taking up golf and
   tennis. You would like to learn, but remember the difficulty you had
   that time you tried to ski. You think to yourself, "I couldn't learn skiing
   so I doubt if I can learn to play tennis."
   This thought is:

almost exactly like I would think	a lot like I would think	somewhat like I would think	a little like I would think	not at all like I would think

5. You and your spouse recently went to an office party at the place
   where your spouse works. You didn't know anybody there and had a
   terrible time. When your spouse asks you if you want to go to the
   neighbors to visit, you think, "I'll have a terrible time just like at that
   office party."
   This thought is:

almost exactly like I would think	a lot like I would think	somewhat like I would think	a little like I would think	not at all like I would think

6. You just finished spending three hours cleaning the basement. Your
   spouse however, doesn't say anything about it. You think to yourself,
   "(S)he must think I did a lousy job."

This thought is:

almost exactly like I would think	a lot like I would think	somewhat like I would think	a little like I would think	not at all like I would think

7. Last night, your spouse said (s)he thought you should have a serious discussion about sex. You think to yourself, "(S)he hates the way we make love."
This thought is:

almost exactly like I would think	a lot like I would think	somewhat like I would think	a little like I would think	not at all like I would think

8. You have been working for six months as a car salesperson. You had never been a salesperson before and were just fired because you had not been meeting your quota. You thought, "Why try to get another job, I'll just get fired."
This thought is:

almost exactly like I would think	a lot like I would think	somewhat like I would think	a little like I would think	not at all like I would think

9. Your job requires a lot of travel. You had hoped to drive 400 miles today but you hit bad weather that slowed you down. When you stopped for the night, you thought, "I didn't make that 400 miles; today was a complete waste."
This thought is:

almost exactly like I would think	a lot like I would think	somewhat like I would think	a little like I would think	not at all like I would think

10. You have just finished nine holes of golf. Totaling your score, you recall that although you got par on seven holes, you got two over par on the last two holes. You think to yourself, "Today I really played poorly."
This thought is:

almost exactly like I would think	a lot like I would think	somewhat like I would think	a little like I would think	not at all like I would think

11. You went fishing for the first time today with some of your friends who love fishing. Nobody got anything, and the group seemed to be

→

discouraged. You thought to yourself on the way home, "I guess I made too much noise or did something that scared the fish off." This thought is:

almost exactly like I would think	a lot like I would think	somewhat like I would think	a little like I would think	not at all like I would think

12. Your friends are all going out to ride their snowmobiles. Last time you went, you ran out of gas, and you think to yourself, "What if I run out gas again; I'll freeze to death." This thought is:

almost exactly like I would think	a lot like I would think	somewhat like I would think	a little like I would think	not at all like I would think

13. You have three children who generally do quite well in school. One of your children came home today and told you that he had to stay after school because he got into a fight. You think to yourself, "He wouldn't have gotten that detention if I disciplined him more." This thought is:

almost exactly like I would think	a lot like I would think	somewhat like I would think	a little like I would think	not at all like I would think

14. You are taking your coffee break when your boss stops by and reminds you of some work that has to get done today. You think to yourself, "If I don't start getting back to work earlier, I'm going to lose this job." This thought is:

almost exactly like I would think	a lot like I would think	somewhat like I would think	a little like I would think	not at all like I would think

15. You have noticed that many of your friends have begun playing tennis and are now urging you to play too. You had taken golf lessons with your spouse last year and had difficulty learning to play golf. You think to yourself, "I had so much trouble learning golf, I doubt if I could learn tennis." This thought is:

almost exactly like I would think	a lot like I would think	somewhat like I would think	a little like I would think	not at all like I would think

16. Your seven-year-old son normally does very well in school. Last week, he brought home a paper which he had done incorrectly and was supposed to do over. You think to yourself, "Oh no, now he's having trouble in school. I better make an appointment with his teacher."
This thought is:

almost exactly like I would think	a lot like I would think	somewhat like I would think	a little like I would think	not at all like I would think

17. Earlier today, your spouse asked to have a serious talk with you after work about some things that were troublesome at home. You have no idea what's going on and you think, "We don't communicate enough; our marriage is going to fall apart."
This thought is:

almost exactly like I would think	a lot like I would think	somewhat like I would think	a little like I would think	not at all like I would think

18. On your last job, you had not received a raise even though a co-worker with similar experience had. You are now up for a raise in your present job and think, "I didn't get a raise the last time and I probably won't now."
This thought is:

almost exactly like I would think	a lot like I would think	somewhat like I would think	a little like I would think	not at all like I would think

19. Your teenage daughter has just asked if two of her friends can stay overnight. You recall that you got very upset when your son had some friends over for pizza several weeks ago and they had made a lot of noise. You think, "If they come over, I'll get upset again."
This thought is:

almost exactly like I would think	a lot like I would think	somewhat like I would think	a little like I would think	not at all like I would think

20. You run a day care center. Today, the mother of a child you have been having difficulty with calls and notifies you that she has quit work and will be withdrawing her child from your program. You think, "She probably thinks I wasn't handling him as well as I should."

→

This thought is:

almost exactly like I would think	a lot like I would think	somewhat like I would think	a little like I would think	not at all like I would think

21. You took your children to the neighborhood pool for the afternoon. Although your kids urged you to swim with them, you were enjoying laying in the sun. Later you look up and see them arguing over a float. You think to yourself, "If I had gone in the water, they probably wouldn't be fighting now."
This thought is:

almost exactly like I would think	a lot like I would think	somewhat like I would think	a little like I would think	not at all like I would think

22. You went shopping for some new clothes today and were unable to find anything you liked. You think, "What a waste of a day."
This thought is:

almost exactly like I would think	a lot like I would think	somewhat like I would think	a little like I would think	not at all like I would think

23. You met with your boss today to discuss how you have been doing on your job. He said that he really thought you were doing a good job, but asked you to try to improve in one small area. You think to yourself, "He really thinks I'm doing a lousy job."
This thought is:

almost exactly like I would think	a lot like I would think	somewhat like I would think	a little like I would think	not at all like I would think

24. Last time you went skiing, you took a hard fall and got shook up. You're supposed to go skiing this weekend but think, "I'll probably fall and break my leg and there will be no one to help me."
This thought is:

almost exactly like I would think	a lot like I would think	somewhat like I would think	a little like I would think	not at all like I would think

---

Reprinted with permission of Dr. Mark F. Lefebvre.

REFERENCES

Andrasik, R., Heimberg, R. G., Edlund, S. R., & Blankenberg, R. (1981). Assessing the readability levels of self-report assertion inventories. *Journal of Consulting and Clinical Psychology, 49*, 142–144.

Baker, A. L., & Wilson, P. H. (1985). Cognitive-behavior therapy for depression: The effects of booster sessions on relapse. *Behavior Therapy, 16*, 335–344.

Beatty, M. J., Plax, T. G., & Kearney, P. (1984). Communication apprehension and the Rathus Assertiveness Schedule. *Communication Research Reports, 1*, 130–133.

Beck, J. G., & Heimberg, R. G. (1983). Self-report assessment of assertive behavior. *Behavior Modification, 7*, 451–487.

Benton, M. K., & Schroeder, H. E. (1990). Social skills training with schizophrenics: A meta-analytic evaluation. *Journal of Consulting and Clinical Psychology, 58*, 741–747.

Berotti, D., Heimberg, R. G., Holt, C. S., & Liebowitz, M. R. (1990). Irrational beliefs among social phobics: An examination of the validity of the Belief Scale. Unpublished manuscript, Center for Stress and Anxiety Disorders: Albany, NY.

Biaggio, M. K. (1980). Assessment of anger arousal. *Journal of Personality Assessment, 44*, 289–298.

Biaggio, M. K., & Maiuro (1985). Recent advances in anger assessment. In C. D. Spielberger & J. N. Butcher (Eds.), *Advances in Personality Assessment: Vol 5* (pp. 71–111). Hillsdale, NJ: Lawrence Erlbaum.

Biaggio, M. K., Supplee, K., & Curtis, N. (1981). Reliability and validity of four anger scales. *Journal of Personality Assessment, 45*, 639–648.

Bonner, R. L., & Rich, A. R. (1987). Toward a predictive model of suicidal ideation and behavior: Some preliminary data in college students. *Suicide & Life-Threatening Behavior, 17*, 50–63.

Bouman, T., & Luteijn, F. (1986). Relations between the Pleasant Events Schedule, depression, and other aspects of psychopathology. *Journal of Abnormal Psychology, 95*, 373–377.

Bouvard, M., Cottraux, J., Mollard, E., & Messy, P. (1986). Validation et analyse factorielle de l'echelle d'affirmation de soi de Rathus. *Psychologie Medicale, 18*, 759–763.

Brown, G. T., & Carmichael, K. (1992). Assertiveness training for clients with psychiatric illness: A pilot study. *British Journal of Occupational Therapy, 55*, 137–140.

Buss, A. H., & Durkee, A. (1957). An inventory for assessing different types of hostility. *Journal of Consulting Psychology, 21*, 343–349.

Buss, A. H., & Perry, M. (1992). The Aggression Questionnaire. *Personality Processes and Individual Differences, 63*, 452–459.

Chandler, T. A., Cook, B., & Dugovics, D. A. (1978). Sex differences in self-reported assertiveness. *Psychological Reports, 43*, 395–402.

Chiles, J. A., Strosahl, K. D., Ping, Z. Y., Michael, M. C., Hall, K., Jomelka, R., Senn, B., & Reto, C. (1989). Depression, hopelessness, and suicidal behavior in Chinese and American psychiatric patients. *American Journal of Psychiatry, 146*, 339–344.

Connell, D. K., & Meyer, R. G. (1991). The Reasons for Living Inventory and a college population: Adolescent suicidal behaviors, beliefs, and coping skills. *Journal of Clinical Psychology, 47*, 485–489.

Dankberg, G. (1991). Degree of cognitive distortions and level of depression in bulimic patients. *Issues in Mental Health Nursing, 12*, 333–342.

DeRubeis, R., Evans, M., Hollon, S., Garvey, M., Grove, W., & Tuason, V. (1990). How does cognitive therapy work? Cognitive change and symptom change in cognitive therapy and pharmacotherapy for depression. *Journal of Consulting and Clinical Psychology, 58*, 862–869.

Dobson, K. S., & Joffe, R. (1986). The role of activity level and cognition in depressed mood in a university sample. *Journal of Clinical Psychology, 42,* 264–271.

Ellis, J. B., & Smith, P. C. (1991). Spiritual well-being, social desirability and reasons for living: Is there a connection? *International Journal of Social Psychiatry, 37,* 57–63.

Evans, D. R., & Hearn, M. T. (1973). Anger and systematic desensitization: A follow-up. *Psychological Reports, 32,* 569–570.

Evans, D. R., & Stangeland, M. (1971). Development of the Reaction Inventory to measure anger. *Psychological Reports, 29,* 412–414.

Flores-Galaz, M., Diaz-Loving, R., & Rivera-Aragon, S. Mera: Una medida de rasgos asertivos para la cultura mexicana. *Revista Mexicana de Psicologia, 4,* 29–35.

Galeazzi, A. (1989). Uno strumento per l'assessment comportamentale: Il Questionario di Assertivita di Rathus (R.A.S.). *Bollettino di Psicologia Applicata, 190,* 3–12.

Gustafson, R. (1992). A Swedish psychometric test of the Rathus Assertiveness Schedule. *Psychological Reports, 71,* 479–482.

Harrell, T. H., & Ryon, N. B. (1983). Cognitive behavioral assessment of depression: Clinical validation of the Automatic Thoughts Questionnaire. *Journal of Consulting and Clinical Psychology, 23,* 721–725.

Hearn, M. T., & Evans, D. R. (1972). Anger and reciprocal inhibition therapy. *Psychological Reports, 30,* 943–948.

Hill, C., Oei, T., & Hill, M. (1989). An empirical investigation of the specificity and sensitivity of the Automatic Thoughts Questionnaire and Dysfunctional Attitudes Scale. *Journal of Psychopathology and Behavioral Assessment, 11,* 291–311.

Hoberman, H. (1990). Behavioral treatments for unipolar depression. In B. B. Wolman & G. Stricker (Eds.), *Depressive Disorders: Facts, Theories, and Treatment Methods* (pp. 310–342). New York: Wiley.

Hollandsworth, J. G. (1976). Further investigation of the relationship between expressed fear and assertiveness. *Behaviour Research and Therapy, 14,* 85–87.

Hollon, S. D., & Kendall, P. C. (1980). Cognitive self-statements in depression: Development of an automatic thoughts questionnaire. *Cognitive Therapy and Research, 4,* 383–249.

Hollon, S. D., & Kendall, P. C., Lumry, A. (1986). Specificity of depressotypic cognitions in clinical depression. *Journal of Abnormal Psychology, 95,* 52–59.

Hull, D. B., & Hull, J. H. (1978). Rathus Assertiveness Scale: Normative and factor analytic data. *Behavior Therapy, 9,* 673.

Ingram, R., Atkinson, J., Slater, M., Saccuzzo, D., & Garfin, S. (1990). Negative and positive cognition in depressed and nondepressed chronic-pain patients. *Health Psychology, 9,* 300–314.

Kauth, M., & Zettle, R. (1990). Validation of depression measures in adolescent populations. *Journal of Clinical Psychology, 46,* 291–295.

Kimble, C. E., & Musgrove, J. I. (1988). Dominance in arguing mixed-sex dyads: Visual dominance patterns, talking time, and speech loudness. *Journal of Research in Personality, 22,* 1–16.

Kralik, K. M., & Danforth, W. J. (1992). Identification of coping ideation and strategies preventing suicidality in a college-age sample. *Suicide & Life-Threatening Behavior, 22,* 167–186.

Kwon, S., & Oei, T. (1992). Differential causal roles of dysfunctional attitudes and automatic thoughts in depression. *Cognitive Therapy and Research, 16,* 309–328.

Lefebvre, M. F. (1981). Cognitive distortion and cognitive errors in depressed psychiatric and low back pain patients. *Journal of Consulting and Clinical Psychology, 49,* 517–525.

Linehan, M. M., Goodstein, J. L., Nielsen, S. L., & Chiles, J. A. (1983). Reasons for staying alive when you are thinking of killing yourself: The Reasons for Living Inventory. *Journal of*

Consulting & Clinical Psychology, 51, 276–286. MacPhillamy, D., & Lewinsohn, P. (1976). *Manual for the Pleasant Events Schedule.* Unpublished manual.

MacPhillamy, D., & Lewinsohn, P. (1982). The Pleasant Events Schedule: Studies on reliability, validity, and scale intercorrelation. *Journal of Consulting and Clinical Psychology, 50,* 363–380.

Malouff, J. M., & Schutte, N. S. (1986). Development and validation of a measure of irrational belief. *Journal of Consulting and Clinical Psychology, 54,* 860–862.

Malouff, J. M., Valdenegro, J., & Schutte, N. S. (1987). Further validation of a measure of irrational belief. *Journal of Rational-Emotive & Cognitive-Behavior Therapy, 5,* 189–193.

Mann, R. J., & Flowers, J. V. (1978). An investigation of the reliability and validity of the Rathus Assertion Scale. *Psychological Reports, 42,* 632–634.

Master, S., & Miller, S. (1991). A test of RET theory using an RET theory-based mood induction procedure: The rationality of thinking rationally. *Cognitive Therapy and Research, 15,* 491–502.

Mayhew, R., & Edelman, R. J. (1989). Self-esteem, irrational beliefs and coping strategies in relation to eating problems in a non-clinical population. *Personality and Individual Differences, 10,* 581–584.

McCormick, I. A. (1985). A simple version of the Rathus Assertiveness Schedule. *Behavioral Assessment, 7,* 95–99.

McIntyre, J. T., Jeffrey, D. B., & McIntyre, S. L. (1984). Assertion training: The effectiveness of a comprehensive cognitive-behavioral treatment package with professional nurses. *Behaviour Research and Therapy, 22,* 311–318.

McNamara, K. (1992). Depression assessment and intervention: Current status and future directions. In S. Brown & R. Lent, *Handbook of Counseling Psychology* (pp. 691–718). New York: Wiley.

Meehl, P. E., & Rosen, A. (1955). Antecedent probability and the efficiency of psychometric signs, patterns, or cutting scores. *Psychological Bulletin, 52,* 194–216.

Morgan, W. G. (1974). The relationship between expressed social fears and assertiveness and its treatment implications. *Behaviour Research and Therapy, 12,* 255–257.

Muran, E., & Motta, R. (1993). Cognitive distortions and irrational beliefs in post-traumatic stress, anxiety, and depressive disorders. *Journal of Clinical Psychology, 49,* 166–176.

Neimeyer, R., & Feixas, G. (1992). Cognitive assessment in depression: A comparison of some existing measures. *European Journal of Psychological Assessment, 8,* 47–56.

Nevid, J. S., & Rathus, S. A. (1978). Multivariate and normative data pertaining to the RAS with the college population. *Behavior Therapy, 9,* 675.

Neyra, C. J., Range, L. M., & Goggin, W. C. (1990). Reasons for living following success and failure in suicidal and nonsuicidal college students. *Journal of Applied Social Psychology, 20,* 861–868.

Nezu, A. M., Nezu, C. M., & Nezu, V. A. (1986). Depression, general distress, and causal attributions among university students. *Journal of Abnormal Psychology, 95,* 184–186.

Nottingham, E. J., & Neimeyer, R. A. (1992). Evaluation of a comprehensive inpatient rational-emotive therapy program: Some preliminary data. *Journal of Rational-Emotive & Cognitive-Behavior Therapy, 10,* 57–77.

Osman, A., Gifford, J., Jones, T., Lickiss, L., Osman, J., & Wenzel, R. (1993). Psychometric evaluation of the Reasons for Living Inventory. *Psychological Assessment, 5,* 154–158.

Osman, A., Gregg, C. L., Osman, J., R., & Jones, K. (1992). Factor structure and reliability of the Reasons for Living Inventory. *Psychological Reports, 70,* 107–112.

Pasquali, L., & Gouveia, V. V. (1990). Escala de Assertividade Rathus—RAS: adaptacao brasileira./Rathus'Assertiveness Scale. *Psicologia Teoria e Pesquisa, 6,* 233–249.

Prezant, D., & Neimeyer, R. (1988). Cognitive predictors of depression and suicide ideation. *Suicide and Life Threatening Behavior, 18,* 259–264.

Range, L. M., Hall, D. L., & Meyers, J. (1993). Factor structure of adolescents' scores on the Reasons for Living Inventory. *Death Studies, 17,* 257–266.

Rathus, S. A. (1973). A 30-item schedule for assessing assertive behavior. *Behavior Therapy, 4,* 398–406.

Rathus, S. A., & Nevid, J. S. (1977). Concurrent validity of the 30-item Assertiveness Schedule with a psychiatric population. *Behavior Therapy, 8,* 393–397.

Rehm, L. (1987). The measurement of behavioral aspects of depression. In A. J. Marsella, R. M. A. Hirshfeld, & M. M. Katz (Eds.), *The Measurement of Depression* (pp. 199–239). New York: Guilford.

Rich, A. R., & Bonner, R. L. (1987). Concurrent validity of a stress-vulnerability model of suicidal ideation and behavior: A follow-up study. *Suicide & Life-threatening Behavior, 17,* 265–270.

Rose, G., & Staats, A. (1988). Depression and the frequency and strength of pleasant events: Exploration of the Staats–Heiby theory. *Behaviour Research and Therapy, 26,* 489–494.

Sahin, N., & Sahin, N. (1992). Reliability and validity of the Turkish version of the Automatic Thoughts Questionnaire. *Journal of Clinical Psychology, 48,* 334–340.

Smith, T., Peck, J., Milano, R., & Ward, J. (1988). Cognitive distortion in rheumatoid arthritis: Relation to depression and disability. *Journal of Consulting and Clinical Psychology, 56,* 412–416.

Simons, A. D., Garfield, S. L., & Murphy, G. E. (1984). The process of change in cognitive therapy and pharmacotherapy for depression. *Archives of General Psychiatry, 41,* 45–51.

Starke, M. D. (1987). Enhancing social skills and self-perceptions of physically disabled young adults: Assertiveness training versus discussion groups. *Behavior Modification, 11,* 3–16.

Strosahl, K., Chiles, J. A., & Lineman, M. (1992). Prediction of suicide intent in hospitalized parasuicides: Reasons for living, hopelessness, and depression. *Comprehensive Psychiatry, 33,* 366–373.

Templeman, T. L. (1990). Relationship of M. S. Belief Scale scores to depression and anxiety in hospitalized patients. *Journal of Rational-Emotive & Cognitive-Behavior Therapy, 8,* 267–274.

Warren, R., & Zgourides, G. (1989). Further validity and normative data for the Malouff and Schutte Belief Scale. *Journal of Rational-Emotive & Cognitive-Behavior Therapy, 7,* 167–172.

Wertheim, E., & Poulakis, Z. (1992). The relationships among the General Attitude and Belief Scale, other dysfunctional cognition measures, and depressive or bulimic tendencies. *Journal of Rational-Emotive & Cognitive-Behavior Therapy, 10,* 219–233.

Wierzbicki, M., & Rexford, L. (1989). Cognitive and behavioral correlates of depression in clinical and nonclinical populations. *Journal of Clinical Psychology, 45,* 872–877.

Chapter 15

Measures of Global Functioning

BRIEF PSYCHIATRIC RATING SCALE

Nature and Uses

The Brief Psychiatric Rating Scale provides clinicians with a method for the quick assessment of major dimensions of psychopathology. It was first developed as a 16-item interview-based rating scale by Overall and Gorham (1962) and later expanded to its present 18-item form (Overall, 1983). The scale items were designed to cover a broad range of symptoms and were based on factor analytic studies of earlier scales as well as the clinical expertise of mental health professionals (Hedlund & Vieweg, 1980; Overall, 1983; Overall & Gorham, 1962). The scale is widely used for diagnosis of severe psychopathology and evaluation of treatment related changes in individuals with severe psychopathology. It is most commonly used with schizophrenics; however, it has also been used with depressed, manic, and demented clients. Several researchers (e.g., Bech, Kastrup, & Rafaelsen, 1986) have proposed slight modifications in the scale, but since the Overall (1983) version seems to be most commonly used, we will report on that version.

Hedlund and Vieweg (1980) reviewed a large number of factor analytic studies of the scale and found that very similar factors emerged in the different studies. Hedlund and Vieweg (1980) and Overall (1983) described the five main factors that have emerged in many studies as thinking disturbance, withdrawal–retardation, anxious depression, hostile suspiciousness, and agitation excitement. Overall and Hollister (1986) report that the scale has been translated into many languages, including Spanish, French, German, Italian, Japanese, Dutch, and Russian.

Administration, Scoring, and Classification Profiles

The assessor first conducts a clinical interview, which should include an introduction and explanation of the purpose of the interview, an initial history, a mental status exam, approximately 10 minutes of nondirective discussion of the client's perceptions of his or her problems, and follow-up questions directed at specific issues not covered during the previous portion of the interview. Overall and Hollister (1986) suggest asking some specific questions that relate to the content of the scale if these areas are not spontaneously addressed during the nondirective portion of the interview; these questions include "Have you ever had any unusual experiences such as seeing or hearing things that others do not? Many people who are nervous or depressed have such experiences at times. When was the last time this happened to you? Tell me more about what you thought while that was going on" (p. 162). The total interview should take approximately 20 minutes.

Based on the information obtained during the interview the assessor then rates each of the 18 symptoms on a 7-point scale of severity. A rating of 0 on any symptom indicates absence of the symptom. These ratings may be used in several different ways (Overall, 1983, Overall & Hollister, 1986; Hedlund & Vieweg, 1980; Beller & Overall, 1984).

First, the 18 ratings may be summed for a total maladjustment score. Second, subscale scores may be arrived at as follows: items 4, 12, and 15 are summed for the Thinking Disturbance subscale; items 3, 13, and 16 are summed for the Withdrawal Retardation subscale; items 2, 5, and 9 are summed for the Anxious Depression subscale; items 10, 11, and 14 are summed for the Hostile Suspiciousness subscale; and items 6 and 17 are summed for the Agitation Excitement subscale.

Third, the ratings may be used for a phenomenological classification into the following eight types of psychopathology: anxious depression, retarded depression, agitated depression, hostile depression, florid thinking disorder, withdrawn disorganized thinking disturbance, agitation excitement syndrome, and paranoid hostile suspiciousness. Table 1 presents the classification into these types following a flowchart format adapted from Overall (1983) and Overall and Hollister (1982). The sums of pairs of items are calculated, one point is added to the pair sums under A, and one point is subtracted from the pair sum under G. The one greatest pair sum indicates the diagnostic category. If two sums are equal, the sum higher in the flow chart (e.g., closer to A) determines the diagnosis.

Table 1

Flow Chart for Classifying Psychopathology
Using the Brief Psychiatric Rating Scale

A. Paranoid-Hostile-Suspiciousness
   item 10 + item 11 + 1 =   ———
   item 10 + item 14 + 1 =   ———
   item 11 + item 14 + 1 =   ———
B. Florid Thinking Disorder
   item 4 + item 12 =   ———
   item 4 + item 15 =   ———
   item 12 + item 15 =   ———
   item 11 + item 15 =   ———
C. Withdrawn Disorganized Thinking Disturbance
   item 3 + item 4 =   ———
   item 3 + item 16 =   ———
   item 4 + item 16 =   ———
D. Retarded Depression
   item 3 + item 9 =   ———
   item 9 + item 13 =   ———
E. Agitated Depression
   item 9 + item 10 =   ———
F. Hostile Depression
   item 9 + item 10 =   ———
G. Anxious Depression
   item 2 + item 9 − 1 =   ———
H. Agitation Excitement Syndrome
   item 6 + item 17 =   ———

Fourth, Beller and Overall (1984) suggest a somewhat different decision path for diagnosing geriatric psychiatric clients. Using the scale, they identified the following five profile types: agitated dementia, retarded dementia, anxious depression, withdrawn depression, and paranoid psychosis. If an individual is considered demented on the basis of high scores on conceptual disorganization (item 4) and disorientation (item 18), then the relative strength of ratings on tension and excitement (items 6 and 17) versus ratings on withdrawal and retardation (items 3 and 13) determines a diagnosis of agitated dementia or retarded dementia. If the individual is not demented, then the possibility of paranoid psychosis should be examined by checking the ratings on items tapping thinking disturbance and perceptual distortion. If paranoid psychosis is ruled out and depressive mood is evidenced, then anxiety and tension versus withdrawal and retardation determine the classification of anxious depressed or withdrawn depressed.

Sample Scores

Jaeger, Bitter, Czobor, and Volavka (1990) reported scale scores for 92 acutely exacerbated newly admitted inpatients with schizophrenia and 26 outpatients with a diagnosis of schizophrenia or schizoaffective disorder. Table 2 shows their scores.

Reliability

Hedlund and Vieweg (1980) reviewed the reliability findings of a number of studies of the Brief Psychiatric Rating Scale. They report that across studies the median interrater reliability for the total psychopathology score was .85. The median interrater reliabilities were .94 for the Thinking Disturbance subscale, .86 for the Withdrawal Retardation subscale, .92 for the Hostile-Suspiciousness subscale, and .92 for the Anxious Depression subscale. Median interrater reliabilities for each of the 18 items ranged from .63 to .88. Flemenbaum and Zimmermann (1973) found that three- to six-month test–retest reliability for each of the 18 items ranged from near 0 to .91.

Validity

Well over a thousand studies provide validity-related information regarding the Brief Psychiatric Rating Scale. The scale has become a standard rating instrument for diagnoses and treatment assessment against which new instruments are often compared.

Hedlund and Vieweg (1980) wrote a comprehensive review of the many validity studies of the Brief Psychiatric Rating Scale. They reported that diagnoses made on the bases of the scale tend to be highly associated with diagnoses made by other means and that the scale is sensitive to treatment related changes in psychopathology. They also pointed out that although there are some diagnostic differences across cultures, studies using the different language versions of the scale have found basically the same results. Recent studies have confirmed the validity of the scale. For example, it has been found to be related to other measures of psychopathology such as depression (e.g., Faustman, Moses, Csernansky, & White, 1989; Margo, Dewan, Fisher, & Greenberg, 1992; Shagass & Roemer, 1992) and schizophrenia (e.g., Faustman et al., 1989; Hafkensheid, 1991) and to be sensitive to change in the symptoms of schizophrenia, depression, and mania (e.g., Heresco-Levy, Greenberg, Lerer, Dasberg, & Brown, 1993; Levinson, Singh, & Simpson, 1992; Lenox, Newhouse, Creelman, & Whitaker, 1992).

TABLE 2
Scores on the Brief Psychiatric Rating Scale (Jaeger et al., 1990)

Group	Total		Thinking disturbance		Withdrawal retardation		Anxious depression		Hostile suspiciousness		Agitation excitement	
	M	SD	M	SD	M	SD	M	SD	M	SD	M	SD
Inpatients	49.0	12.6	14.3	5.2	10.1	3.3	8.5	3.6	8.3	3.5	6.9	2.8
Outpatients	32.6	7.2	8.8	4.0	7.3	2.7	6.2	2.0	5.4	2.2	4.9	2.3

Several studies provide evidence that the profiles derived from the scale have resulted in diagnoses that agree with diagnoses made by other means (e.g., Overall & Hollister, 1980; Chan & Lai, 1993; Beller & Overall, 1984) and that individuals who fit different profiles respond to different types of treatment (e.g., Raskin, Schulterbrandt, Reatig, Crook, & Odle, 1974; Beller & Overall, 1984).

Brief Psychiatric Rating Scale

Directions: Place the number that best represents the level of severity of each symptom next to the item describing that symptom.

0 = Not Present
1 = Very Mild
2 = Mild
3 = Moderate
4 = Moderately Severe
5 = Severe
6 = Extremely Severe

_____ 1. *Somatic Concern*—preoccupation with physical health, fear of physical illness, hypochondriasis

_____ 2. *Anxiety*—worry, fear, overconcern for present or future

_____ 3. *Emotional Withdrawal*—lack of spontaneous interaction, isolation, deficiency in relating to others

_____ 4. *Conceptual Disorganization*—thought processes confused, disconnected, disorganized, disrupted

_____ 5. *Guilt Feelings*—self-blame, shame, remorse for past behavior

_____ 6. *Tension*—physical and motor manifestations of nervousness, overactivation, tension

_____ 7. *Mannerisms and Posturing*—peculiar, bizarre, unnatural motor behavior (not including tic)

_____ 8. *Grandiosity*—exaggerated self-opinion, arrogance, conviction of unusual power or abilities

_____ 9. *Depressive Mood*—sorrow, sadness, despondency, pessimism

_____ 10. *Hostility*—animosity, contempt, belligerence, disdain for others

_____ 11. *Suspiciousness*—mistrust, belief others harbor malicious or discriminatory intent

_____ 12. *Hallucinatory Behavior*—perceptions without normal external stimulus correspondence

_____ 13. *Motor Retardation*—slowed, weakened movements or speech; reduced body tone

_____ 14. *Uncooperativeness*—resistance, guardedness, rejection of authority

_____ 15. *Unusual Thought Content*—unusual, odd, strange, bizarre thought content

_____ 16. *Blunted Affect*—reduced emotional tone, reduction in normal intensity of feelings, flatness

_____ 17. *Excitement*—heightened emotional tone, agitation, increased reactivity

_____ 18. *Disorientation*—confusion or lack of proper association for person, place or time

---

Reprinted with permission of Dr. John E. Overall.

Clinical Global Impressions

Purpose and Development

The Clinical Global Impressions measure (Guy, 1976) was developed by the National Institute of Mental Health (NIMH) for use in pharmacological treatment studies and was included in the Early Clinical Drug Evaluation program (ECDEU), a major research initiative. It consists of a single clinician-rating for each of three concepts: Severity of Illness, Global Improvement (improvement over time), and Efficacy (therapeutic effect in relation to side-effects). In theory, clinicians may use it for any measurable form of maladjustment. Rabkin and Klein's (1987) comment that it is routinely used as an outcome measure in treatment studies was confirmed by our finding many published studies that have recently used the Severity or Global Improvement items.

Administration and Scoring

The measure includes only three items, which are considered separate and are not combined in any way. Any one or all of the items may be used. For the Severity and Efficacy items, the rating time-span is now or the prior week. For Improvement, the rating time span is from admission to the present.

The instructions for the measure do not direct that any specific information be collected, but interviews and a review of records would seem appropriate. The instructions provide only minimal information about how to decide what rating to give.

Clinicians use separate 7-point scales to make the Severity and Improvement ratings and a 2-variable grid to make the Efficacy rating. To determine Efficacy, therapeutic effect and side-effects are each rated on a 1–4 scale, and then therapeutic effect is divided by side-effects for an Efficacy score that can range from 0.25 to 4.0, with higher scores indicating more therapeutic effect in relation to side-effects.

Researchers often dichotomize the Improvement item into responders and nonresponders. Rabkin and Klein (1987) recommended characterizing responders as patients who receive scores of 1 or 2, indicating they are at least "much improved."

The third item, Efficacy, is the most unusual, may be the least valuable (Beneke & Rasmus, 1992), and appears to be the least used of the items. It asks clinicians to rate "drug effect only," but that may be difficult to do because of the possibility of natural recovery and situational changes producing an improvement.

Sample Scores

Typically Severity scores average between 4 (moderately ill) and 5 (markedly ill) at baseline in treatment studies (e.g., Claghorn, Kiev, Rickels, Smith & Dunbar, 1992; Schweizer, Rickels, Csanalosi, London, & Turner, 1990). In many published studies, the mean Severity score decreases by about a point with an active treatment but decreases only slightly in the placebo group (Claghorn et al., 1999; Schweizer et al. 1990).

In published treatment studies, the Improvement score often shows a mean of 2 (much improved) to 3 (minimally improved) for the active treatment and a mean of 3 to 4 (no change) for the placebo (e.g., Claghorn et al., 1992; Kiev, 1992).

Reliability

Beneke and Rasmus (1992) calculated 8-week test–retest rank-order correlations for the German version of the Clinical Global Impressions in several clinical groups and found correlations of .20 to .81 for Severity, .15 to .78 for Improvement, and .21 to .80 for Therapeutic Effects and Side-Effects.

Validity

Perhaps because of the strong face validity of the Global Impressions items, few efforts have been made specifically to validate the items. Indeed, the Severity item is sometimes used as a validity standard for new measures.

Beneke and Rasmus (1992) found that intercorrelations of change scores on the Severity item and scores on the Improvement item and therapeutic effects rating ranged from .47 to .93, suggesting that the three ratings were measuring the same construct. Fieve, Goodnick, Peselow, Barouche, & Schlegel (1986) found that Improvement ratings correlated .83 to .95 with change scores on the Hamilton Rating Scale for Depression and with patient ratings of improvement. Rabkin and Klein (1987) reported that Severity and Improvement scores each correlated over .80 with Hamilton Depression Rating Scale scores during treatment.

Gotesdam (1981) found that Severity item scores correlated significantly with 23 items from three geriatric rating scales and appeared to be most associated with items rating the communication and helpfulness of the client. Kay, Opler, & Lindenmayer (1988) found significant correlations between Severity scores and well-validated measures of positive and negative symptoms of schizophrenia. Ahmed & Laffferty (1982) found that

Severity ratings completed by nurses correlated highly with psychiatrist ratings on a manic rating scale.

Many studies have shown that the Severity and Improvement items are sensitive to treatment effects. Recent studies have found that group means on the Global Impressions Severity and Improvement items showed the same pattern of improvement in different experimental conditions as group means on other validated measures of anxiety (e.g., Laakmann, Blaschke, Hippius, & Schewe, 1989), depression (e.g., Carmen, Ahdieh, Wyatt-Knowles, Warga, & Panagides, 1991), and schizophrenia (e.g., Kane, Honigfeld, Singer, Meltzer, & Clozaril Collaborative Study Group, 1989). These other measures have included client self-reports (e.g., Claghorn, 1992) and clinician ratings based on highly structured interview schedules (e.g., Siris, Bermanzohn, Gonzalez, Mason, White, & Shuwall, 1991).

It is much more difficult to point to evidence that the Efficacy item is valid. The item's matrix format does not translate well into a number that can be analyzed statistically (Beneke & Rasmus, 1992). That may be a major reason that Efficacy ratings are rarely mentioned in research reports.

In a critical review of the Clinical Global Impressions, Beneke and Rasmus (1992) reported that the Severity and Improvement items had nonnormal score distributions in clinical samples and therefore concluded that with these items nonparametric (e.g., rank order) statistics will usually be more appropriate for data analysis than parametric (e.g., analysis of variance).

CLINICAL GLOBAL IMPRESSIONS

1. *Severity of Illness*—Considering your total clinical experience with this particular population, how mentally ill is the patient at this time?

   1 = Normal, not at all ill   5 = Markedly ill
   2 = Borderline mentally ill   6 = Severely ill
   3 = Mildly ill   7 = Among the most extremely ill
   4 = Moderately ill   patients

2. *Global Improvement*—Rate total improvement whether or not in your judgment it is due entirely to drug treatment. Compared to his condition at admission to the project, how much has he changed?

   1 = Very much improved   5 = Minimally worse
   2 = Much improved   6 = Much worse
   3 = Minimally improved   7 = Very much worse
   4 = No change

3. *Efficacy Index*—Rate this item on the basis of *drug effect only*. Select the terms that best describe the degrees of therapeutic effect and side-effects and make a mark in the box where the two items intersect.

   EXAMPLE: Therapeutic effect is rated as "Moderate" and side effects are judged "Do not significantly interfere with patient's functioning." Mark the area where the two intersect.

	Side-effects			
	None	Do not significantly interfere with patient's functioning	Significantly interfere with patient's functioning	Outweigh therapeutic effect
Therapeutic effect	1	2	3	4
4. *Marked*—Vast improvement. Complete or nearly complete remission of all symptoms	4.00	2.00	1.33	1.00

3. *Moderate*—Decided improvement. Partial remission of symptoms	3.00	1.50	1.00	0.75
2. *Minimal*—Slight improvement which doesn't alter status of care of patient	2.00	1.00	0.67	0.50
1. *Unchanged or Worse*	1.00	0.50	0.33	0.25

Scale in public domain.

REFERENCES

Ahmed, A., & Lafferty, D. (1982). Scales for measuring mania. *Canadian Journal of Psychiatry*, 27, 659–662.

Bech, P., Kastrup, M., & Rafaelsen, O. J. (1986). Mini-compendium of rating scales for states of anxiety, depression, mania, schizophrenia, with corresponding DSM-III syndromes. *Acta Psychiatrica Scandinavica*, Vol 73 (*suppl. no 326*), 5–37.

Beller, S. A., & Overall, J. E. (1984). The Brief Psychiatric Rating Scale (BPRS) in geropsychiatric research: II. Representative profile patterns. *Journal of Gerontology, 39*, 194–200.

Beneke, M., & Rasmus, W. (1992). "Clinical Global Impressions" (ECDEU): Some critical comments. *Pharmacopsychiatry, 25*, 171–176.

Carmen, J., Ahdieh, H., Wyatt-Knowles, E., Warga, E., & Panagides, J. (1991). A controlled study of mianserin in moderately to severely depressed outpatients. *Psychopharmacology Bulletin, 27*, 135–139.

Chan, D. W., & Lai, B. (1993). Assessing psychopathology in Chinese psychiatric patients in Hong Kong using the Brief Psychiatric Rating Scale. *Acta Psychiatrica Scandinavica, 87*, 37–44.

Claghorn, J. (1992). The safety and efficacy of paroxetine compared with placebo in a double-blind trial of depressed outpatients. *Journal of Clinical Psychiatry, 53*, 33–35.

Claghorn, J., Kiev, A., Rickels, K., Smith, W., & Dunbar, G. (1992). Paroxetine versus placebo: A double-blind comparison in depressed patients. *Journal of Clinical Psychiatry, 53*, 434–438.

Faustman, W. O., Moses, J. A., Csernansky, J. G., & White, P. A. (1989). Correlations between the MMPI and the Brief Psychiatric Rating Scale in schizophrenic and schizoaffective patients. *Psychiatry Research, 28*, 135–143.

Fieve, R., Goodnick, P., Peselow, E., Barouche, F., & Schlegel, A. (1986). Pattern analysis of antidepressant response to fluoxetine. *Journal of Clinical Psychiatry, 47*, 560–562.

Flemenbaum, A., & Zimmermann, R. L. (1973). Inter- and intra-rater reliability of the Brief Psychiatric Rating Scale. *Psychological Reports, 32*, 783–792.

Hafkensheid, A. (1991). Psychometric evaluation of a standardized and expanded Brief Psychiatric Rating Scale. *Acta Psychiatrica Scandinavica, 84*, 294–300.

Hedlund, J. L., & Vieweg, B. W. (1980). The Brief Psychiatric Rating Scale (BRS): A comprehensive review. *Journal of Operational Psychiatry, 11*, 48–65.

Heresco-Levy, U., Greenberg, D., Lerer, B., Dasberg, H., & Brown, W. A. (1993). Trial maintenance neuroleptic dose reduction in schizophrenic outpatients: Two-year outcome. *Journal of Clinical Psychiatry, 54*(2), 59–62.

Gotesdam, K. G. (1981). A geriatric rating scale empirically derived from three rating scales for geriatric behavior. *Acta Psychiatrica Scandinavica, 64* (*Supplementum 294*), 54–63.

Guy, W. (1976). *ECDEU Assessment Manual for Psychopharmacology*. Rockville, MD: National Institute of Mental Health.

Jaeger, J., Bitter, I., Czabor, P., & Volavka, J. (1990). The measurement of subjective experience in schizophrenia: The Subjective Deficit Scale. *Comprehensive Psychiatry, 31*, 216–226.

Kane, J., Honigfeld, G., Singer, J., Meltzer, H., & Clozaril Collaborative Study Group (1989). Clozapine for the treatment-resistant schizophrenic: Results of a US multicenter trial. *Psychopharmacology, 99*, 60–63.

Kay, S. R., Opler, L. A., & Lindenmayer, J. (1988). Reliability and validity of the positive and negative syndrome scale for schizophrenics. *Psychiatry Research, 23*, 99–110.

Kiev, A. (1992). A double-blind, placebo-controlled study of paroxetine in depressed outpatients. *Journal of Clinical Psychiatry, 53*, 27–27.

Laakmann, G., Blaschke, D., Hippius, H., Schewe, S. (1989). Double-blind study of metaclazepam versus diazepam treatment of outpatients with anxiety syndrome. *Pharmaco-psychiatry, 22,* 120–125.

Lenox, R. H., Newhouse, P. A., Creelman, W. L., & Whitaker, T. M. (1992). Adjunctive treatment of manic agitation with lorazepam versus haloperidol: A double-blind study. *Journal of Clinical Psychiatry, 53*(2), 47–52.

Levinson, D. F., Singh, H., & Simpson, G. M. (1992). Timing of acute clinical response to fluphenazine. *British Journal of Psychiatry, 160,* 365–371.

Margo, G. M., Dewan, M. J., Fisher, S., & Greenberg, R. P. (1992). Comparison of three depression rating scales. *Perceptual and Motor Skills, 75,* 144–146.

Overall, J. E. (1983). Brief Psychiatric Rating Scale and Brief Psychiatric History Form. In P. A. Keller & L. G. Ritt (Eds.), *Innovations in Clinical Practice: A Source Book* (pp. 307–316). Sarasota, FL: Professional Resource Exchange.

Overall, J. E., & Gorham, D. R. (1962). The Brief Psychiatric Rating Scale. *Psychological Reports, 10,* 799–812.

Overall, J. E., & Hollister, L. E. (1980). Diagnosis and the phenomenology of depressive disorders. *Journal of Consulting and Clinical Psychology, 48,* 626–634.

Overall, J. E., & Hollister, L. E. (1982). Decision rules for phenomenological classification of psychiatric patients. *Journal of Consulting and Clinical Psychology, 50,* 535–545.

Overall, J. E., & Hollister, L. E. (1986). Assessment of depression using the Brief Psychiatric Rating Scale. In N. Satorius & T. A. Ban (Eds.), *Assessment of Depression* (pp. 159–178). New York: Springer Verlag.

Rabkin, J. G., & Klein, D. F. (1987). The clinical measurement of depressive disorders. In A. J. Mareslla, R. M. Hirshfeld, & M. M. Katz (Eds.), *The measurement of Depression* (pp. 30–83). New York: Guilford.

Raskin, A., Schulterbrandt, J. G., Reatig, N., Crook, T. H., & Odle, D. (1974). Depression subtypes and response to phenelzine, diazepam, and a placebo. *Archives of General Psychiatry, 30,* 66–75.

Shagass, C., & Roemer, R. A. (1992). Evoked potential topography in major depression: II. Comparisons between subgroups. *International Journal of Psychophysiology, 13,* 255–261.

Siris, S., Bermanzohn, P., Gonzales, A., Mason, S., White, C., & Shuwall, M. (1991). The use of antidepressants for negative symptoms in a subset of schizophrenic patients. *Psychopharmacology Bulletin, 27,* 331–335.

Schweizer, E., Rickels, K., Csanalosi, I., London, J., & Turner, D. (1990). A placebo-controlled study of enciprazine in the treatment of generalized anxiety disorder: A preliminary report. *Psychopharmacology Bulletin, 26*(2), 215–217.

Index